OXFORD MEDICAL PUBLICATIONS

Psychological Medicine of HIV Infection

Psychological Medicine of HIV Infection

José Catalán
Reader in Psychiatry and Honorary Consultant Psychiatrist, Charing Cross and Westminster Medical School and Riverside Mental Health Trust, London

Adrian Burgess
Lecturer in Psychology as Applied to Medicine, Charing Cross and Westminster Medical School, London

and

Ivana Klimeš
Consultant Clinical Psychologist, Warneford Hospital, Oxford

with the collaboration of

Brian Gazzard
Consultant Physician and Clinical Director of HIV Services, Chelsea and Westminster Hospital, London

Oxford New York Toronto
OXFORD UNIVERSITY PRESS
1995

Oxford University Press, Walton Street, Oxford OX2 6DP
Oxford New York
Athens Auckland Bangkok Bombay
Calcutta Cape Town Dar es Salaam Delhi
Florence Hong Kong Istanbul Karachi
Kuala Lumpur Madras Madrid Melbourne
Mexico City Nairobi Paris Singapore
Taipei Tokyo Toronto
and associated companies in
Berlin Ibadan

Oxford is a trade mark of Oxford University Press

Published in the United States
by Oxford University Press Inc., New York

A catalogue record for this book is available from the British Library

Library of Congress Cataloging in Publication Data
Catalán, José, 1949–
Psychological medicine of HIV infection/José Catalán, Adrian Burgess, and Ivana Klimeš.
p. cm. – (Oxford medical publications)
Includes bibliographical references and index , Alk. paper
1. AIDS (Disease) – Psychological aspects. I. Burgess, Adrian. II. Klimes, Ivana. III. Title. IV. Series.
[DNLM: 1. HIV Infections – psychology. 2. HIV Infections – physiopathology. 3. HIV Infections – therapy. WC 503.7 C357p 1995]
RC607.A26C378 1995 616.97'92'0019 – dc20 95–15496
DNLM/DLC for Library of Congress
ISBN 0 19 262202 1

Typeset by Footnote Graphics, Warminster, Wilts
Printed in Great Britain on acid-free paper by
Bookcraft (Bath) Ltd, Midsomer Norton, Avon

Foreword

Professor Jonathan Mann, Director, François-Xavier Bagnoud Center for Health and Human Rights, Harvard School of Public Health

The World Health Organization defines health as a state of 'physical, mental, and social well-being'. Yet in contrast to the prodigious energy and resources spent on the physical dimensions of health (even if generally limited to diseases, disability, and death rather than well-being), much less is done about the equally vital dimensions of mental and social well-being.

This book is an important part of a growing effort to redress this balance. This book does not seek to do so by denying either biomedical realities or the strengths of the scientific method. In fealty to its title, Catalán and colleagues have written a complete, extremely well organized book which bridges the biomedical and the psychosocial. It is particularly accessible and suited to the health professional audience; with clarity and intellectual coherence it brings to the reader the full range of what is known regarding the psychological medicine of HIV/AIDS.

It is fitting that such a well organized and creative book be written about HIV/AIDS. For while HIV/AIDS has underscored the limited value of geographical borders, it has also helped to bring about greater cross-disciplinary understanding and mutual respect. The pandemic has shaken many disciplinary and intellectual 'givens', just as it has challenged societal organization and purpose.

It is hoped that readers of this book will be inevitably drawn to go even beyond the psychological dimensions and perspective on mental well-being which is its primary focus. How we define a problem determines what we do about it. The ultimate challenge to all who are concerned with promoting and protecting health is to integrate physical, mental, and societal aspects of the global phenomenon of HIV/AIDS, and of health itself. This book is a sensitive and eminently successful contribution to those who seek this path.

Foreword

Preface

The psychological, social, and neuropsychiatric implications of what we now call HIV infection were recognized from very early in the epidemic, and over the last decade and a half there has been a substantial growth in the awareness of the importance of the mental aspects of HIV infection, both in terms of provision of care and in the prevention of its transmission. As HIV infection has continued its seemingly relentless spread throughout many communities, often affecting individuals already stigmatized and disadvantaged, the complexity of the psychological and social reactions to the infection and the difficulties involved in changing attitudes and behaviour have become even more apparent. At the same time, the literature on the psychological and neuropsychiatric manifestations of HIV has grown fast and extensively, making it hard for people with HIV infection and for professionals and volunteers caring for them to keep up with a constantly expanding body of publications.

Faced with this daunting picture, we have attempted what in restrospect looks to us like an overambitious task: to provide a critical and comprehensive review of the mental health manifestations of HIV infection and of some of its legal and ethical consequences, while still maintaining a practical perspective which could be of value to those working in the front line. Throughout the book, we have aimed at balancing the role of psychological, neurobiological, and social factors in HIV infection. The first three chapters cover the general psychological reactions to HIV infection, the more specific psychiatric syndromes, and brain-related manifestations. The systematic assessment of mental health problems and the range of interventions available to deal with them are the subject of Chapters 4 and 5. Prevention strategies to reduce the spread of infection and the possible contribution of psychological and behavioural factors to the prevention of disease progression are reviewed in Chapter 6. The burden of care on professionals and volunteers is discussed next, and Chapter 8 reviews legal and ethical issues of relevance to mental health. The final chapter contains an update of the general clinical and treatment aspects of HIV infection.

We are indebted to many who, directly or indirectly, have helped us to maintain our enthusiasm and commitment during the long gestation of the book. First of all, we acknowledge the contribution of the many people with HIV infection we have known over the last ten years or so. Their fortitude, determination, and humour, as well as their sadness, have been our main source of inspiration, and they have taught us much about how to cope with adversity. We are also grateful to many collaborators in clinical and research work over the years, among them Torsten Baldeweg, Alexandra Beckett, Alison Bond, Ann Day, Rob Flynn, Adrienne Garrod, Brian Gazzard, John Gruzelier, David

Hawkins, Andrea Pergami, Kate Pugh, Massimo Riccio, Peter Scragg, Ashok Singh, Richard Starmans, Sue Thornton, and Sonya Wood. David Erskine provided valuable help on pharmacological aspects. Librarians Reinhard Wentz, Tracy Cox, and Tricia Gwynn-Jones coped admirably with our request for literature searches and kept us well supplied with papers and research reports. Michael Gelder was the source of support and advice at the outset, and Steven Hirsch gave sound advice in the last few years. Gloria Davies and Paula Bowman gave valuable secretarial assistance. Finally, we are particularly grateful to our partners Harry, Lesley, and Ivan who gave much encouragement and complained little during the long struggle to get the manuscript into shape. While all those named above and many others have contributed to the final product, its shortcomings are ours alone.

We hope that this book will prove useful to professional and voluntary workers involved in caring for people with HIV, and to researchers working to minimize the adverse mental health effects of HIV infection and to those attempting to reduce its spread. Furthermore, we hope that the experience gained and lessons learnt in the provision of psychological, medical, and social care for people with HIV infection will influence the attitudes towards and care given to people with other serious diseases.

London and Oxford J. C.
June 1995 A. B.
I. K.

Contents

1 Psychological consequences of HIV infection

1.1 Introduction

Finding that one has HIV infection can have psychologically devastating consequences. It is therefore surprising to realize that the majority of people with HIV infection cope remarkably well with the consequences of their condition for much of the time. Such positive coping is not achieved without much effort and a substantial minority of people will experience psychological problems at some stage, and a few will suffer severe and persistent difficulties.

Notification of a diagnosis of HIV infection is usually followed by adverse psychological consequences, but the intensity, duration and specific characteristics of the psychological response will vary from person to person, and many factors will influence the development of subsequent emotional reactions and the use of different coping mechanisms. These factors include the way the news about HIV infection was broken, the person's previous experience of coping with adversity, past history of psychological problems, and degree of current social supports, to mention only the most obvious (Sensky, 1990). The pattern of psychological reactions that can develop in response to the knowledge of a diagnosis of HIV disease is comparable to the range of reactions seen in other potentially life-threatening conditions, such as cancer, especially those involving a good deal of uncertainty over their outcome, unpleasant symptoms and complications, and complex and painful treatment.

Responses to a diagnosis of HIV infection include in the first instance shock, denial, distress, followed by gradual acceptance. Anger directed towards others including partners, friends, medical advisers, or self-recrimination and feelings of guilt, are common. Decompensation and persistent distress, denial with accompanying behavioural correlates, and in a number of cases, major psychiatric disorder, may follow. Most of these are predictable responses, which for the most part will fall within the range of what could be regarded as statistically normal. Normal response, however, does not mean that it has to be endured alone, without recourse to psychological support from partners, friends, or voluntary and professional agencies. It does mean, though, that for most people the period of distress will be self-limited, and that only a proportion will experience severe and prolonged difficulties.

While the problems are similar to those seen in other severe physical disorders, HIV disease does not happen in a vacuum or without a social context. In developed countries, individuals who develop HIV infection often belong to groups that have experienced previous social rejection and problems, psychological difficulties, and chronic physical disease, all of which increase vulnerability to further psychological problems. Furthermore, a link has been established between HIV disease and poverty, both in developing and developed countries (Mann et al, 1992), and there is also evidence that low socioeconomic status may adversely affect HIV disease progression (Schechter et al, 1994). The development of HIV disease can lead to major changes in family and social structure particularly in developing countries with high rates of heterosexual infection (Mann et al, 1992), which in turn can have adverse consequences for the surviving children. All these features which are characteristic of HIV disease will, therefore, tend to magnify the psychological and social impact of the disorder.

In this chapter, the psychological impact of HIV infection is reviewed, describing first the psychological consequences for the person with HIV at different stages of infection: at the time of testing for HIV infection, during the asymptomatic stage, when symptoms develop, and in terminal stages. The specific problems of children are considered next, and finally the consequences for partners, carers and relatives.

1.2 Psychological problems at the time of HIV testing

Laboratory testing for HIV antibodies has been routinely available to clinicians since 1985, and the techniques currently in use are reliable and can give results fairly promptly, even on the same day of testing (Squire et al, 1991). False positive results are exceedingly rare, although when they occur they can cause major psychological and social problems (Sullivan et al, 1993). Prior to 1985, it was possible for someone to be concerned about being infected with HIV, but there was no way of confirming it, unless AIDS-related symptoms developed. It was this uncertainty that lead to the concept of 'the worried well' (Forstein, 1984; Morin et al, 1984), which in those early days was applied to people exhibiting fears of AIDS, sometimes as a result of sexual contact with a person who subsequently went on to develop the disease. In other cases, fear of AIDS was a result of hypochondriasis or other psychiatric disorder involving pathological fears or abnormal beliefs about health. It is likely that many of those who in the pre-HIV test era were described as 'worried well', were in fact already infected with HIV. The term 'worried well' has been used in more recent years in rather a different sense, to refer to people with minimal or no risk of HIV infection, but who are persistently preoccupied with thoughts and fears of HIV infection, often in spite of multiple negative HIV test results. The problems of this group of individuals are discussed later in this chapter.

HIV testing can be performed in recognized testing sites in hospitals, for example in genitourinary and antenatal clinics, drug dependency units, haemophilia and blood transfusion centres, as well as in community-based facilities, such as general practice. In fact, it is possible for any doctor with access to laboratory facilities to request a test. Official guidelines endorsed by the WHO make it clear that testing for HIV should only be carried out with the person's full and informed consent, save in exceptional circumstances. It has also been stressed by statutory and voluntary agencies that HIV testing should not be carried out without discussion and careful consideration of the implications of the results of the test, which can be very grave, even in the case of a negative test result (Miller et al, 1986a). This process is usually known as pre-test counselling, and is considered in detail later in this chapter, while the ethical and legal matters concerned with HIV antibody testing are discussed in Chapter 8.

It is true, however, that official guidelines are sometimes disregarded or not fully adhered to, so that individuals are on occasion tested without their prior knowledge and consent, with potentially serious consequences for the person's psychological and social status. Testing without consent also places the professional who requested the test in a legally exposed situation. Similarly, the nature and quality of the pre- and post-test counselling can vary considerably, depending on the setting where it is carried out, the attitudes and training of the counsellor, and the extent to which the individual is prepared to ask questions or challenge the counsellor.

Psychological characteristics of people seeking HIV testing

The clinical experience of those working in the field is that most people requesting HIV testing show moderate to mild levels of distress, which is dispelled either by counselling without the need for testing, or on learning of a negative test result. If the result is positive, the process of coming to terms with its implications may be associated with greater psychological morbidity, either short- or long-term (Seidl and Goebel, 1987; Miller, 1987).

Many factors influence a person's decision to seek HIV testing: perception of risk, fear of consequences, impact of publicity (Thompson and McIver, 1988; Beck et al, 1990), degree of knowledge of HIV infection and attitudes about it, as well as psychological distress and social pressures (Lewin and Williams, 1988). Among pregnant women, the factors which influence the decision to be tested include perceived benefits of the test to the woman, partner and baby, perceived risk of HIV infection, and being unmarried (Meadows et al, 1993a).

Perry et al (1990a) studied over 200 people who regarded themselves at risk of HIV infection and requested antibody testing in New York. The sample included gay and bisexual men, injecting drug users, and non-drug using heterosexual men and women who were partners of people thought to be at risk of infection. Levels of psychopathology at the time of testing were low and not very different from those found in a comparable sex- and age-matched community sample, but the most striking finding was the much higher than expected rates of lifetime psychopathology in this group of individuals seeking HIV testing. For example, a history of mood disorders, mostly depression, was found in more than 40 per cent of the patients, and this was about seven times higher than expected. About 20 per cent had a history of alcohol dependence, and 30 per cent of dependence on other substances, even after injecting drug users had been excluded from this analysis. Interestingly, those who subsequently were found to be HIV positive did not differ from negatives in current or past levels of psychopathology. Similar results have been reported from London by

Riccio et al (1993) in a study of over 100 gay men seeking HIV testing. In this study, current levels of psychopathology and distress were generally low, and there were no differences between those subsequently found to be seropositive and those who were seronegative.

Suicidal ideation around the time of HIV testing is discussed in detail in Chapter 2. One of the most important findings is that sucidal thoughts are very common among people seeking HIV test prior to the results being known regardless of whether they turn out to be seropositive or not. This is consistent with the reports quoted above showing marked similarities in current and past psychopathology. In view of the relationship between suicidal ideas and subsequent suicide and reports of increased risk of suicidal behaviour in AIDS, individuals coming forward for HIV testing need to be regarded as vulnerable to psychological problems. This is particularly important when the pre- and post-test counselling facilities available are less sophisticated than those described in research reports, as is often likely to be the case.

Not all those who come forward for HIV testing return to learn the results. Catania et al (1990a) found that 28 per cent of people attending a free anonymous testing facility in California failed to return to collect their test results. They found that those not returning for the results were less well informed about the significance of the HIV test, had more AIDS-related anxiety, were less well educated and were more likely to be young people who had had a blood transfusion, than those who came back. It is likely that anxiety played a part in their failure to return, and in addition to having public health implications concerning use of resources and prevention of spread, these results highlight the need for adequate and sensitive counselling of people attending HIV testing sites. A study from the US, involving more than half a million participants, found that about one-third of people failed to return for their test result. Those least likely to return for post-test counselling included young people, African-Americans and those pre-test counselled and tested in genitourinary medicine or family planning clinics were (Valdiserri et al, 1993).

Psychological status after HIV testing

In most instances, the distress associated with notification of a positive HIV test result is short-lived, as discussed above in relation to the prevalence of suicidal ideas before and after testing. However, there have been anecdotal reports of major psychological disturbance following a positive HIV test result, including suicide (Pierce, 1987). The role of mental illness in people who commit suicide is sometimes difficult to establish. In one case known to us, a 62-year-old retired physician committed suicide by hanging himself two weeks after learning of his positive serostatus. He was well informed about HIV infection, had received good pre- and post-test counselling. It appears, however, that he had for some years maintained that he would end his life should he develop cancer or other serious condition, and on learning his HIV serostatus, made careful plans to kill himself.

The effects of disclosure of HIV test results on mental health were studied by Ostrow et al (1989a), who investigated a cohort of gay men enrolled in the

Multicenter AIDS Cohort Study (MACS), some of whom wished to know the result of their HIV test. HIV positive individuals who chose to be told the result showed a decline in their mental health, while those who were ignorant of their results showed improvement over comparable periods. In contrast, those who were HIV seronegative, regardless of whether they knew the results or not, improved their psychological functioning over time. Interestingly, disclosure of HIV test results had minimal effects on sexual behaviour (see Chapter 6).

Work carried out in the United Kingdom, on the other hand, has produced contrasting findings. Pugh et al (1994), studying the cohort of gay men seeking testing at a London site mentioned above (Riccio et al, 1993), found significant reductions in psychological morbidity six and 12 months after testing and there were no differences in mental health between those who were HIV seropositive and those who were HIV seronegative. It is important to stress that all patients entered in the investigation had received detailed pre- and post-test counselling, which is likely to have been an important factor in the reduction in distress levels for both groups. Similar findings were reported by Perry et al (1993) who followed-up 328 individuals after HIV testing, including 106 people who were HIV seropositive and 222 who were HIV seronegative. At 12 months, over a third had significant levels of psychological morbidity, which could be predicted by several baseline factors: high scores for psychological morbidity, low socio-economic status, female sex, history of injecting drug use and heterosexual risk factors for HIV infection. Interestingly, HIV status was not associated with levels of psychological morbidity.

Disclosure of the test result is only one factor influencing the psychological response: how the results are given, and the nature of the counselling used can also play a part. Perry et al (1991) evaluated three different counselling interventions to reduce the distress associated with HIV testing. All patients received standard pre- and post-test counselling, but in addition, following notification of the results, patients were randomly allocated to standard counselling alone, six weekly individual 'stress prevention training' sessions, or three weekly 'interactive video programme' sessions. Three months later, there were significant reductions in distress levels for all patients, regardless of HIV status or post-test result intervention, although HIV positive individuals who had received 'stress prevention training' showed greater reductions in stress. Again, it is important to emphasize that all had come forward voluntarily and had received detailed pre- and post-test counselling of a fairly sophisticated nature, including the group receiving standard counselling only.

Mandatory HIV tests, with pre- and post-test counselling, have been performed on US military personnel, and Pace et al (1990) have described the psychological profile of those who were HIV seropositive assessed a few months after test notification. A sample of 95 seropositive individuals, half of whom had known their HIV status for less than 4 weeks and the rest for periods ranging between 9 and 14 months, were assessed. More than a quarter were found to have had major psychiatric disorders, according to DSM-III-R axis I. When psychiatric disorders regarded as minor were included (e.g. simple phobias, adjustment disorders, or loss of sexual interest), more than 60 per cent were found to have a psychiatric diagnosis. Interestingly, about a third of those with HIV infection met the criteria for a retrospective diagnosis of major psychiatric disorder at some stage in their lives. No adequate control group was available for comparison and so it is difficult to generalize from this sample of individuals belonging to a particular social and employment group, who were tested compulsorily, but the substantial prevalence of psychological morbidity after the test is a cause for concern, while the previous history of psychiatric disorder highlights once more the pre-morbid vulnerability of this group of people found to be HIV positive.

Partner notification in HIV infection is controversial although there is now a good deal of experience about it both in the US and in Europe (see Chapter 6). One particular concern is whether individuals who are notified and counselled about having had sexual or needle-sharing contact with a seropositive person are at particular risk of psychological or social problems, and also whether the index person may also suffer as a result of guilt or other problems. There is little research on these matters, but what there is suggests that provided contact is made by trained staff, with counselling skills and sensitivity, and that efforts are made to maintain confidentiality, adverse consequences are minimal (Jones et al, 1990; Giesecke et al, 1991; Spencer et al, 1993).

Some individuals are at particular risk of experiencing difficulties following notification of a positive HIV test result. At particular risk are those who discover their HIV status at the same time as they develop HIV-related complications, usually leading to hospitalization. Typically, the person will have been admitted to hospital with a severe chest infection which turns out to be *Pneumocystis carinii* pneumonia, and the patient's serostatus is established after investigation of the cause of the disease. Not infrequently, the patient had experienced some concerns in the past about the possibility of being HIV positive, but had decided against testing on the grounds that it would be better not to know. There is some evidence to suggest that such individuals tend to use avoidance as an habitual coping strategy (Katz, 1992). The double blow of discovering the positive serostatus and the diagnosis of AIDS takes a greater psychological toll, and may require intensive work on the part of staff involved in the patient's care. The situation is even more complicated when HIV testing had been carried out without the patient's consent, as sometimes happens.

Subjective experience of having a positive test result

The anonymous writer of the *British Medical Journal* article 'Don't tell me on a Friday' sums up nicely in the title the immediate impact of notification of the results (Richards, 1986) and the need for support in the next few hours and days after the result is disclosed. There are many detailed and moving descriptions of the range of initial responses available in the literature, as in Grimshaw (1987) and Miller (1987).

A detailed interview study of 16 HIV seropositive gay and bisexual men carried in Sweden (Mansson, 1990) where a large proportion of the population has been tested voluntarily, shows the subtle and less subtle pressures individuals regarded at risk of HIV infection can face. It also highlights the distress experienced while waiting for the result, or when being given the news by doctors who may be poorly trained in the process of communicating bad news to patients, or when the medical team is not supported by professionals or volunteers able to provide psychological support. McCann and Wadsworth (1991) asked 265 HIV positive gay men about their experience of being tested and their responses to being notified of their results. More than 70 per cent were satisfied with the way the news was given, but 20 per cent felt they were treated in an insensitive way. Similar findings were reported by Pergami et al (1994a) in a survey of 30 gay men, who also identified the quality of information given and the attitude of the doctor giving the results as important factors affecting satisfaction with the consultation.

In a study including 46 women attending a central London clinic, 23 of whom were HIV seropositive, Beevor and Catalán (1993) examined the reasons why women came forward for HIV testing. They found that perception of risk was the most common reason for seeking testing in those who were uninfected. In contrast, health problems that frequently turned out to be HIV-related, led to seeking testing in amongst those women who were HIV seropositive, and in a number of instances this occurred during pregnancy. An alarmingly high number of women claimed not to have received adequate pre-test counselling, and some had been tested without consent. After notification of the result, one-fifth of the HIV seropositive group did not tell anyone for some time, and a similar number expressed regret about knowing they were positive. It is difficult to know how general these findings are, but it is a cause for concern that poor counselling and few supports were available for this vulnerable group.

Abnormal beliefs in people seeking testing

Amongst people seeking HIV testing, there are some who present with distress about being infected and remain concerned about HIV infection, or may be convinced that they are infected, even after one or more negative HIV tests. Reassurance and basic counselling of the kind usually offered at testing sites provide transient or minimal relief and the person soon returns to a state of preoccupation and concern about being infected. Not infrequently, such individuals return for further testing, or move on to another testing facility, sometimes under an assumed name.

Many different terms, some of them novel, have been used in clinical practice and in the literature to describe this group of individuals or the psychiatric syndrome some of them suffer: the 'worried well' (Miller, 1986), AIDS-phobia (Jacob et al, 1987), pseudo-AIDS (Miller et al, 1985) and AIDS panic (Windgassen and Soni, 1987). As is often the case, new words have tended to obscure, rather than clarify the problem, and terminology has not always kept pace with developments in knowledge about HIV, so that terms which were useful before HIV tests became available, such as 'worried well' (Forstein, 1984; Morin et al, 1984), have now acquired a new and misleading meaning. People with persistent concerns about having venereal diseases, notably syphilis, cancer, or other conditions with high social and media profiles, are not new. Genitourinary physicians, family and hospital doctors, and mental health workers are familiar with these recurrent attenders (Frost, 1985). What appears to be different in this case is the nature and content of the concerns, rather than the form the psychopathological problem takes, or the psychological processes involved.

Concerns about HIV infection which do not subside after notification of a negative test result and appropriate counselling about its significance should be regarded as a *symptom*, rather than a diagnosis: in other words, irrational worries about HIV infection are seen in a wide range of different kinds of psychological disorders, and it is undesirable to categorize them all under some superficially appealing label, before making an attempt at sorting out what the specific problem is and what factors contribute to its development (Riccio and Thompson, 1987; Segal, 1988). Irrational concerns about health can be the result of inadequate information and mistaken attitudes; they may be part of a neurotic disorder, such as an adjustment reaction, obsessional disorder, somatization disorder or hypochondriasis (Appleby, 1987; Lewin and Williams, 1988; Kamlana and Gray, 1988; Miller et al, 1988; Warwick, 1989), or they may be delusional in nature, resulting from an affective disorder, such as major depression or mania, or schizophrenia (Rapaport and Braff, 1985; Jenike and Pato, 1986; Valdiserri, 1986; Lawlor and Stewart, 1987; Altamura et al, 1988; Mahorney and Cavenar, 1988; Todd, 1989; Frierson, 1990). Accurate assessment is essential, as many of these syndromes can be treated successfully, and failure to identify and treat can have major adverse consequences (see Chapters 4 and 5 on psychiatric assessment and management).

People with hypochondriasis have received a good deal of attention in the HIV literature (Davey and Green, 1991), compared with those with delusional or other disorders, and this is consistent with clinical experience which suggests that neurotic disorders are more common in this setting than psychotic conditions (psychotic disorders in HIV disease are discussed in Chapter 2). Miller et al (1988) described 19 individuals attending a genitourinary department with persistent concerns about HIV infection. The large majority were men, of whom two-thirds were gay or bisexual. All manifested anxiety symptoms and obsessional thoughts involving HIV disease, and in particular related to situations they regarded as having placed them at risk of acquiring the infection. Many exhibited rituals involving washing, checking for lesions, or compulsive reading of newspaper articles or books about HIV. A primary diagnosis of depression was given to 14 of the 19 patients. Background problems showed a good degree of consistency: sexual guilt, involving marital infidelity or difficulties accepting homosexuality was common. Interestingly, as a group, they were characterized by having no or very low risk of HIV infection, as their persistent fears had prevented them from taking part in risky activities. More than half of the patients in this series had a past psychiatric history, commonly anxiety or depression, and less frequently eating or obsessional disorders. The prevalence of abnormal beliefs about infection in the context of HIV is not known, although their repeated presence at genitourinary clinics and other facilities, makes patients with persistent concerns appear more numerous than they really are.

1.3 Psychological problems in asymptomatic HIV infection

After seroconversion, a period of asymptomatic HIV infection follows. The duration of this stage of infection is 10 or more years for most individuals (see Chapter 9), although this average figure hides a wide range of individual variability, and therefore prediction in a particular person's case is very difficult. Attempts to predict progression are made even more complicated by the fact that the date of seroconversion is not usually known, except when it has followed a clearly identifiable event, such as a blood transfusion, or when a previous HIV seronegative test result can help to locate the time of infection accurately.

For the majority of individuals, this asymptomatic stage brings into focus many threats and fears about the present and the future, but fortunately for some, this happens at a time when it is still possible to remain somewhat distanced and detached from the possibility of ill-health and the implications of treatment choices. This period of respite and freedom from the urgency of sickness allows most people to start confronting a possibly bleak future in such a way that some positive effects follow. For example, priorities can become clearer, important decisions faced, and the support of friends and relatives can become more precious. Sadly, not everyone is able to cope in this positive and successful manner, and for many this is a troubled and painful time, when old unresolved problems come to the surface again, and maladaptive ways of coping threaten to take over.

In this section, the evidence concerning psychological and social adjustment and problems of asymptomatic individuals is reviewed. Information will be presented first from work based on relatively unselected populations, such as people attending clinics for HIV disease or volunteers involved in cohort studies, and then by describing the psychosocial problems of HIV asymptomatic individuals referred for specialist mental health care. Research into the psychological and social implications of HIV infection raises many methodological issues which, while not new, highlight the need to proceed with caution in the interpretation of results.

1.3.1 Research surveys

Most of the research publications available concern samples from developed countries, and many involve gay/bisexual men. For these reasons, the results obtained cannot be generalised to all populations with HIV infection, or to individuals from developing countries with major economic and social difficulties and where the hospital and community care systems are very different. The results of those studies which compare the psychological status of people with asymptomatic HIV infection with comparable HIV seronegative controls are summarized in Table 1.1.

Gay/bisexual men

Controlled investigations of the psychosocial status of gay/bisexual men with asymptomatic infection have given contradictory results but most studies,

Table 1.1 Summary of studies comparing psychological status in those with asymptomatic HIV infection with uninfected controls

	No difference	Difference
Gay/bisexual men	Ostrow et al, 1986, 1989b Atkinson et al, 1988 Blaney et al, 1990 Williams et al, 1991 Fell et al, 1993 Pugh et al, 1994 Gala et al, 1993 Perkins et al, 1994 Maj et al, 1994a	Kurdeck and Siesky, 1990 Rabkin et al, 1990a Joseph et al, 1990 Catalán et al, 1992a Perkins et al, 1993a
Injecting drug users	Silberstein et al, 1987 Egan et al, 1992 Maj et al, 1994a	Pakesch et al, 1992 Gala et al, 1993
Men with hæmophilia	Dew et al, 1990	Parish et al, 1989 Catalán et al, 1992b Pasqual-Marsettin et al, 1992
Heterosexual men and women	Gala et al, 1993 Pergami et al, 1994b Beevor et al, 1991 Mellers et al, 1991 Pergami et al, 1993	

though by no means all, have found that asymptomatic infection has little if any impact on mental health after the initial adjustment reaction to the diagnosis. Some of these reports are summarized below.

The largest study of this type reported to date comes from the preliminary report on a Chicago cohort of over 3000 patients involved in the Multicenter AIDS Cohort Study (MACS) (Ostrow et al 1986). One problem with this study, and the subsequent reports with over 5000 participants on the same cohort, is that it is unclear how many participants knew their HIV status at the time (Ostrow et al, 1989b). Atkinson et al (1988) in a cross-sectional study of 17 people with asymptomatic infection and 11 HIV seronegatives controls carried out in San Diego, California, found no differences between groups in current psychological morbidity or levels of lifetime psychopathology, which was as high as 80 per cent, regardless of HIV status. Blaney et al (1990) in Miami compared 45 people with asymptomatic infection and 13 HIV seronegative individuals cross-sectionally and found no differences in emotional distress or coping strategies, in spite of the fact that those with HIV infection reported more negative life events and worse perceived impact. Williams et al (1991) in a New York cross-sectional investigation of 124 people with HIV infection and 84 HIV seronegative individuals, the baseline stage of a prospective cohort study (Gorman et al, 1991) also failed to find differences in current and lifetime psychopathology between the groups. Fell et al (1993) in London studied 59 people with asymptomatic HIV infection and 26 uninfected gay men at baseline and about 11 months later, and found no differences between groups regarding overall psychiatric morbidity, anxiety and depression at both stages of assessment, although those with asymptomatic HIV infection showed a decline in their levels of anxiety over time. In another London study, Riccio et al (1993) found no differences between 68 individuals with HIV infection and 32 HIV seronegative controls at the cross-sectional baseline stage of a prospective investigation, and at the subsequent 12-month follow-up (Pugh et al, 1994). Gala et al (1993) found no differences between 94 HIV seropositive individuals and 38 HIV seronegative gay men in a cross-sectional study from Milan. Perkins et al (1994) detected no differences in current or past psychopathology in a sample of 98 HIV positive asymptomatic and 71 seronegative gay men, although major depression was common in both groups. Finally, no differences were found in psychiatric status between asymptomatic and seronegative patients in the cross-sectional phase of the large multicentre WHO neuropsychiatric study, which included gay/bisexual men from Munich, São Paulo, Kinshasa, Nairobi, and Bangkok (Maj et al, 1994a).

In contrast, fewer studies have reported significant differences between HIV asymptomatic and seronegative gay/bisexual men. More death anxiety, lower levels of optimism and more distress were found by Kurdek and Siesky (1990) in a study of 27 people with asymptomatic HIV infection compared with and 15 HIV seronegative controls in Ohio. Rabkin et al (1990a) reported lower levels of hope in a study of 124 HIV seropositive and 84 seronegative gay men in New York. Joseph et al (1990) in a 3-year follow-up of Chicago men involved in the MACS found that AIDS-specific distress was higher in HIV seropositive gay men and tended to increased over time, while other measures of psychological morbidity were comparable between groups. All participants, regardless of HIV status had higher levels of psychological morbidity than the general population, although not as high as that of psychiatric out-patients. Catalán et al (1992a) compared 19 HIV seropositive asymptomatic and 24 HIV seronegative gay men in a cross-sectional study and found the HIV seropositive group to have worse overall levels of morbidity to experience more sexual dysfunction although there were no differences on other measures of psychological adjustment. A higher prevalence of personality disorder was reported by Perkins et al (1993a) in people with asymptomatic HIV infection compared with uninfected controls. Furthermore, those individuals with HIV infection and personality disorders had more severe mood disturbance, were more likely to experience social conflict, and to use denial and helplessness as ways of coping.

A number of investigations which have not used HIV negative controls have provided further information. Chuang et al (1989) described 65 people who were seropositive for HIV at various stages of disease: 24 with asymptomatic infection, 22 with AIDS-Related complex (ARC) and 19 with AIDS. Group comparisons showed that those men living with AIDS had better scores than the other two groups for depression, Profile of Mood States total and anxiety scores. Suicidal ideation was rare in all groups. King (1989a) studied over 60 asymptomatic gay/bisexual men receiving care for HIV infection in London, as part of a cross-sectional study involving 192 men at various stages of disease. About one third had significant levels of psychiatric morbidity, a proportion comparable to reports from other studies of out-patient attenders at genito-urinary medicine clinics. No differences in levels of distress were found between patients at different stages of HIV infection. Cazzullo et al (1990) studied 92 HIV people with asymptomatic HIV infection from Italy, including drug users, gay men, and heterosexuals, and found that their depression and anxiety levels were comparable to those of the general population, and no differences were found between groups. Kelly et al (1991a), in a report from Brisbane, Australia, studied 30 gay and bisexual men with asymptomatic HIV disease using the General Health Questionnaire (GHQ) and found 'psychiatric caseness' rates comparable to published figures for general hospital in-patients.

Injecting drug users

Silberstein et al (1987) found no differences in psychological measures when comparing 70 HIV seropositive and 141 HIV seronegative injecting drug users attending a methadone service in New York. In contrast, Pakesch et al (1992), in a study of 42 HIV seropositive and 31 HIV seronegative drug users in Vienna found more depressive symptoms in HIV seropositive group. Egan et al (1992) in a prospective cohort study from Edinburgh, compared 125 injecting drug users with asymptomatic infection with 27 who were uninfected. They found no differences in anxiety and depression either at baseline or at 16-month follow-up.

Somewhat surprisingly, Gala et al (1993), in a cross-sectional study of injecting drug users from Milan, found HIV seronegative ($n = 91$) drug users to have higher levels of psychological morbidity than those who were HIV seropositive ($n = 157$) . In addition, injecting drug users, regardless of serostatus had poorer psychological adjustment than other gay/bisexual men and non-injecting drug using heterosexuals with HIV infection, although this finding was not confirmed in another, uncontrolled study from Italy (Cazzullo et al, 1990). Maj et al (1994a) found no differences between asymptomatic and seronegative drug users in the WHO study referred to above.

Men with haemophilia

HIV infection HIV infection has added to the difficulties experienced by people with haemophilia (Agle et al, 1987; Wilkie et al, 1990a; Catalán and Klimes, 1991), and in some cases contributed to the development of major psychological problems. Parish et al (1989) studied 351 men with haemophilia in Los Angeles and found those with HIV infection reported higher levels of stress, greater difficulty in close relationships and greater fear of stigmatization. Dew et al (1990) compared 31 asymptomatic men and 44 negatives, finding no significant differences in levels of psychological distress, which were generally low. Contrasting findings have been reported by Catalán et al (1992b). In a cross-sectional study from Oxford using standardized interview and self-report measures, they compared 31 men with asymptomatic HIV infection and 36 who were uninfected.

They found that the seropositive group had higher overall levels of psychological morbidity, greater levels of hopelessness, and more sexual difficulties.

Rather unexpected results were reported by Pasqual-Marsettin et al (1992) from Bari, Italy, who found higher levels of anxiety and depression in HIV seronegative men with haemophilia over a two-year period. It is possible that the people who were HIV seropositive might have started to develop successful coping mechanisms to minimize their concerns about health, while those who were seronegative continued to see themselves at risk of infection and did not trust their doctors about the safety of blood products.

Heterosexual men and women

Gala et al (1993) and Pergami et al (1994b) found no differences between 28 people with asymptomatic HIV infection and 30 uninfected individuals from Milan studied cross-sectionally. Similar results were reported by Beevor et al (1991), Mellers et al (1991), and Pergami et al (1993) in controlled investigations of psychological adjustment of women with HIV infection.

Uncontrolled studies of women with HIV infection have provided details about their characteristics and problems. James (1988) described 15 asymptomatic women identified during pregnancy: the majority were Black and almost half injected drugs. Mood disorders were present in 20 per cent, adjustment disorders in 53 per cent, personality disorders in 73 per cent, and 26 per cent had a history of attempted suicide. Brown and Rundell (1990) described 18 women with asymptomatic HIV infection in the United States Air Force, 50 per cent of whom were Black. Half were given a psychiatric diagnosis including hypoactive sexual desire (20 per cent), adjustment disorders (15 per cent), and subtle cognitive impairments (10 per cent). Concerns about confidentiality, pre-existing problems and care of the children were highlighted in the series described by Sherr et al (1993).

Brown et al (1992) have reported the results of an uncontrolled study of 442 men in the United States Air Force with HIV infection, the large majority in the earliest stages of the infection. No information was provided in the report about history of risk behaviours, and so it is not possible to determine to which transmission category the men belonged. Major depression and anxiety disorders and sexual dysfunction were more common in this sample than would have been expected in a matched general population control group, and, in addition, the HIV seropositive men had an increased lifetime prevalence of major depression and alcohol misuse prior to HIV infection compared with population norms.

1.3.2 Referral to specialist mental health services in asymptomatic HIV infection

Several reports of patients with HIV disease referred to liaison psychiatry services have been reported and most have included individuals with asymptomatic infection, as well as those with AIDS. The majority of people in these series, however, had symptomatic disease and relatively few are asymptomatic.

Psychosocial reactions and depressive disorders are more common in those with asymptomatic infection whereas organic brain syndromes are more often seen in symptomatic disease.

Sno et al (1989) reported on 51 HIV medical in-patients referred to psychiatrists between 1983 and 1988 in Amsterdam, representing 19 per cent of all HIV medical admissions. Only 6 (12 per cent) were asymptomatic, and the diagnoses given included: atypical psychosis, delirium, major depression, panic disorder and bereavement. Ayuso-Mateos et al (1989) described 100 HIV patients referred to the psychiatric service of a Madrid teaching hospital between 1984 and 1989, most of whom were in-patients at the time (90 per cent) and only a third were asymptomatic. The most common diagnoses were substance misuse (51 per cent), adjustment disorder (15 per cent) and delirium (12 per cent), although no information is given about psychiatric diagnoses by disease stage. Seth et al (1991) described 60 patients referred to the liaison psychiatry service at St. Mary's Hospital, London, over a 12-month period, 21 (35 per cent) of whom were asymptomatic. Psychiatric diagnoses included: adjustment reactions ($n = 7$), paranoid reactions ($n = 5$), depressive disorders ($n = 4$), schizophrenia ($n = 2$), personality change ($n = 2$), and mania ($n = 1$). Affective disorders and dementia were more common in the symptomatic group.

In our own liaison psychiatry service (Douzenis et al, 1991), we studied the first 200 referrals, 42 (21 per cent) of whom were asymptomatic. In contrast with previous reports, only a minority, 74 (37 per cent), were medical in-patients at the time of referral. The most common diagnoses were: adjustment reactions ($n = 11$), depressive disorders ($n = 8$), substance misuse ($n = 6$), and personality disorder ($n = 5$). All cases of organic brain syndromes ($n = 19$) and psychotic illnesses ($n = 6$) occurred in individuals with symptomatic disease.

1.3.3 Summary and methodological problems

Several points arise from this review of published research reports about the psychological adjustment of people with asymptomatic disease, the personal descriptions of those with HIV, and the experience of liaison psychiatrists.

(a) The large majority of controlled studies show that there are very few differences in levels of distress and psychological morbidity between people with asymptomatic HIV infection and comparable HIV seronegative controls. This applies to gay/bisexual men, injecting drug users, and heterosexual men and women. Although most studies find no differences, a few do report poorer psychological well-being in those with HIV infection, while others paradoxically, find that, uninfected individuals have poorer mental health.

(b) Levels of distress in individuals at risk of HIV infection, whether actually infected or not, are generally of mild severity, although they are somewhat higher than expected for general population samples.

(c) A substantial proportion of individuals at risk of HIV infection, regardless of HIV status, have a history of psychiatric disorder and treatment, prior to HIV infection.

(d) Injecting drug users, whether HIV infected or not, have higher levels of psychiatric morbidity than other groups of individuals with HIV infection, such as gay/bisexual men and men with haemophilia.

(e) Substance misuse, adjustment reactions, and depression are the most common psychiatric diagnoses given to people with asymptomatic HIV infection referred to psychiatric services. Organic brain syndromes and psychotic illnesses are seen very infrequently.

The finding that individuals with HIV who remain healthy do not differ significantly from comparable people who are HIV seronegative is somewhat puzzling, as it is contrary to expectation. There are several possible explanations for these findings. High levels of lifetime psychopathology prior to HIV infection are present in many individuals at risk of infection, regardless of their actual serostatus, and this suggests that those with and without HIV infection have much in common regarding predisposition to psychological problems. There is also evidence that personality disorders are common in populations at risk of HIV infection (Ross et al, 1988) and as well as amongst people with HIV infection (Perkins et al, 1993a; Brooner et al, 1993). Furthermore, it may be that the nature of the psychological and social supports available to people with HIV infection has helped to minimize the adverse psychological consequences of HIV. However, this explanation seems unlikely, as there is evidence of continuing rejection and social difficulties in people with HIV infection (King, 1989b), and in any case it would be surprising if medical and social services could have had such a powerful impact.

Methodological issues, such as sampling and selection of subjects for the various studies, probably account for many of the inconsistencies in the findings reported. Many studies include a preponderance of white, well-educated and financially successful individuals. It can be argued that these socially advantaged people, who volunteer for extensive investigations lasting several years, are not typical of the general population of people with HIV infection and may be better adjusted than a more representative selection of people with HIV infection. Using such unrepresentative groups of people may obscure real differences in psychological status between those with and without HIV infection. In addition, there may be different processes of selection at work in the case of HIV seropositive and HIV seronegative individuals. People with HIV infection may participate in research partly for selfish reasons (they may expect to receive greater care and attention as a result) as well as for altruistic motives (so that others might benefit from research done on them). People without HIV infection, who by definition remain at risk of infection, may choose to participate in research involving HIV testing (sometimes at regular intervals) to seek reassurance that they are healthy. Such self-selection dynamics may mean that research samples of uninfected individuals, as a group, are really not typical of the population they are intended to represent.

Two Italian studies, one involving men with haemophilia (Pasqual-Marsettin et al, 1992) and another with injecting drug users, gay/bisexual men and heterosexuals (Gala et al , 1993) actually found higher levels of distress in the HIV seronegative group. These findings are counter-intuitive and require some explanation. It is tempting to speculate that such findings reflect widespread anxiety about HIV infection in the general population, with high levels of perceived risk amongst those who are HIV seronegative, and mistrust of the health messages provided by doctors and other authority figures.

In summary, it can be concluded that, with some methodological reservations, most people with asymptomatic HIV infection do not show higher levels of psychological morbidity than comparable individuals who remain seronegative. As some people with asymptomatic HIV infection do experience psychological difficulties, the question to be considered is not so much whether there are differences in psychological distress in relation to HIV status, but rather what are the factors that contribute to the development of psychological disorders in this group of individuals. This issue is discussed in detail later in the chapter.

1.4 Psychological problems in symptomatic HIV infection

The words we use to talk about HIV infection have a psychological and social significance of their own, beyond their strictly medical or scientific meaning (see Sontag, 1988, for a subtle discussion of the terminology of illness and its social meanings). HIV researchers tend nowadays to use the terms *HIV disease* or *HIV infection* to cover all stages of disease, including AIDS, while in earlier days, it was common to make a distinction between HIV and AIDS, as if they were two quite distinct and separate entities. Current classifications of HIV infection regard the condition as a continuum, as in the 1987 Center for Disease Control classification (see Chapter 9). Interestingly, this classification has actually done away with the word AIDS completely, using instead a numerical system, with subgroupings to describe the various stages.

It is easy to see how the old approach, making a clear separation between the two categories, would be reassuring to those who are in the healthy, non-AIDS, group, and conversely, how those given the dreaded label of AIDS would become alarmed. A further complication was created by the need to create a new category for those who had not developed AIDS, but could not be said to be healthy either: AIDS-related complex (ARC) came to be seen as the pre-AIDS stage. In contrast with older nomenclatures, contemporary classification systems may impart a sense of confidence, and possibly of false reassurance by seeking to avoid the word AIDS altogether. At the same time, the idea of a continuum, and the role of the CD4 lymphocyte count as an indicator of disease progression, can cancel out the advantage, and may, once more, lead to distress, by highlighting the possibility of a downward slide from a healthy state to the development of increasingly severe symptoms in parallel with a decline in the CD4 count.

Changes in terminology and classification systems are reflected in the psychiatric literature, so that ARC and AIDS feature in earlier publications, while later workers tend to talk in terms of early symptomatic and advanced disease. The term AIDS continues to show remarkable resilience. Comparisons between earlier and later studies are therefore not always strictly legitimate, as the classification of disease stages is not consistent.

As in the case of people with asymptomatic infection, we shall review first the published evidence from research investigations, and then the problems of individuals referred to mental health services with symptomatic disease.

1.4.1 Research surveys

Fewer research investigations have focused on people with symptomatic disease than on those with asymptomatic disease. Often these studies have included relatively small numbers and the groups studied have tended to be more restricted than those involving asymptomatic individuals. In general, levels of psychological morbidity tend to be higher in people with symptomatic disease than in asymptomatic infection (see reviews: O'Dowd, 1988; Catalán, 1988, 1990a; Miller and Riccio, 1990), but the research evidence is not entirely consistent.

Gay/bisexual men

Atkinson et al (1988) studied cross-sectionally 28 gay/bisexual men with a diagnosis of ARC or AIDS and compared them with 17 gay men with asymptomatic infection and 31 uninfected individuals of whom 11 were gay. Those people with symptomatic disease were more likely to experience anxiety symptoms or misuse alcohol in comparison with controls. Viney et al (1989) found that patients with symptomatic disease but without AIDS showed more distress and anger than patients with other disorders, although they also tended to manifest more positive feelings. Catalán et al (1992a) compared 24 people with HIV infection, 5 of whom had symptomatic disease, with 25 seronegative gay/bisexual men in a cross-sectional study. In spite of small numbers, those patients with symptomatic disease had significantly poorer mental health, and 40 per cent were classifiable as psychiatric cases. There was also a tendency for those individuals with symptomatic disease to have an external health locus of control (i.e. they attributed their health state to factors outside of their own control) and to have lower scores on the challenge dimension of the Hardiness scale (a measure of the extent to which health problems are perceived as a challenge to be overcome).

In contrast, Kurdek and Siesky (1990), in another cross-sectional study, found that people with symptomatic HIV infection had more favourable scores than those with asymptomatic infection. Fell et al (1993) in the prospective study referred to above found that people with symptomatic HIV infection had higher levels of psychological disturbance than either people with asymptomatic disease or those who were uninfected. Over time, they found that people with asymptomatic infection showed a decline in their levels of mood disturbance and those with symptomatic disease showed no improvement. Maj et al (1994a) in the multicentre WHO neuropsychiatric study compared the psychological status of representative selections of people with HIV infection at five different centres around the world, most of which included significant numbers of gay/bisexual men. In two of the centres, they found greater psychological morbidity in people with symptomatic infection compared with those who had asymptomatic disease or were seronegative. Interestingly, there were no significant differences between the groups in terms of their psychological status in the other three centres.

The difficulties raised by HIV infection classification systems are illustrated in the MACS report by Hoover et al (1993). They compared 916 gay men who were not close to developing AIDS and presumed to be asymptomatic with 2161 seronegative controls. The 'asymptomatic' group reported significantly more symptoms of ill-health, had lower haemoglobin and body mass index than the HIV seronegative group. In addition the asymptomatic group reported higher levels of depression prior to notification of serostatus and this deteriorated further over time, while no such change was seen in the seronegative group.

Although people with symptomatic HIV disease tend to report poorer mental health than those with asymptomatic infection, it should not be assumed that the further advanced the disease is, the poorer the psychological well-being is likely to be. Indeed, there are several reports suggesting that people with early symptomatic disease, or ARC, have higher levels of psychological morbidity than those with AIDS (Perry and Markowitz, 1986; Temoshok et al, 1986). Tross et al (1987) studied hospitalized patients in New York and reported high levels of distress in 63 per cent of patients with ARC, compared with 52 per cent in those with AIDS and 31 per cent in controls. King (1989a) in an uncontrolled London study found patients with ARC to have the worst levels of psychological morbidity, although the differences did not reach statistical significance. Chuang et al (1989), quoted above, found the best psychological status in people with AIDS, compared with other groups, although all showed evidence of distress.

Injecting drug users

In the Edinburgh study cited above, Egan et al (1992) found no significant differences in terms of anxiety or depression between a group of injecting drug users with symptomatic HIV infection and one consisting of uninfected individuals. These groups were followed up for 16 months, and although those with symptomatic infection tended to have higher depression scores than the other group, the difference was not significant.

Men with haemophilia

In the cross-sectional study from Oxford of men with haemophilia, (Catalán et al, 1992b), men with symptomatic HIV disease were found to have higher overall levels of psychological morbidity, more depression and greater levels of hopelessness than those who were HIV seronegative. The men with symptomatic disease generally reported poorer mental health than those with asymptomatic disease.

Heterosexual men and women

There is remarkably little work on the psychological impact of symptomatic HIV infection in heterosexuals and none including hetrosexual men. Bialer (1992) studied 62 women attending out-patient medical care services in New York. The majority had symptomatic disease, were injecting drug users and Hispanic or Black. More than a third had pathological levels of anxiety, and moderate to severe depression was present in 45 per cent. In this population it is difficult to separate demographic characteristics and drug use from HIV infection itself when considering the aetiology of the psychological difficulties.

1.4.2 Referral to specialist mental health services in symptomatic HIV infection

Referral of patients with HIV disease or any other condition for psychiatric consultation is influenced by many factors. Some are related to the patient's own mental state while others are related to the availability of mental health personnel and services, and the expertise and skills of the medical team. This means that referral rates to different hospitals are likely to reflect this range of factors, rather than the true prevalence of psychiatric disorders.

Perry and Tross (1984) in a study involving 52 patients, mostly gay and bisexual men, found that 19 per cent of in-patients with AIDS receiving medical care at the New York Hospital were referred for psychiatric consultation. The majority were referred as a result of management problems, and the rest for diagnostic assessment or self-referral. Retrospective examination of the case-notes revealed that mood disturbance had been identified in more than 80 per cent and signs of organic brain disorders in over 65 per cent of patients with AIDS. Dilley et al (1985) in San Francisco described 13 (33 per cent) patients with AIDS referred for psychiatric consultation, out of total of 40 in-patients most of whom were gay or bisexual men. Assessment of mood was the most common reason for referral (10 cases). All except one were given psychiatric diagnoses which included adjustment disorder ($n = 7$), major depression ($n = 2$), dementia ($n = 1$), delirium ($n = 1$) and panic disorder ($n = 1$). Buhrich and Cooper (1987) reported from Sydney a lower psychiatric consultation rate amongst in-patients with ARC and AIDS, over a 16-month period. Twenty-two (15 per cent) out of 150 patients were referred and all were gay or bisexual men. The authors stressed that these patients represented those suffering the most severe psychological problems, as patients with milder disorders were appropriately managed by the medical and nursing teams. Organic brain disorders were the most common diagnoses. Ten presented with acute or sub-acute syndromes, one suffered long standing epilepsy and another had a low IQ. Other diagnoses included Adjustment disorder with depressive symptoms ($n = 4$) patients, psychotic illness ($n = 2$), mania ($n = 1$), schizophreniform disorder ($n = 1$), drug dependency-related problems ($n = 3$) and major depression ($n = 1$).

Lyons et al (1989) found that psychiatric consultations were requested for 22 (24 per cent) out 90 medical in-patients with AIDS admitted to the Northwestern Memorial Hospital in the US. Adjustment and neurotic disorders were the most common diagnoses ($n = 12$), followed by organic brain syndromes ($n = 9$), substance misuse ($n = 5$), major depression ($n = 4$), and psychotic disorders (one mania and one schizophrenia). Interestingly, referral for psychiatric consultation or to social workers was predictive of longer hospital stay, even when severity of illness was controlled for. The conclusion from this is that psychiatric morbidity has implications for the cost of hospitalization.

Ayuso-Mateos et al (1989) described 100 HIV patients referred for psychiatric consultation in Madrid and found the majority to be symptomatic (69 per cent belonging to CDC group IV). The psychiatric diagnoses quoted above (1.3.2; see also Table 9.2), reflect the predominance of drug users in HIV patients in Spain, although the report does not provide information for psychiatric diagnoses by disease stage.

In the report by Sno et al (1989), 45 (88 per cent) of all HIV patients referred for consultation had symptomatic disease, the majority having AIDS. Organic brain syndromes were the most common diagnosis ($n = 20$), followed by major depression ($n = 11$), adjustment disorder ($n = 5$) and psychosis ($n = 4$).

O'Dowd and McKegney (1990) compared patients with AIDS with patients who were not HIV seropositive who had been referred for psychiatric consultation at the Montefiore Medical Center in New York over a 12-month period. Patients with AIDS represented only 6 per cent of all cases, and compared with non-HIV patients of similar age, they were found to include more Hispanics and be more severely symptomatic and disabled. Patients with AIDS were statistically more likely to have organic brain disorders, including dementia. There were trends suggesting that drug misuse and adjustment disorder were more common and alcohol misuse, schizophrenia and personality disorder less common in those with AIDS.

In the report by Seth et al (1991) affective disorders were present in 30 (77 per cent) of all symptomatic patients (CDC group IV) referred for consultation, while dementia was diagnosed in only 4 (10 per cent).

Our experience (Douzenis et al, 1991) with 200 HIV patients referred for psychiatric consultation, including 152 (76 per cent) with symptomatic disease (CDC group IV), is comparable to that described in other reports with significant numbers of adjustment and mood disorders. The main diagnoses were adjustment disorders were seen in 44 (29 per cent); major depression in 24 (16 per cent); organic brain syndromes in 19 (13 per cent); alcohol-related problems in 17 (11 per cent); and psychotic illness in 6 (4 per cent).

Symptomatic HIV patients requiring psychiatric hospitalization are likely to be those with the most severe psychiatric syndromes. Baer (1989) described 60 patients with AIDS or ARC admitted to the psychiatric department at San Francisco General Hospital. Most were white, male and gay or bisexual. A diagnosis of depression was given to 20 (33 per cent) of patients, including 13 (22 per cent) cases of adjustment disorder and 7 (12 per cent) of major depression; dementia was present in 18 (30 per cent), often in association with other syndromes; psychotic illnesses, including schizophrenia, brief reactive psychosis and mania, were diagnosed in 16 (27 per cent) patients.

In summary, reports of HIV symptomatic individuals belonging to a variety of transmission categories tend to indicate that psychiatric morbidity is increased in this group when compared with people with asymptomatic infection or with people who are HIV seronegative. Organic brain disorders, major depression, psychotic illnesses and adjustment disorders, as well as worsening of substance misuse are not uncommon in symptomatic patients. The association between symptomatic HIV disease and psychiatric morbidity is consistent with the experience of liaison psychiatrists dealing with conditions other than HIV infection. One practical consequence of the increased prevalence of mental health problems in symptomatic patients is the need to ensure that physicians and nurses involved in their care have the skills to recognize and manage such problems (see Chapter 4).

1.5 Psychological problems in the final stages of HIV infection

In AIDS it can be difficult to decide at what point the word 'terminal illness' should be used, as efforts to predict survival are unreliable, and the complexity of medical conditions and treatments required can mean that active treatments are sometimes continued until shortly before death (Andersen and MacElveen-Hoehn, 1988). It is not surprising to find that severe deterioration in health is often associated with psychological and neuropsychiatric problems. For some, who until then had coped well, the final stages may lead to distress or major problems related to poor symptom control, major physical complications or sudden awareness of the proximity of death. For others, depression and fear may have been present since the diagnosis was made. The dividing line between *normal* and *pathological* fear, or between understandable suicidal thoughts and suicide risk in the context of severe depression may be difficult to draw, and may even be of little relevance. The main issue is how to enable the person to remain in control and as comfortable and pain-free as possible. Furthermore, neuropsychiatric problems, including HIV-associated dementia and manic disorders, are not uncommon in the late stages of the disorder, adding to the problems that individuals and their relatives face.

1.5.1 Emotional and social changes in terminal illness

Before HIV disease became a problem, much of the knowledge about the psychological aspects of terminal illness was based on the experience of people with cancer, in particular those receiving care in hospices. It is instructive to read this literature as it is of great relevance to the problems seen in HIV disease (Kubler-Ross, 1970; Stedeford, 1984, Parkes, 1986; Vachon, 1993). Kubler-Ross in particular has been influential in describing the stages that people facing death often go through, such as denial, anger, bargaining, depression, and acceptance. It should not be assumed, however, that there is a right way of dying which requires a progression through phases which culminates in some form of peaceful and contented state. People vary enormously in the way they confront their end, some denying until the end their approaching death, while others may switch and alternate modes of coping within a short period of time. The awareness of approaching death brings about changes in help-seeking and social support. Catania et al (1992a) have shown how in gay men, disease progression is associated with an increased involvement with the person's biological family, and with a reduction in death-related anxiety, often leading to an improvement in communication and relations with parents and other relatives. As George (1992) has argued, such changes in social relations may well reflect the individual's efforts to make sense of approaching death by seeking reconciliation and meaning.

In the UK, palliative care hospices are now well established, and they provide a wide range of facilities from residential to home care and support. McCarthy (1990) in a pilot study of nearly 200 patients in 12 hospices in the UK, found the majority of residents to be suffering from cancer, with only 4 per cent having AIDS. In all cases, the need for emotional support was the second most common reason for referral, after symptom control. Emotional problems included anxiety (62 per cent), depression (36 per cent), withdrawal (26 per cent), denial (21 per cent) and mental confusion (21 per cent). Empirical research has shown that patients with terminal cancer and their families regard emotional difficulties, in particular anxiety, as a very important problem (Higginson et al, 1990). There is also evidence that most people with cancer would prefer to die at home, although this does not always happen (Townsend et al, 1990).

Ramsay (1992) has described the work of a psychiatrist attached to a hospice dealing mostly with cancer patients. About 10 per cent of patients cared for over a 12-month period were referred for psychiatric consultation. Depression was the most common reason for referral (46 per cent), followed by behavioural problems and paranoia (15 per cent each), intractable pain (12 per cent) and anxiety (8 per cent). A diagnosis of depression was made in most cases (54 per cent), and an organic brain syndrome was found in almost a quarter. In most cases intervention was brief, and only a minority of patients required more prolonged care over a period of weeks or longer.

1.5.2 Mental health problems in the terminal stages of HIV infection

The pattern of psychological reactions in the terminal stages of AIDS are largely the same as those seen in other diseases. There are some important differences, however. People dying with AIDS tend to be relatively young (compared with those with cancer) and background social and family factors, including the social reactions to a diagnosis of AIDS can make the situation harder to confront. There is, for example, some evidence to suggest that terminally ill patients with AIDS show lower levels of hope than similarly ill patients with cancer, and this difference may well be related to fears of isolation and rejection (Herth, 1990).

Baker and Seager (1991) compared the psychosocial needs of patients with and without AIDS cared for in a hospice in Iowa, US. Patients with AIDS had fewer community supports and required more involvement from hospice staff, who also reported finding their work more demanding than that involving patients with other diseases. The social isolation of people with AIDS and the presence of unresolved issues related to drug use or sexuality were identified by staff as contributors to their difficulties. Volunteers working in an AIDS-dedicated hospice were found to experience a greater sense of health threat than those working in a traditional hospice (Shuff et al, 1991), and Malcolm and

Sutherland (1992) have also highlighted the possible impact on staff looking after people with AIDS of the risks of infection with HIV as well as tuberculosis and hepatitis B and C, and its effect on the care provided. Sims and Moss (1991), a nurse and a doctor with enormous experience in dealing with the problems of terminal care in a hospice for people with AIDS, have provided a moving and clear account of the emotional, social and physical needs of people faced with the final stages of illness. Fears of loss of control, dignity or physical integrity; loss of hope; fear of the mode of death; and powerful emotions, like anger and guilt, are common. In addition, organic brain syndromes with confusion, memory impairment and personality changes are often present.

Detailed empirical studies of the mental health problems that arise in the terminal stages of AIDS are few, but there are accounts of the main psychiatric problems that may arise at this stage, including mood disorders, such as depression and anxiety, concerns about body image, psychotic illness such as schizophrenia-like disorders and mania (see Chapter 2) and organic brain syndromes (see Chapter 4), (Wells, 1987; Schofferman, 1987; Carr, 1989; Cole, 1991). Fernandez et al, (1989a) found organic brain syndromes to be present in nearly 60 per cent of patients who were severely ill with AIDS referred for psychiatric consultation, delirium being the most common form of disorder.

Ethical issues become prominent here too. Decisions as to when to provide active treatment as opposed to palliative care (George, 1991; Martin, 1991), the use of advance directives, what provision to make for people with HIV infection rather than for those suffering from other diseases (Miller, 1991), and the complex question of euthanasia (Morissette, 1990; Beckett, 1991) (see Chapter 8).

1.5.3 Subjective experience of living and dying with AIDS

Moving accounts of the process of coping with declining health and death are available in publications dealing with the emotional and practical aspects of the infection. Thus Sims and Moss (1991) have illustrated the problems seen in hospice-based palliative care. Martelli et al (1987) provide very practical insights into the problems of people with AIDS and their carers, and Teguis (1992) and Puentes (1992) give personal accounts and descriptions of different ways of coping with advanced AIDS. Kirkpatrick (1994) has provided a moving example of the process of death and adjustment to it.

1.6 Psychological impact on children

1.6.1 Epidemiological and clinical aspects

By the beginning of January 1992 more than 1 million children had been infected with HIV world-wide, representing about 8 per cent of all cases of HIV infection (Mann et al, 1992). The large majority of cases came from sub-Saharan Africa (over 900 000), Latin America (about 40 000) and South-east Asia (24 000). Epidemiological projections indicate that 1.2 million more children will become infected by 1995. It is likely that global gains in child survival recently achieved will be reversed, in particular in areas where HIV infection is common in childbearing women (Mann et al, 1992). The majority of children with HIV infection have been infected perinatally (about 85 per cent of cases of paediatric AIDS in the US), the rest having been infected through contaminated blood products or during treatment for haemophilia). The rate of mother-to-child transmission appears to vary between cohorts from 7 to 42 per cent (Mann et al, 1992). There is growing evidence that in a proportion of cases HIV infection is the result of child sexual abuse (see Chapter 3).

HIV infection in children has a poorer outcome than in adults, the large majority of children with congenitally acquired infection not surviving beyond 5 years of age. Diagnosis of infection in children born to HIV positive mothers can be problematic, as maternal antibodies can persist for up to 18 months, and clinical assessment may be unreliable (Sherr, 1991). New techniques to identify HIV in children have been developed, such as the DNA or RNA polymerase chain reaction (PCR), and *in vitro* antibody production. Unfortunately, these methods are still not routinely available (Gibb and Newell, 1992).

1.6.2 The psychological impact of HIV infection on children

As argued by Bailey (1992), HIV infection threatens children not just through the consequences of direct infection, illness and death, but as a result of infection in the child's parents. Children with HIV infection progress to disease and death more quickly than adults, and the infection is usually associated with delayed growth and development. On the other hand, the effects of HIV infection in the parents, whether the child is also infected or not, are likely to include periods of parental hospitalization and eventual death. Chronic and progressive illness will be associated with severe emotional and practical pressures on the rest of family members, compounding the difficulties in the future care of the orphaned children (Canosa, 1991; Sherr, 1991).

The child with HIV infection

Melvin and Sherr (1993) studied 18 children with HIV infection being cared for at a London hospital. Half of the children were under the age of two, only one being over 12 years old. The mothers were positive in all but one case, and almost half of the fathers were infected, the rest being uncertain about their HIV status. In most cases, other relatives were unaware of the situation, and only the oldest child in the cohort knew of his and his parents' status. Financial and practical difficulties were common, including language and economic problems. The authors identified complex areas of need related to the children's own developmental and health needs, maternal isolation and lack of supports, and the competing health care needs of mothers and children.

Schooling will raise particular difficulties for older children in relation to confidentiality, their right to education, and fears of rejection by other children, their families and the educational authorities, in addition to the children's own health care and educational needs (Ginzburg and Hanlon, 1990; Sherr, 1991;

Claxton and Harrison, 1991). Children with haemophilia and other disorders such as thalassaemia can face specific difficulties, which are influenced by the severity of the pre-existing disorder and parental attitudes to it, and by the nature and quality of the relationships between the child and the parents (Anastasopoulos and Tsiantis, 1990; Tsiantis and Meyer, 1992), although psychological problems are not inevitable in this group of children (Logan et al, 1990). Fostering and adoption may be required and confidentiality about the children's status and whom to inform, as well as selection and training of foster parents will be important issues (Skinner, 1991).

The uninfected children of HIV infected parents

While developed countries are also facing this issue (Weil-Halpern, 1989; Giaquinto et al, 1992; Michaels and Levine, 1992; Ronald et al, 1993), it is in developing countries where the consequences for the family are the most dramatic (Hunter, 1990). Ankrah (1993) has described graphically the African situation, stressing how as the parents become progressively unwell, their children may be required to take a 'parental' role, with adverse consequences in terms of their schooling and psychological and social development, and with major effects on the family structure and on the surviving orphaned children, which now form part of a family headed by grandparents, who may in turn be frail and unable to provide economic support.

Siblings of HIV infected children

Children with HIV infection are not the only ones to suffer the effects of the disease: their uninfected siblings may also be affected. Behavioural problems are not uncommon in this group of children, although the aetiological factors may be difficult to separate. Pre-existing problems, family disruption as a result of HIV infection, parental ill-health, competition for affection and care, guilt and anticipated bereavement may all contribute (Sherr, 1991).

Children facing death

Severe illness and death in children raise complex problems concerning what to discuss with the child and when, who should talk with the child about it and in what way. Notification of the infection and its meaning, reasons for investigations and treatment, and answering questions about the likely consequences of the illness may have to be dealt with at some stage. As in the case of other life-threatening illnesses (Woolley et al, 1989), the way the surrounding adults and health professionals respond will play an important part in the process (Sherr, 1991; Kuykendall, 1991).

The effects of parental or sibling loss on a child will be modulated by many factors, including the age of the child, the subsequent mothering experience and the family's approach to coping with death. While little has been published about HIV-related bereavement in children, there is a body of literature about child bereavement in general, showing an initial increase in psychological symptoms and behavioural problems, sometimes of a persistent nature (Raphael, 1977a; Van Eerdewegh et al, 1982). In the case of HIV infection, the fact that the remaining family may not be in a good position to provide emotional support and stability will add to the risk of longer-term problems.

1.7 Psychological impact on partners and relatives

HIV infection is not simply an individual matter: illness in one person will have effects on those close to him or her, and their response in turn may enhance or inhibit adequate coping and influence the person's physical and psychological well-being (Maj, 1991; Bor et al, 1993a). Those close to the person with HIV infection include primarily partners, relatives and informal carers.

1.7.1 The psychological impact on partners

The presence of HIV infection in one person will have important effects for the couple, and these effects will change over time, as the emotional and practical needs of the infected individual increase with disease progression. Initially, concerns about infecting the other person may be paramount, on occasions becoming a major obstacle. Worries about the health of the infected partner and about the couple's ability to cope with the stresses of possible illness may be prominent. Issues of contraception and fertility will have to be confronted by heterosexual couples. The relationship may well be strengthened as a result of these pressures, but often pre-existing problems and difficulties may become more severe, threatening the survival of the relationship (Ussher, 1990). Mutual interdependence may become more marked (Bor et al, 1990). Loss and bereavement may be complicated and prolonged by unresolved difficulties in the relationship, and by exposure to repeated grief over HIV-related deaths.

Studies of gay couples have shown that partners of HIV infected men have substantial levels of anxiety and depression (Church et al, 1988; Maj, 1991). When both partners are HIV infected, it may be difficult to be clear as to who is the 'sick' partner and who is the 'carer', and indeed these roles may be reversed from time to time, highlighting the complementarity of the relationship (Bor et al, 1990). Sometimes a pattern of overidentification may occur, leading the uninfected partner to put himself at risk of infection as a way developing a closer bond and to lose himself in the relationship. Dependence, low self-esteem and social isolation are common themes in such couples (Morgan and Jones, 1993). The carers themselves often are aware of their need for emotional and practical support (McCann and Wadsworth, 1992). Partners who themselves are HIV positive are likely to show higher levels of distress than those who are uninfected (Hamel et al, 1991b). It is not unusual for partners not to know their serostatus: dealing with the consequences of one person being infected may be regarded as sufficiently stressful, without having to face the possibility of further bad news.

In contrast to gay couples, female partners of men with haemophilia and HIV infection do not appear to have worse levels of psychological morbidity than female partners of seronegative men with haemophilia (Dew et al, 1991; Klimes et al, 1992). Both groups of women, however, report poorer mental health than demographically comparable women. It seems, therefore, that HIV infection, in particular in the early stages, may not add to the stresses that these women already face when dealing with haemophilia in their partners.

Fears of infecting partners are common both in gay and heterosexual couples, and these fears may play a part in the sexual difficulties they often report (George, 1990; Catalán et al, 1992a, b; Klimes et al, 1992). In heterosexual couples, wish for children will raise complex ethical and practical problems (Smith et al, 1991; Goldman et al, 1992, 1993a), which have been highlighted by reports that show that insemination of seronegative women with processed semen of HIV infected men may result in conception without maternal infection (Semprini et al, 1992).

1.7.2 The psychological impact on relatives

Parents, children, siblings and other relatives will be affected by HIV infection in one family member. Coping with fears of infection, concerns over confidentiality, facing grief and stigma, adapting to changes in the family structure as the disease progresses are common tasks for families with AIDS (Gibb et al, 1991; Lippmann et al, 1993; Ankrah, 1993). A graphic illustration of the family consequences in developing countries is given by McGrath et al (1993) who studied in detail 22 families in Kampala, Uganda, showing the psychosocial impact on individuals in the family and the direct effect on family functioning. Shock and distress reactions were common. Feelings of isolation from other families and neighbours were frequent both in the infected persons and their relatives, and fears of rejection were associated with the appearance of outward signs of illness. Financial problems resulting from inability to travel and seek work because of ill-health were very common, often leading to family rationing of limited resources. Lack of mobility in turn would lead to reduction in support from other social networks.

The consequences are no less striking in developed countries. Atkins and Amenta (1991) found that families dealing with AIDS experienced significantly more stress, lower levels of trust and more illness, and reported more rules prohibiting emotional expression than other families in a hospice setting. Families with haemophilia and thalassaemia experience specific problems, in particular dealing with adolescent children and with the wider social network (Miller et al, 1989; Anastasopoulos and Tsiantis, 1990; Tsiantis and Meyer, 1992; Brown and DeMaio, 1992; Goldman et al, 1993b). In a study of 30 natural caregivers of children with HIV infection, Reidy et al (1991) identified economic difficulties and the need to confide in others as important unmet needs, in spite of good medical care provision. Levels of psychological functioning in caregivers have been found to be largely related to the HIV infected person's own levels of psychological distress, although the presence of physical problems and lack of social support are also important contributors (Stewart et al, 1993). In a study of parents of gay sons with AIDS, Takigiku et al (1993) identified parental attitudes to homosexuality and the family ethos regarding affection/obligation as important determinants of parental stress.

1.8 Summary

In this chapter research and clinical findings concerning the psychological consequences of HIV infection was reviewed. The impact of HIV testing was considered first. Surveys of people seeking testing show that a substantial proportion have a past history of psychological difficulties, and that the process of undergoing testing generates distress and suicidal ideation in some individuals. While notification of a negative test result is associated with improvement in psychological status, those found to be HIV positive tend to have more persistent levels of distress. People with abnormal beliefs associated with concerns about HIV infection in the absence of evidence of infection are present among those seeking testing, and it is important to assess their psychopathology carefully before planning how best to help.

Research on the psychological status of individuals with asymptomatic and symptomatic disease belonging to various transmission categories was also discussed. Overall, most studies comparing people with asymptomatic HIV infection with those who are seronegative do not find substantial differences, but there are important methodological problems which complicate the interpretation of research in this area. There is less debate about individuals with symptomatic disease. Most reports suggest that decline in health is associated with increase in psychological morbidity, and this is particularly relevant at the first development of symptoms and in the terminal stages of the disease.

The psychological impact of HIV infection on children can be devastating. HIV not only affects those children who are themselves infected, but also the children of infected parents and the siblings of an infected child. HIV may also have marked negative impact on the mental health of partners, carers and relatives.

2 Special mental health problems in HIV infection

2.1 Introduction

In the previous chapter the general psychological impact of HIV infection and the pattern of psychological reactions that can occur at different stages of disease was reviewed. In this chapter, the focus is on specific mental health problems which can develop in association with HIV infection. While some of these syndromes are not common, they all have important practical implications for the care and management of people with HIV infection.

2.2 Suicidal behaviour and HIV infection

Suicidal preoccupations and suicidal acts (completed suicide and deliberate self-harm) are not uncommon in people who suffer serious physical disorders or in those facing the terminal stages of their illness. Indeed, it would be surprising not to find such self-destructive thoughts and actions at a time when concerns about pain, fear of increased dependence on others, and worries about physical decay may be prominent in the person's mind.

Studies of patients with cancer have shown an increased risk of suicide in comparison with matched populations (Louhivuori and Hakama, 1979; Fox et al, 1982; Allebeck and Bolund, 1991), and a history of significant physical illness is present in a substantial number of individuals who commit suicide (Robins et al, 1959; Whitlock, 1986; Barraclough and Hughes, 1987). In the case of HIV infection, a combination of vulnerability factors, both social and psychological, are often present. In addition to risk factors seen in other groups, people with HIV infection not only have to deal with a potentially life-threatening disorder but also with the negative social consequences of the disease.

2.2.1 Suicidal ideas and suicide risk

Suicidal ideas

Suicidal ideation is relatively common in people with HIV infection and in those tested for HIV. As many as 30 per cent of people seeking HIV testing at a New York hospital (a sample including gay men, injecting drug users and non-drug-using heterosexuals of both sexes), disclosed suicidal ideas at the time of pre-test counselling. One week after notification of the test results there was little change among those found to be HIV seropositive, while only 17 per cent of those who were seronegative reported suicidal thoughts. Two months later, after having received post-test counselling, about 15 per cent of people, regardless of HIV status, still reported such thoughts (Perry et al, 1990b). Schneider et al (1991a) studied suicidal ideation over the previous six months in a cohort of Los Angeles gay men participating in the Multicenter AIDS Cohort Study (MACS), and found 27 per cent, regardless of HIV serostatus, to have had suicidal ideas over that period of time. Individuals with high suicidal ideation scores were more likely to have depressive symptoms, describe feelings of loneliness and lack of social support. They also reported more negative HIV related experiences, such as recent ARC/AIDS-related death of a partner, were more likely to have close friends with ARC, and more likely to have been given a recent diagnosis of ARC (Schneider et al, 1991b).

Controlled studies from the UK have usually found lower proportions of patients with HIV infection reporting suicidal ideas than are found in the US. In a controlled cross-sectional study of gay men who had known their status for about two years, 8 per cent of those with HIV infection reported suicidal ideas in the previous month, compared with 4 per cent of those uninfected. A prospective study of gay men seeking HIV testing at a London genitourinary clinic found no differences in the proportions of men reporting having had suicidal thoughts in the preceding month between those who turned out to be HIV seropositive (3 per cent) and those who were seronegative (6 per cent) (Riccio et al, 1993). At the 12-month follow-up none of the subjects reported suicidal ideas (Pugh et al, 1994).

Similar results were obtained in investigations of men with haemophilia. A cross-sectional study of men who had known their serostatus for about two years found suicidal ideas in only 3 per cent of those who were HIV seropositive and none of those who were seronegative. A second, prospective investigation of men with haemophilia who had known their serostatus for at least three years, found 7 per cent of the HIV seropositive group to have suicidal ideas at study entry and 4 per cent 12 months later. Again, none of the seronegative group reported suicidal ideas at entry and only 3 per cent did so a year later (Catalán, 1991a).

Thoughts about death and suicidal ideas are reported frequently by long-term AIDS survivors. In a study of 60 gay men with a history of AIDS-defining illnesses of at least three years (Rabkin et al, 1993), a third admitted to thoughts about wanting to die at some point after their AIDS diagnosis, and a quarter considered suicide as an option for the future, when circumstances became intolerable. Interestingly, this group of long-term survivors did not report a history of deliberate self-harm after diagnosis of HIV infection and, as a group, they showed low levels of psychological morbidity.

Suicide risk

Suicide risk in patients with HIV infection referred to a psychiatric consultation service gives a somewhat different pattern. McKegney and O'Dowd (1992) assessed 'suicidality' (a term which the authors did not operationally define) in a large number of patients with HIV at different stages of disease referred to a

New York psychiatric service over a 3-year period, and compared them with a group of patients without HIV infection referred to the same service. Of 322 patients with AIDS, 9 per cent were considered suicidal by psychiatrists, compared with 18 per cent ($n = 82$) of the group without AIDS and 9 per cent ($n = 1086$) in a group of patients who were HIV seronegative or had not been tested. The lower proportion of AIDS patients manifesting suicidality compared with others is intriguing. Organic brain syndromes (delirium and dementia) were the most frequent diagnosis in AIDS patients, possibly masking psychological disorders, or simply altering the order of care priorities. In addition, for some patients with AIDS the diagnosis might have helped to focus attention on survival and increased their efforts to cope successfully with their condition.

Hopelessness

In studies involving non-HIV samples, hopelessness has been found to predict subsequent suicide in people with depressive disorders and in those who have made suicide attempts (Beck et al, 1975, 1985). Rabkin et al (1990a) found higher levels of hopelessness in gay men with HIV infection than in comparable seronegative controls, although the authors argued that hopelessness was more likely to be a function of depressed mood than of HIV serostatus. Men with both haemophilia and HIV infection, whether symptomatic or not, have been found to have significantly higher hopelessness levels than comparable HIV seronegative men with haemophilia (Catalán et al, 1992b). A similar investigation involving gay men failed to find significant differences in hopelessness in relation to serostatus, with both HIV seropositive and seronegative gay men showing levels of hopelessness similar to those of HIV seropositive haemophiliacs (Catalán et al, 1992a). Hopelessness was found to be an independent predictor of psychiatric morbidity in both gay men and men with haemophilia, but not HIV status. There is evidence to suggest that different factors contribute to the presence of high levels of hopelessness in seropositive compared with seronegative individuals. In a cross-sectional study of 61 HIV seropositive gay men and men with haemophilia compared with a similar number of controls, predictors of hopelessness were found to differ in relation to serostatus. In the men with HIV infection, 59 per cent of the variance of the hopelessness score was accounted for by four factors: low internal locus of control, poor social adjustment, lack of an intimate partner, and poor self-regulating beliefs. In those who were HIV seronegative, three factors accounted for 34 per cent of the variance of the hopelessness score: family psychiatric history, not having a confidant and having low self-regulating beliefs (Catalán et al, 1992c).

In the study by Schneider et al (1991a) quoted above, suicidal ideation in people without HIV infection was associated with current levels of depression and hopelessness. In contrast the key factors in those who were HIV seropositive included mood disturbance, loneliness, lack of perceived control over risk of developing AIDS, and AIDS-related life events.

2.2.2 Completed suicide

Surveys of suicide in people with HIV

Several studies have provided evidence to support the view that AIDS is associated with an increased risk of suicide. The methodology used has included descriptions of clinical series of suicides in people with HIV infection, prospective and retrospective surveys, and post-mortem research. See Table 2.1 for a summary of some of the published reports.

The first detailed series of people with AIDS committing suicide was published by Marzuk et al (1988), who identified 12 men in New York city in 1985. The authors showed that the relative risk of suicide in men with AIDS aged between 20 and 59 was 36 times that of men without the diagnosis and in the same age group, and 66 times the general population risk. Describing the characteristics of the 12 identified suicides, the study showed that all had died within eight months of receiving an AIDS diagnosis, rather than in the very late stages of the disease. Violent methods had been chosen by 10 individuals, including falls from heights, hanging and use of firearms. In three cases, the fall had occurred from a medical ward where the patient was receiving treatment at the time. A history of previous suicidal behaviour was known in four of the men. In five of the cases, individuals had seen a psychiatrist in the previous four days, and in two of these cases the person had been receiving in-patient psychiatric care until a few days before suicide. Thirty additional cases were reported for 1986–7 (Marzuk, 1991), showing a similar suicide rate to the earlier series, and indicating a greater use of self-poisoning and higher percentage of Blacks and Hispanics. A fifth of cases occurred in medical wards.

Other researchers have published similar results, indicative of increased suicide risk in AIDS, but with a variable range of rates. Kizer et al (1988) identified 13 suicides in men with AIDS in California during 1986, which represents a relative risk 16 times that of comparable men without AIDS in California. Plott et al (1989) identified five suicides in people with AIDS in Texas over a 20 month period, representing a rate of 221.7/100 000, compared with 13.6/100 000 for the general population. Cote et al (1992) used official US statistics to identify suicides in persons with AIDS from 1987 through 1989 in 45 US states and the

Table 2.1 Increase in suicide rates compared with age- and sex-matched controls

Author	Location	Increase in suicide risk
Marzuk et al, 1988	New York	36 times
Kizer et al, 1988	California	16 times
Plott et al, 1989	Texas	16 times
Cote et al, 1992	45 US states	7.4 times
Pugh et al, 1993	London	10 times
Wedler, 1991	Germany	11 times

District of Columbia. A total of 165 suicides were identified, all but one being men. Compared with demographically similar men in the general population, people with AIDS had a suicide rate 7.4 times higher, although a statistically significant decline in the relative risk was seen over time. Suicides were predominantly white (87 per cent) with a median age of 35 years (range 20 to 69) and comparable, in demographic terms, to all people with AIDS alive during the study period.

Researchers outside the US have also found an increase in the risk of suicide amongst people with HIV infection. Pugh et al (1993) found six cases of suicide in men with HIV infection in a central London hospital service over a two-year period. The relative risk amongst HIV cases was 10 (95 per cent confidence interval 4 to 26 times) compared with that of a sex- and age-matched population residing in the same district. At least five had received an AIDS diagnosis. Two died within 6 months of receiving a positive HIV test, and the rest between 13 and 25 months after the diagnosis of AIDS. A history of psychiatric treatment was present in four and in two, the psychiatric history predated the HIV diagnosis. Violent methods were common, falling from a height occurring in three cases, including one person who jumped from his hospital room. Preliminary reports from Germany (Wedler, 1991) suggest a similar pattern, with a suicide rate in people with HIV 11 times greater than that of a sex- and age-matched population.

Most studies have involved people with AIDS, although an early brief report from Miami referred to seven suicides occurring shortly after HIV testing (Pierce, 1987) and other anecdotal reports have highlighted the risk of suicide following HIV testing (Miller et al, 1986a, b). In contrast, Hull et al (1988) have reported the absence of suicides after HIV testing in New Mexico, possibly reflecting the nature and quality of the support services available.

HIV-associated suicides have also been reported in people who were HIV seronegative but who were afraid of having become infected. Halttunen et al (1991) described 28 cases in Finland, a country with a high suicide rate, in people who considered themselves at risk of acquiring the infection. All appeared to have been suffering from psychiatric disorders, mostly depression, and 60 per cent had been in contact with the health services in the week prior to their death.

A different approach to the study of suicide in HIV infection was used by Rajs and Fugelstad (1992), who studied all medico-legal autopsies in Stockholm (performed when death occurred outside hospital as a result of external violence, poisoning, or in unclear or suspicious circumstances), over a five year period (1985–90). There were 85 HIV seropositive cases (68 men and 17 women), representing 0.50 per cent of all autopsies during the study period. A verdict of suicide was given in 21 (25 per cent) cases, including 12 gay men, 8 injecting drug users and 1 blood transfusion recipient. Six suicides had an AIDS diagnosis, the rest were asymptomatic. Death occurred at home in 17 cases, in hospital in one case, and the remainder outdoors. Methods used included overdose of drugs in 12 cases, drowning in 2, and a variety of other methods, mostly violent, in the rest. Toxicological analysis indicated that all except one case were under the influence of medicinal or narcotic drugs or alcohol at the time of death.

Interestingly, in addition to the suicide cases, 47 (55 per cent) deaths in people with HIV infection were the result of accidental overdose by intravenous injection of drugs.

Does HIV infection increase the risk of suicide?

While most of the papers quoted support the view that AIDS is associated with an increased suicide risk, there are complex methodological questions which make certainty in this area difficult (for reviews see Marzuk, 1991, Platt, 1991; and Marzuk and Perry, 1993). For example, proper matching of suicides with comparison groups should include such variables as injecting drug use and sexual orientation, so as to be able to compare 'like with like', and to avoid underestimating the suicide risk in the control populations (Hull et al, 1988). Furthermore, there are problems establishing the true extent of suicide in people with HIV infection ('numerator') as well as the number of HIV infected individuals in a particular district ('denominator'). For example, in the context of severe or terminal illness it is not always possible to decide on the cause of death. In particular with suicide, many relatives and carers may not be willing to disclose information which might attract further stigma. Deaths involving injecting drug use may be classified as accidental or as overdoses, rather than be given a suicide verdict (Raj and Fugelstad, 1992). For obvious reasons of confidentiality, there are no comprehensive data banks holding details of HIV infected individuals of the kind that would allow follow-up and estimation of risk over time. HIV infection has been considered as one possible contributing factor to the increase in the suicide rate in young men (Hawton, 1992). This is unlikely (Buehler et al, 1990), as the numbers involved are very small, representing about 3 per cent of male suicides in New York in 1985 (Marzuk et al, 1988) and 0.2 per cent in Texas (Plott et al, 1989).

Whether suicide risk is increased in persons with HIV infection, compared with other populations, will continue to be a matter for debate and further research. Whatever the answers are to the research questions, clinicians and others involved in providing care to people with HIV infection will encounter instances of suicide, and so it is important to know more about this group of individuals, establish the factors that contribute to suicide in HIV, and most importantly, to develop effective ways of assessing and providing care for those at risk (see Chapters 4 and 5).

Discussion of suicide inevitably raises complex ethical and legal questions about physician-assisted suicide, euthanasia, and advance directives (Glass, 1988) and these are addressed in Chapter 8.

2.2.3 Deliberate self-harm

People involved in acts of deliberate self-harm (also known as attempted suicide and parasuicide) include two groups of individuals. First, there are those with high suicidal intent who survived as a result of medical treatment or the early identification of risk factors. Second, there are those with low or ambivalent suicidal intent, but who are motivated by a wish to express their distress, communicate anger or other feelings, or who desire to escape from their predicament for a time. The latter group represents the majority of cases of deliberate self-harm. Deliberate self-harm is much more common than completed suicide, and has reached epidemic proportions in many countries (Hawton and Catalán, 1987).

There are important differences between individuals involved in deliberate self-harm and those who commit suicide in terms of their demographic characteristics, psychiatric status, social difficulties and methods of self-harm used, but there are also areas of overlap between the two groups (for review see Hawton and Catalán, 1987). The complexities of the relationship between suicidal intent, method used and motivation are illustrated in the case described by O'Donnell et al (1992). In this case, a man with AIDS decided to end his life by jumping in front of a train on the London Underground and, by good fortune, survived the attempt with minimal injuries. In spite of having shown high suicidal intent at the time of the act, a few days later he showed a remarkably positive attitude.

Several authors have described examples of people who deliberately attempted to become infected with HIV as a way of committing suicide. In the cases described by Frances et al (1985) and Flavin et al (1986) the three gay men in question were dependent on alcohol and only one of them appeared to have become infected with HIV. Papathomopoulos (1989) described the case of a young woman who, following break-up of a relationship, had unprotected sexual intercourse with a man whom she knew to be HIV seropositive with the aim of becoming infected. As in the previous cases, the decision to seek infection occurred against a background of emotional distress, negative feelings about herself, and self-destructive ideation.

Studies of US military personnel with HIV infection carried out by Rundell et al (1988) have provided information on the frequency of suicide attempts in this particular population. In a retrospective case-control study of 147 HIV people with asymptomatic infection, 7 (5 per cent) cases of deliberate self-harm were identified over a period of 11 months, giving an attempt rate of 4500 per 100 000 person-years. Social isolation and lack of social support, use of denial as a way of coping, multiple psychosocial stressors and alcohol misuse were amongst the factors that contributed to the act (Rundell et al, 1988). A 37-fold increased risk of attempted suicide was reported by Brown and Rundell (1989) in women with HIV infection in the United States Air Force.

Gala et al (1992a) followed-up 213 HIV individuals with asymptomatic infection (168 men and 45 women) for 42 months. The sample included 123 injecting drug users, 68 gay men, and 22 non-drug using heterosexuals. A past history of deliberate self-harm prior to notification of the HIV test result was present in 13 per cent (16 per cent of drug users, 9 per cent of gay men, and 9 per cent of heterosexuals). Following HIV diagnosis, 12 (5.6 per cent) went on to make further attempts, eight within 6 months of notification and the remaining four between 4 and 36 months. Psychotropic drugs were used in half of the cases, heroin in 3, superficial wrist-cutting in 2 and ingestion of bleach in one case. The risk of deliberate self-harm in this population was increased in those with a past psychiatric history (7.7-fold) or a past history of deliberate self-harm (5-fold).

Clinical studies of people with HIV infection referred to the mental health services give some idea of the practical aspects of deliberate self-harm in HIV. In an effort to identify predictors of deliberate self-harm, O'Dowd et al (1992) studied the features of individuals making suicide attempts while receiving out-patient psychiatric care in a New York service dealing mostly with injecting drug users and heterosexuals with HIV infection. Over a 4½ year period, 9 suicide attempts were made by 7 (3.3 per cent) patients out of a total of 210. This surprisingly small group of patients differed from non-attempters in that they were more likely to be female, white, younger, and to have become infected through heterosexual intercourse or by injecting drugs. Substance misuse and a diagnosis of personality disorder were more common in attempters, and they were also more likely to report previous attempts and have a history of psychiatric treatment. Further comparisons were made between attempters and a matched group of non-attempters (matching included sex, age, race and HIV transmission category). Attempters had made more previous attempts and, when first assessed as out-patients, had shown higher levels of psychological distress as measured by the General Health Questionnaire.

In a study carried out in central London, 22 individuals who were HIV seropositive (64 per cent of whom were symptomatic) were referred over an 18 month period to a general hospital service for the psychosocial assessment of individuals involved in deliberate self-harm. People who were HIV seropositive represented 3.4 per cent of all referrals to the service, and they included a much greater proportion of men. Ninety-five per cent of those with HIV infection were men compared with 55 per cent amongst the rest, reflecting the pattern of HIV infection in London, where a majority of cases are gay men. Further comparisons were made between people with HIV infection and a sex- and age-matched control group of uninfected attempters in order to identify their distinguishing features. Demographically, those who were HIV seropositive were more likely to be gay/bisexual and to be unemployed. They were also more likely to receive a diagnosis of depressive disorder, but less likely to be misusing alcohol. There were no differences between groups regarding a previous history of deliberate self-harm, but there were differences in previous psychiatric care. HIV seropositive individuals were more likely to have received out-patient treatment, while more seronegatives had a history of in-patient psychiatric treatment, possibly in connection with their greater misuse of alcohol. The most important difference regarding methods used in the attempt concerned the use of anti-HIV medication, which was employed by 10 per cent of HIV individuals. The risks involved in the overdosage of drugs like zidovudine (ZDV) have been well documented (Spear et al, 1988; Routy et al, 1989; Terragna et al, 1990) and highlight the need for assessment of risk of suicidal behaviour when medication is being prescribed. There were few differences between groups regarding current social or other problems, except for the predictable presence of concerns about physical health which were mentioned by half of those who were HIV seropositive.

2.2.4 Conclusion

Suicidal behaviour and ideas are not uncommon in people with HIV infection. Indeed, suicidal thoughts are probably a universal phenomenon at some stage among people with the infection. For most people, such thoughts will be transient, not seriously distressing and of limited significance. For some, however, thoughts of suicide may become a source of distress and may suggest that a severe psychiatric disorder, such as major depression, is developing. Whether suicide and deliberate self-harm are more common or not in people with HIV infection, and if so to what extent, are still matters for debate, but whatever the answer, it is clear that a proportion of people with HIV infection will commit suicide and a somewhat larger group will be involved in non-fatal acts of deliberate self-harm. It is the responsibility of those involved in the care of people with HIV infection to ensure that the risk of suicidal behaviour is recognized and that appropriate psychiatric and social care are provided.

2.3 Psychotic disorders

Major psychiatric disorders, such as mania and schizophrenia, can occur in people with HIV infection. While their prevalence is not high, their development can lead to difficult diagnostic and management problems, and referral to the psychiatric in-patient services for further assessment and care is common in the case of people with both HIV and a psychotic disorder.

Here we shall review the clinical syndromes included under the term psychosis, discuss their prevalence and possible aetiological factors, and describe their clinical characteristics. Issues of assessment and management are covered in Chapters 4 and 5.

2.3.1 Diagnostic terminology

The term psychosis is a generic label which generally includes, using DSM-III-R terminology, manic episodes, schizophrenia and other conditions such as delusional disorder, brief reactive psychosis, schizophreniform disorder and atypical psychosis. Sometimes there is sufficient evidence to make a diagnosis of organic delusional or mood disorder, but organic syndromes like delirium and dementia, or major depression with delusions and/or hallucinations, are not usually included under this rubric. The principal clinical features of psychosis are delusions, hallucinations, and abnormal mood, in the absence of an acute brain syndrome (delirium) or of gross structural brain disease (see Chapter 4).

The use of the term psychosis in relation to HIV infection should not be regarded as implying that a new disease entity or diagnostic category has been identified (Vogel-Scibilia et al, 1988). The syndromes included under the term are well known, and when they develop in people with HIV infection, efforts should be made to clarify the clinical features and to establish their aetiology, which may well be on occasions unrelated to HIV.

2.3.2 Prevalence

There are problems in attempting to establish the frequency with which psychotic disorders develop in HIV infection. The term tends to be used in the literature in an imprecise way, with limited use of operational definitions, and so it is sometimes difficult to be sure what specific syndrome is being described. Published descriptions usually consist of case reports or small series, and the size of the population of HIV individuals from whom they are drawn is not always clear. A further problem concerns the question of whether psychotic syndromes are increased in HIV. Although it has been claimed that the prevalence of mania is increased in people with HIV infection (Kieburtz et al, 1991b), there are methodological problems involved in comparing rates of mania in HIV with those of a matched population. As in the case of suicide, matching should include variables like history of substance misuse, socioeconomic factors, and past psychiatric history, as well as sex and age, to avoid overestimating the prevalence of psychosis in people with HIV. Unfortunately, data about such control populations are not readily available.

Psychosis in patients with HIV infection

Most reports suggest a relatively low frequency of psychotic disorders in people with HIV. Amongst patients admitted to hospital for treatment of HIV-related disease, between 1 and 2 per cent have been reported to develop psychosis (Buhrich and Cooper, 1987; Sno et al, 1989; Lyketsos et al, 1993a), while Halstead et al (1988) estimated that under 1 per cent of all individuals who were HIV positive living in a central London district suffered such disorders. In contrast to these low figures, Harris et al (1991) found psychotic disorders in 9.7 per cent of HIV asymptomatic individuals, although only 3.2 per cent had a new onset psychosis not due to substance misuse. The reasons for the higher prevalence in this report are unclear, but methodological factors and differences in subject selection might have played a part.

Psychosis in HIV referrals to psychiatric services

There is a wide range in the published proportions of patients with HIV infection referred to psychiatrists with a psychotic disorder. The proportions range from 2 per cent (Ayuso-Mateos et al, 1989) through 3 per cent (Douzenis et al, 1991, Catalán, 1992), 5 per cent (Alexius, 1991), 9 per cent (Buhrich and Cooper, 1987; Lyketsos et al, 1993a), 10 per cent (Sno et al,1989), 18 per cent (Seth et al,1991) to a high of 21 per cent (Harris et al, 1991). Such variation is likely to be the result of many factors. The kind of psychiatric service available and the degree of access to other sources of psychological support will be particularly important in determining whether all patients with psychological problems are referred to the psychiatrist, or only those with severe forms of mental illness, and so affect the relative proportion of referred patients with psychosis.

Patients with psychotic illnesses represent a substantial proportion of all people with HIV who require psychiatric hospitalization. In surveys, at least 30 per cent of all admissions of patients with HIV infection are for psychotic illnesses (Baer, 1989; Smith, 1990). In a report by Douzenis et al (1991), where the existence of comprehensive out-patient and community care meant admission to psychiatric hospital was required only for the most severe disorders, the large majority of admissions (83 per cent) involved psychotic illnesses.

2.3.3 Aetiological factors

It should not be assumed that psychotic disorders in HIV infected individuals are always the direct result of the infection, and it is important to exclude pre-existing or contemporary contributing factors. See Table 2.2 for summary of aetiological factors.

Pre-existing psychotic disorders

Mania and schizophrenic disorders are relatively common conditions. The lifetime prevalence of schizophrenia has been estimated to be about 1–2 per cent and that of mania about 1 per cent (Robins et al, 1984). It is, therefore, inevitable that some people with a history of psychosis will also acquire HIV infection. Indeed, it is conceivable that the sexual disinhibition associated with a manic episode might lead to sexually unsafe behaviour and to an increased risk of HIV. In the report by Harris et al (1991) 5 (42 per cent) out of 12 patients with psychosis had a past history of schizophrenia or schizoaffective disorder, and in our centre 4 (18 per cent) out of 22 had a previous history. There was, however, a difference by syndrome. Only 1 (6 per cent) person with mania had a past history of bipolar affective disorder, while 3 (50 per cent) of those with schizophrenia had a pre-existing schizophrenic condition (Catalán, 1992). As many as half had a personal or family history in the series of patients with HIV infection reported by Lyketsos et al (1993a).

Substance misuse

Amphetamines, cocaine and other psychostimulants can precipitate psychotic syndromes. In the survey by Baer (1989) of patients admitted to a psychiatric unit, amphetamines and cocaine were implicated in 4 (20 per cent) out of 20 cases of psychosis, Harris et al (1991) found amphetamine misuse in 2 (17 per cent) out of 12, and substance misuse is mentioned in 2 (15 per cent) of 13 in the report by Alexius (1991).

Table 2.2 Aetiological factors in HIV-associated psychotic disorders

Aetiology	Reported prevalence
Pre-existing psychotic disorders	18–42%
Substance misuse	15–20%
Psychogenic reaction	25%
Iatrogenic factors	none reported
HIV-related brain disease	21–61%

Psychogenic reaction to HIV infection

The distress often associated with HIV infection can lead on occasions to unusual and severe psychological reactions. There is evidence that life events can be associated with the onset of psychotic symptoms (Bebbington et al, 1993), and the concept of psychogenic psychosis has a long tradition in the history of psychiatry, although at present its use is largely restricted to Scandinavian countries (Stromgren, 1974). Unsurprisingly, the only mention of this aetiology is contained in a report from Stockholm (Alexius, 1991), where psychogenic psychosis accounted for a quarter of cases of psychosis in HIV patients.

Iatrogenic causes

A variety of therapeutic drugs and treatments can cause psychotic symptoms as a side-effect or adverse reaction, and in a medical condition as complex as HIV affecting multiple organs, and requiring a variety of treatments, it is important to evaluate the possible role of medication in leading to psychiatric complications (see Chapter 4).

There has been concern about the possible contribution of anti-retroviral medication to the causation of psychotic disorders. A number of reports have implicated zidovudine (ZDV) in the development of mania. Maxwell et al (1988) described two cases of mania in gay/bisexual men who had AIDS for several months. In one case, mania developed within three days of starting zidovudine, improved on its discontinuation, and recurred again within a few hours of starting zidovudine. In the second case, manic symptoms occurred after 16 months on zidovudine, improved after discontinuation but reappeared on re-introduction of the anti-retroviral. Both patients were able to tolerate zidovudine subsequently when neuroleptics and lithium were added. Similar cases were reported by O'Dowd and McKegney (1988) and Schaerf et al (1988), and interestingly all four patients had either a history of affective disorder or evidence of cognitive impairment. Cognitive decline is also a feature in the two manic patients described by Wright et al (1989): one developed dementia within six months, and the other had some cognitive impairment when started on zidovudine. Kieburtz et al (1991b) found 5 (62 per cent) out of 8 manic patients to be on zidovudine at the time of developing psychiatric disease, and in our series of 22 psychotic patients, 7 (31 per cent) were on zidovudine at the time, but this proportion was similar to that of a control group of contemporary patients, matched in terms of sex, age, and CD4 count (Catalán, 1992).

Dideoxyinosine (ddI) has also been associated with psychotic disorders. Orth et al (1991) described two patients who developed a manic syndrome after 3 months on ddI and who recovered on discontinuation of the drug. In our case-control study involving 22 psychotic patients there was a non-significant trend towards those patients with mania being more likely to have used ddI.

It is possible that some people with HIV infection who are predisposed to the development of manic syndromes or whose brain function is compromised by the disease are at risk of developing psychotic disorders when receiving zidovudine or ddI, but the small number of cases reported in the literature in spite of the widespread use of these drugs suggests that the risks are small, and that other factors account for the majority of cases of psychosis.

HIV-related brain disease

In view of the prevalence of neuropsychiatric syndromes in HIV infection, one likely cause of psychotic disorders to be considered is the presence of *structural* brain disease, as opposed to a *non-structural* disorder (Rogers, 1992). A number of reports have provided detailed information about the neurological and cognitive status of psychotic patients with HIV, and its clear that in a proportion of cases brain disease was present, although this was not invariably the case (Kermani et al, 1985; Perry and Jacobsen, 1986; Gabel et al, 1986; Thomas and Szabadi, 1987; Beckett et al, 1987; Buhrich et al, 1988; Schmidt and Miller, 1988; Milner, 1989; McGowan et al, 1991). Meningeal enhancement on MRI has been described in mania (Kieburtz et al, 1991b; Kieburtz and Caine, 1992), and Ronchi et al (1992) found neurological and neuroradiological abnormalities in one-third of their cases. Harris et al (1991) reviewed the evidence for organic disease in published reports and found 33 per cent of cases had abnormal clinical neurology, 48 per cent abnormal brain imaging, 28 per cent abnormal cerebrospinal fluid (CSF), 50 per cent abnormal electroencephalogram (EEG), and 61 per cent abnormal neuropsychology. Sewell et al (1994) in their series involving 20 cases of psychosis found a trend towards greater neuropsychological impairment than controls, but magnetic resonance imagin (MRI), CSF, and neuropathological investigations failed to provide conclusive evidence for organic brain involvement.

In the series reported by Lyketsos et al (1993a), patients with mania without a personal or family history of mood disorder were more likely to be given a diagnosis of cognitive impairment at the time of their presentation, which also tended to occur at a more advanced stage of HIV disease. In contrast, subjects with a past history of mood disorder presented at earlier stages of HIV infection, and were less likely to show cognitive impairment. While these figures indicate that in some cases of psychosis significant structural brain disease is likely to be present, as has been reported in patients with multiple sclerosis and psychotic illness (Feinstein et al, 1992), it is unclear what the exact prevalence of abnormalities is in these didorders. In many of the reports included in the review only some patients had detailed neurological investigations and it is likely that they were the more severely ill or those with a clinical picture suggestive of organicity. Furthermore, many of the patients were suffering from advanced HIV disease, and neurological abnormalities would have been expected in a substantial number of patients at this stage of disease, regardless of whether a psychosis was present. The fact that psychotic symptoms can develop in AIDS in the absence of significant brain disease is illustrated by the case described by Dening et al (1992) of a man with haemophilia without a psychiatric history who, as participant in a cohort study of the neuropsychological consequences of HIV, had serial detailed neuropsychological assessments before and after his psychotic disorder showing only mild functional impairments and no evidence of deterioration three months after the episode. The involvement of the dopaminergic system in cases of HIV-related psychosis has been postulated in view of AIDS patients sensitivity to dopamine-blocking agents (Hollander et al, 1985; Maccario and Scharre, 1987; Hriso et al, 1991), which may be due to subclinical nigral degeneration (Reyes et al, 1991).

2.3.4 Clinical features

Most of the information available in the literature comes from a few series and case reports including small numbers of patients. Particularly useful are the review of published cases by Harris et al (1991) and the series by Sewell et al (1994).

Psychiatric syndromes

In the 31 cases of new-onset psychosis reviewed by Harris et al (1991), delusions were present in 87 per cent, mood disturbance in 81 per cent, hallucinations and thought disorder in 61 per cent, bizarre behaviour in 52 per cent, and cognitive impairment in 35 per cent. In Sewell and co-workers' series (1994), all patients had delusions, 18 (90 per cent) reported hallucinations, and 13 (65 per cent) had mood abnormalities: depression, euphoria, and mixed depression and euphoria. The authors stressed the difficulty reaching a diagnostic formulation. If the assumption was made that the syndrome was related to HIV–brain involvement, the diagnosis would be one of organic delusional or organic mood syndrome, while if no aetiological assumption was made the diagnosis would be major depression, bipolar disorder, psychotic disorder, and schizophrenia.

Manic syndromes have been described in early disease (Gabel et al, 1986) but mostly in advanced symptomatic disease (Kermani et al, 1985; Perry and Jacobsen, 1986; Buhrich et al, 1988; Schmidt and Miller, 1988; Dauncey, 1988; Maxwell et al, 1988; O'Dowd and Kegney, 1988; Schaef et al, 1988; Milner, 1989; Kieburtz et al, 1991b; McGowan et al, 1991). In our London series of 22 psychotics, 16 (73 per cent) had manic syndromes, and of these 2 (12 per cent) were asymptomatic, 2 (12 per cent) had early symptomatic disease and the rest, 12 (75 per cent), had AIDS (Catalán, 1992).

Schizophrenic syndromes have been described also in early disease (Thomas et al, 1985; Maccario and Scharre, 1987; Halevie-Goldman et al, 1987; Halstead et al, 1988), but the majority of reports involve patients with ARC/AIDS (Perry and Jacobsen, 1986; Jones et al, 1987; Thomas and Szabadi, 1987; Halstead et al, 1988; Buhrich et al, 1988; Gawlitza and Reuter, 1988). Schizophrenic patients represented only 27 per cent of our London series of psychotic patients, 2 (33 per cent) with asymptomatic disease, 1 (17 per cent) with early sypmtomatic disease and 3 (50 per cent) with a diagnosis of AIDS (Catalán, 1992).

Some reports have included under the rubric of psychosis delusional disorders with depressed mood (Beckett et al, 1987; Heyman and Fahy, 1992).

HIV disease characteristics

In the review by Harris et al (1991), slightly more patients with psychosis were asymptomatic than had ARC or AIDS. In our London series, however, the group mean CD4 count was 69.8 cells/mm^3 (sd = 98.3), and 68 per cent had an

AIDS diagnosis, 14 per cent had early symptoms, and only 18 per cent were asymptomatic (Catalán, 1992). These findings are comparable to those reported by Alexius (1991), whose patients included 54 per cent with AIDS, and only 30 per cent with asymptomatic infection. Most patients in Sewell's series belonged to CDC group IV. While psychotic disorders can occur at all stages of disease, it is likely that the aetiology will vary with degree of illness, so that organic factors may well be more common in patients with AIDS, and pre-existing disorders or substance misuse more common in early disease, as in the series reported by Lyketsos et al (1993a).

Demographic and social characteristics of patients

Most reports have been published in North America and Northern European countries, and the characteristics of patients described reflect the epidemiology of HIV infection in the populations studied, so that middle-aged gay/bisexual men and male injecting drug users are usually included, although women (Gabel et al, 1986) and men with haemophilia (Gawlitza and Reuter, 1988; Dening et al, 1992) have also been reported. Unfortunately, very little is known about psychotic illnesses in developing countries with high prevalence of HIV infection.

Course and prognosis

In general, most patients show improvement in psychiatric symptomatology, although their clinical prognosis is poor. Many reports describe fairly rapid decline in a substantial proportion of patients (El-Mallakh, 1991), and in a number of cases a dementia syndrome develops (Smith, 1990), or at least cognitive decline without dementia and with neuropathological evidence of encephalopathy (McGowan et al, 1991).

In our London series, we compared survival in 18 new-onset psychotic patients with 87 matched HIV controls (matched for age, sex, CD4 count and date of onset of psychotic illness). The life expectancy of patients with psychosis was significantly shorter (mean = 8.8 months, median = 8.0, sd = 7.2) than for controls (mean = 12.5, median = 10.0, sd = 8.3). One explanation for this could be that those patients with psychosis, while showing similar levels of immune deficiency to the control group, had more widespread and severe HIV disease, possibly involving the central nervous system. Reduced life expectancy for patients with psychotic illnesses has also been reported in other studies (Sewell et al, 1994). It is known that AIDS patients presenting with neurological disease have a shorter survival rate than patients presenting with other disorders (Casabona et al, 1991), and that the presence of poor neuropsychological test performance in both asymptomatic and symptomatic gay men with HIV infection is associated with increased risk of death (Mayeux et al, 1993), suggesting that brain involvement may be an important aetiological factor in psychotic disorders.

2.3.5 Conclusion

Psychotic disorders occur in people with HIV infection, and they can develop at all stages of disease. While they are not very common, it is probable that there is an increased risk for psychosis in people with HIV infection. The presence of psychosis in people with HIV raises important diagnostic questions, and it is essential to try to identify possible aetiological factors, including medication and associated neurological or other disease. The outcome of the psychiatric syndrome is generally favourable in the short term, but some patients manifest evidence of cognitive decline. In addition, psychotic disorders are associated with reduced survival particularly in people without a who have had no previous psychotic episode.

2.4 Sexual dysfunction problems in HIV disease

Sexual problems are common in people with serious physical diseases (Bancroft, 1989; Horton, 1991; Coates and Ferroni, 1991), and a substantial number of people referred to sexual dysfunction clinics suffer from concurrent physical disorders (Catalán et al, 1990). HIV disease is no exception. The psychological reactions to the infection, such as guilt about sexual behaviour, concern about changes in physical appearance and worries about passing on the virus to sexual partners, are important contributors to the development of sexual dysfunction problems. Furthermore, progressive physical disease and its treatment can cause added difficulties. Here we shall review the range of sexual dysfunctions that occur in HIV disease, their prevalence and aetiological factors.

2.4.1 Prevalence of sexual dysfunction

Kaplan et al (1988) reported no sexual partners in 23 per cent of previously sexually active gay men after they developed HIV lymphadenopathy. Brown and Pace (1989), in a preliminary report of the psychological status of HIV asymptomatic United States Air Force personnel, found hypoactive sexual desire in about 13 per cent, a proportion significantly higher than that of a control group. Subsequent work by this group identified an even higher proportion of sexual problems amongst men in the armed forces who had asymptomatic HIV infection. More than a fifth of a sample of 422 men enrolled in the study who had known their HIV status for about three years reported sexual dysfunction problems. Hypoactive sexual desire was the most common problem, occurring in 97 per cent dysfunctional cases. It is of interest to note that although the prevalence of affective disorders was higher in the HIV seropositive group than expected, more than 70 per cent of sexually dysfunctional men had no affective or anxiety disorders, suggesting that in most cases sexual problems were not part of a major psychiatric disorder (Brown et al, 1992). More than half of a sample of people with advanced HIV disease participating in a drug trial reported current sexual dysfunction (Tindall et al, 1992, 1994).

Gay/bisexual men

Surveys of sexual problems in a variety of transmission groups have confirmed the frequent presence of difficulties. In a controlled study of mostly asymptomatic gay men who had known their serostatus for about two years, Catalán et al (1992a) found that 75 per cent had experienced significant loss of sexual interest since discovery of their serostatus compared with 6 per cent of HIV seronegative controls. Both groups experienced erection and orgasm problems, but delayed ejaculation was significantly more common in the HIV seropositive group, who reported it in 38 per cent of cases. A number of uncontrolled investigations have provided similar results. Tindall et al (1992) identified sexual dysfunction in about 50 per cent of symptomatic gay men entering a trial of anti-retrovirals of which erection and ejaculation problems were the most frequent, and they were usually long standing and affecting all sexual situations. Chalmers et al (1992) studied 30 out-patient gay men, 60 per cent of whom were symptomatic. They found that in the previous three months, half had experienced loss of sexual interest, a third had persistent erectile difficulties, and a third had ejaculation problems. Loss of interest and erectile problems were significantly more common in symptomatic individuals. In all, 77 per cent had some sexual dysfunction, while 27 per cent had difficulties establishing relationships which they attributed to their serostatus. Dupras and Morisset (1993) found 57 per cent of a self-selected sample of 88 HIV seropositive gay men to be sexually dysfunctional, with loss of desire, erectile disorders and inhibited ejaculation being the problems most frequently reported.

Women

Significant impact on sexual behaviour and response was reported in 20 non-drug using women in the United States Air Force. Sexual abstinence, loss of interest and reduction in frequency of sexual intercourse was reported in 55 per cent since seroconversion, and 20 per cent met the criteria for new onset hypoactive desire disorder (Brown and Rundell, 1990). We have conducted an investigation involving 49 HIV seropositive women and 43 comparable seronegatives who had sought HIV testing at a genitourinary clinic in central London. A smaller proportion of women with HIV infection were in a relationship, a fact the women attributed to HIV. Loss of sexual interest following the discovery of serostatus was present in 11 per cent of those who were HIV seropositive, all of whom had symptomatic HIV disease, while no seronegative woman experienced loss of interest. In an Italian sample of 57 HIV asymptomatic women and 23 seronegatives, including mostly injecting drug users, Pergami et al (1993) found significant disruption of sexual life in two-thirds of women, although only a relatively small proportion had become abstinent, but there were no differences in relation to serostatus.

Men with haemophilia and their partners

Men with haemophilia, regardless of HIV status, have also had to make sexual adjustments as a result of HIV infection, although those who are HIV seropositive have tended to experience greater difficulties. Loss of interest following HIV testing has been reported in 55 per cent of men with haemophilia with HIV infection (mostly asymptomatic) compared with 33 per cent for those who were seronegative (Catalán et al, 1992b). Erection and ejaculation problems were found in both groups, with premature ejaculation and delayed ejaculation being significantly more common in the seropositive group (Catalán et al, 1992b). The sexual partners of these men were also experiencing difficulties, in particular when the man was HIV seropositive (Klimes et al, 1992).

2.4.2 Causes of sexual dysfunction in HIV disease

In a condition as complex as HIV disease, it is likely that a combination of factors, both psychosocial and organic, will contribute to the development of sexual dysfunction problems.

Psychosocial reactions to HIV infection

In the early stages of discovery of a positive serostatus, feelings of shock and distress will often lead to loss of interest in sex, and to powerful feelings of guilt, contamination and fear of illness. Later, feelings of loneliness and yearning for closeness and intimacy may conflict with concerns about a wide range of possible problems: fear of infecting one's partner, disfigurement due to illness (e.g. Kaposi's sarcoma of the skin), fear of death, concerns about whether to discuss HIV, how to negotiate safer sex without disclosing HIV status, chances of developing or maintaining relationships and the risks and difficulties involved in wishing to have children. It is not surprising that faced with such difficult questions, sex may be pushed into the background, while for others the anxiety involved in sexual contact may lead to unsatisfactory response. The response of the person's partner and the strength of the relationship before and after HIV will also be relevant to the development of sexual problems (George, 1990; Ussher, 1990).

Pre-existing sexual dysfunction and associated disorders

While most reports of sexual problems in HIV infection suggest that the problems were precipitated by discovery of the serostatus or after development of physical complications, it should be remembered that sexual dysfunctions are relatively common, and that research carried out before HIV was identified has shown that sexual dysfunctions and concerns about sexual performance are not rare in people attending clinics for sexually transmitted disease (Catalán et al, 1981), a population rather comparable to those with HIV infection. Alcohol misuse, usually a long-standing pre-existing problem, is seen in people with HIV (Schleifer et al, 1990) and amongst attenders at clinics for sexually transmitted diseases (Catalán et al, 1988), and can also contribute to the development of sexual problems. It is likely that a history of previous difficulties will increase the risk of further sexual problems following HIV infection.

HIV-related organic factors

There is good evidence for testicular and hormonal abnormalities in men with advanced HIV disease. Men with AIDS have been shown to have significantly lower levels of serum testosterone than controls (Dobs et al, 1988; Lefrere et al, 1988; Croxson et al, 1989). Hypergonadotropic hypogonadism (testicular insufficiency) seems the more common form, although hypogonadotropic forms of hypogonadism also occur, suggesting that hypothalamic involvement may important in some cases (Klauke et al, 1990). Abnormalities in the morphology, numbers and motility of sperm have been described in HIV symptomatic men (Brockmeyer et al, 1989; Krieger et al, 1991). Autopsy studies have demonstrated the presence of abnormalities in a majority of cases, with atrophy, lymphocytic infiltration, interstitial fibrosis and, at times, opportunistic infections (Rogers and Klatt, 1988; Paepe and Waxman 1989).

The mechanisms involved are unclear. While hypogonadism and testicular atrophy can happen in chronic, debilitating diseases, it is also possible that HIV may have direct effects both in the gonad and in the hypothalamus, or that immune-mediated mechanisms play a part. It has been suggested that the reduction in serum tryptophan and blood serotonin which occur in HIV infection (Werner et al, 1988; Larsson et al, 1989) could contribute to sexual dysfunction (Dursun, 1993).

Iatrogenic causes

Drugs and other treatments used to deal with HIV disease can contribute to the development of sexual problems. Sometimes the effects are non-specific, as in the case of chemotherapy or radiotherapy causing short-term malaise and tiredness. An example of a more specific aetiology of sexual dysfunction in males is caused by megestrol, a synthetic progesterone which is sometimes used for the treatment of weight loss and cachexia in HIV disease (Von Roenn et al, 1988), and which has been found to be associated with the loss of sexual thoughts and erectile dysfunction (Summerbell et al, 1992).

2.4.3 Conclusions

Sexual dysfunctions are common in people with HIV infection. Psychosocial reactions to the infection, relationship difficulties and concerns about infecting partners all contribute to the development of problems. In addition, physical disorders can also play a part in the causation of sexual problems, in particular in symptomatic disease, when the effects of medication may also be important. Assessment of sexual dysfunction in people with HIV will need to take into account this array of possible causes before deciding what form of intervention may be appropriate.

2.5 Miscellaneous mental health problems

Any form of mental health problem can develop in a person with HIV infection. As discussed in this and in the previous chapter, psychiatric disorder may sometimes be the result of HIV infection itself, but it could also be a chance association, although it is not always easy to clarify the aetiological factors involved in each particular case. In practice, whether HIV causes the problem or not, HIV infection is likely to complicate both the understanding of the psychiatric disorder and in particular its management. Here we review some examples of co-morbidity which may raise problems for those caring for people with HIV infection. The association between substance misuse, including alcohol, and the risk of HIV infection is covered elsewhere (Chapter 6).

2.5.1 Personality problems

There has been no systematic study of the prevalence of personality disorder in people with HIV infection, and it is clear that there are important methodological and conceptual problems in this area of research (King, 1993a). The concept of personality disorder is a rather vague one and it is not surprising that there is great variability in the proportions of individuals reported to suffer from personality disorder in different surveys. King (1993a) found that about a fifth of patients referred to a liaison psychiatry service had a personality disorder and this was the same regardless of HIV serostatus. Perkins et al (1993a) in a study involving 58 HIV asymptomatic and 53 seronegative gay men, found a significantly greater prevalence of personality disorders in those with HIV infection: 33 per cent compared with 15 per cent in the control group. Borderline personality was the most common diagnosis, followed by dependent, passive–aggressive and histrionic personality. The presence of a personality disorder was associated with worse psychological status and dysfunctional coping. Whether there is increased prevalence of personality problems in people with HIV infection or not, in practice people with such problems are likely to create difficulties for those involved in their care and to place heavy demands upon the health and social services. It is in such cases that co-ordination of resources and planning of care delivery will be particularly important (see Chapter 4).

2.5.2 Feigned HIV infection

It is not surprising that a condition of such high profile as HIV infection should be feigned by individuals seeking to benefit from the notoriety and attention given to those with the disease. Deliberate production of symptoms occurs in two kinds of disorders, the difference between them resting on whether the benefit sought is an internal one, fulfilling a psychological need, or an external one, such as financial gain.

Factitious disorders are defined in DSM-III-R as the intentional production or feigning of physical or psychological symptoms, resulting from a psychological need to assume the sick role, rather than from an external incentive, such as economic gain or better care. Munchausen syndrome is a particularly chronic and persistent form of factitious disorder often identified in accident and emergency departments. There is a handful of case reports in the literature involving factitious disorders related to HIV (Miller et al, 1986c; Baer, 1987; Robinson and Latham, 1987; Evans et al, 1988a; Nickoloff et al, 1989; Kavalier, 1989; Frumkin and Victoroff, 1990; Bialer and Wallack, 1990; Cottam et al, 1991; Munckhof and Jenkins, 1993), and they describe people who presented to doctors with detailed accounts of their symptoms and history of infection, and who turned out to be seronegative. Their characteristics, history and subsequent behaviour are typical of those seen in general hospitals and psychiatric clinics in general, suggesting that the choice of HIV infection was incidental, and to some extent influenced by fashion.

It is not always easy to distinguish factitious disorders from malingering, which is defined in DSM-III-R as the intentional production of false or grossly exaggerated symptoms motivated by external incentives, such as money, drugs, or avoidance of situations, as the dividing line between internal and external gain can be difficult to draw. In HIV settings, cases of malingering usually involve seronegative individuals pretending to be seropositive, sometimes to the extent of altering their medical records (Zumwaldt et al, 1987; Parmar et al, 1990), although malingering in a person with AIDS has been described (Gorton et al, 1989).

2.5.3 Eating disorders

Poor appetite, weight loss and concerns about changes in physical appearance are common in HIV infection, usually as a result of medical complications and their treatment, or in the case of concerns about physical appearance, as an understandable reaction to anticipated or actual emaciation or disfigurement. If they are at all concerned about their weight, people with HIV infection tend to worry about becoming too thin, rather than the opposite. Some, however, may develop morbid preoccupations about putting on weight and about their shape, and such concerns may lead to behaviours that complicate their clinical course and management.

Ramsay et al (1992) described four gay men with HIV infection, aged between 25 and 36, referred to a liaison psychiatry service for the treatment of their eating disorders. Two had features of bulimia nervosa (Russell, 1979), in one case long-standing and in the other, following HIV diagnosis and after having stopped substance misuse. A long-standing pattern of restrictive eating without apparent distortion of body image was present in another, and the final case showed marked preoccupation with body image, ambivalent feelings about putting on weight, and episodes of self-induced vomiting. Management was complicated by the conflict between the patient's wish to be thin and the fact that thinness implied decline in health. In addition, medical interventions to restore or increase weight can lead to discomfort about shape and size, and may result in behaviours such as self-induced vomiting, dieting or over-exercising.

It is not clear whether HIV infection is associated with an increased risk for eating disorders, or whether gay men are at particular risk. Bulimia and other eating disorders are relatively common in women (Fairburn and Cooper, 1982) but they have also been described in men (Russell, 1979; Gwirtsman et al, 1984; Herzog et al, 1984; Robinson and Holden, 1986; Dunkeld Turnball et al, 1987). A number of men in these studies were gay (Herzog et al, 1984; Robinson and Holden, 1986), and it has been argued that gay men may be under greater social pressure to be thin than heterosexual men, and thus be at risk of eating disorders (Herzog et al, 1984). While this view seems plausible, to date there is no empirical evidence to support it.

Whether eating disorders are increased in HIV or not is to some extent irrelevant: if eating disorders occur in association with a physical disorder, as has been reported in the case of diabetes (Fairburn et al, 1991; Striegel-Moore et al, 1992; Peveler et al, 1992), the symptoms and associated behaviours are likely to affect the clinical management and possibly the course of the condition, and it is important for clinicians to recognize such problems and ensure that adequate care is given.

2.5.4 Disorders of sexual identity

Male-to-female transsexuals can be at risk of HIV infection as a result of unprotected sexual intercourse or injecting drug use. Before and after surgical sexual reassignment, some male-to-female transsexuals lead a gay lifestyle and may have had unprotected anal intercourse with infected partners. Alternatively, they may have been involved in activities such as prostitution (often having sex with bisexual men) and injecting drug use which are associated with increased HIV risk (Pang et al, 1994). Gattari et al (1991) studied 22 injecting drug using transvestite and transsexual prostitutes and found 19 (86 per cent) to be HIV infected, compared with 32 per cent of male heterosexual injecting drug users attending the same clinic in Rome. A subsequent report (Gattari et al, 1992) including 57 subjects found 42 (74 per cent) to be HIV seropositive. Unsurprisingly, HIV infected subjects were more likely to be injecting drug users, share needles, have greater number of partners, and less likely to use condoms. Modan et al (1992) compared 36 transsexual and 128 female prostitutes in the Tel Aviv area and found 11 per cent and 4 per cent to be HIV seropositive, respectively.

Apart from the obvious implications for prevention when substance misuse and prostitution are implicated, HIV infection in transsexuals undergoing sex re-assignment can raise management problems. Hormonal treatment may contribute to immune suppression and surgery-related infections may be particularly unwelcome in the presence of impaired immune function. Awareness of the risk of future illness and shortened survival will add to the urgency and demands for surgical treatment that many transsexuals experience, leading to genuine feelings of distress and anguish arising out of the sense of living with borrowed time. Such pressures do not assist the process of adjusting to the physical and psychosocial changes involved in sexual re-assignment. Finally, at a time when resources for health care are limited and there is a debate about prioritizing needs, surgery for transsexuals with HIV infection raises practical and ethical problems (Pang et al, 1994).

2.5.5 People with learning difficulties

Concern has been expressed about the risk of HIV infection in people with learning difficulties, both those in institutional care with some contact with the community, but mostly in the case of those who after having spent some time in residential institutions have now moved into smaller units or sheltered housing: it is argued that they may not be fully aware of the risks involved in injecting drug misuse or unprotected sexual intercourse, and as a result they may put themselves at risk of HIV (Robertson et al, 1991). Some of these arguments have been put forward before in relation to the risks of pregnancy and sexual abuse.

Five cases of HIV infection in people with learning disabilities were described by Brown (1991), illustrating the psychosocial and neuropsychological problems they raise. They were all gay or bisexual males, and had mild to moderate degrees of learning difficulties and therefore lived outside institutions. Unprotected sexual intercourse was widespread, and knowledge about HIV infection appeared limited. Neuropsychological deficits became prominent as HIV disease progressed, but their pre-existing impairments made interpretation of neuropsychological test results complex. To date, there is little evidence that HIV infection is a significant problem in people with learning difficulties, although it has to be said that research in this field has been limited. A recent review (Brener and Jadresic, 1992) found little evidence of HIV infection in institutions for people with mental disabilities, a handful of cases having been identified in the US ($n = 11$) and none in European studies. There is concern, however, about the ethical and practical implications of screening people with learning disabilities (Bayer et al, 1986) and about how to obtain informed consent for testing (Kastner et al, 1989). The need for targeted education about HIV prevention for people with learning disabilities and those involved in their care is possibly a greater priority at the present time, requiring the will to discuss difficult issues, such as sexuality, contraception and relationships (Kastner et al, 1989; Hall et al, 1990; McCarthy and Rooney, 1991; Brener and Jadresic, 1992; Dent et al, 1994).

2.5.6 Sexual offenders and survivors of sexual abuse

Sexually transmitted diseases can be acquired as a result of rape (Forster, 1992, 1994), and there is understandable concern about the risk of HIV infection for victims of sexual abuse. Murphy et al (1989) documented the case of a seronegative 24-year-old woman who seroconverted three months after being raped, and made reference to three other possible cases, although other surveys of rape victims have not identified further cases (Estreich et al, 1990; Jenny et al, 1990). Even if the risk of HIV infection following rape appears to be low at present, the possibility of infection will add to the short- and long-term psychosocial difficulties of the survivor, and sensitive psychological and medical care will be required (Murphy, 1990).

An even more disturbing picture is emerging regarding children. Sexual abuse has been identified as the cause of HIV infection in children. Gutman et al (1991) studied 96 HIV seropositive children receiving paediatric care at Duke University, NC, and identified 14 (14.6 per cent) with a history of sexual abuse. Careful investigation established that in four children HIV infection had been the result of sexual abuse, and was the likely cause in another six, indicating that in this particular sample of seropositive children at least four per cent acquired the infection as a result of sexual abuse. The children usually lived in deprived socioeconomic conditions, with alcohol and substance misuse problems and prostitution at home. Two-thirds of cohabiting siblings of the 14 HIV seropositive sexually abused children were found to have been definitely or probably abused, but the suspected perpetrators, often a relative, had not been brought to trial or received therapy, highlighting the need to examine urgently the legal and ethical aspects of the problem to prevent further offences and infections (Gutman et al, 1992). An extensive nation-wide survey carried out by Gellert et al (1993) in the US has provided further evidence about this problem. The authors identified 28 HIV seropositive children where sexual abuse was the only likely method of infection and another 13 where other factors were also implicated. Amongst those who had acquired the infection via sexual abuse, 64 per cent were females and 71 per cent African-American, and their mean age was 9 years. In almost half of the cases, parents were the perpetrators, and another relative in a quarter. While the cases identified represent a small proportion of all cases of child sexual abuse, they point towards the need to be aware of the possible association of two tragic problems. There are complex barriers to the recognition of HIV infection in sexually abused children, as there are barriers to the identification of sexual abuse itself. Gutman et al (1993) have discussed these obstacles at length and have put forward recommendations for the evaluation of children where the possibility of HIV infection as a result of sexual abuse exists.

Survivors of child sexual abuse appear to be subsequently more likely to be involved in behaviours that carry risk of HIV (Zierler et al, 1991) and can grow up to become the perpetrators of further abuse. In this context it is a matter of concern that 19 per cent of patients with HIV infection referred to a specialist psychological service gave a history of sexual abuse before the age of 14 (Burgess and Welch, 1991).

2.6 Factors associated with psychological morbidity

It is to some extent surprising that in spite of the many psychological and social problems that can develop as a result of HIV infection, many infected people cope remarkably well with the problems associated with their declining health. Identifying those likely to deal positively with the consequences of HIV infection and, by implication, those who experience severe difficulties, and recognizing the circumstances that contribute to successful or problematic coping are important tasks. Understanding of the mechanisms that influence the process of adaptation to the possibility of ill-health or to its reality should in turn help those involved in caring for people with HIV infection to be aware of the indicators of risk of psychological problems, and to target resources towards those with the greatest needs.

Research reports and clinical experience indicate that the factors known to contribute to the development of psychological morbidity in general (Goldberg and Huxley, 1992) are also relevant in HIV infection. Some are contemporary,

Table 2.3 Factors associated with psychological morbidity in HIV infection

HIV-related factors	– notification of HIV diagnosis – development of symptoms – start of treatment
Past history of psychological problems	– past psychiatric treatment – personality disorder
Lack of social supports	– few close relationships – poor quality of social supports – loneliness
Coping style	– avoidance – mental and behavioural disengagement – helplessness – poor internal locus of control
Life events	– losses due to AIDS
Demographic features	– age (the very young and the older person) – women – non-white ethnicity – injecting drug use

such as the severity of symptoms and HIV disease stage, the quality of social supports, and the current coping style, while others relate to demographic aspects, such as ethnic characteristics, gender and age, or to pre-existing and long-established traits, such as personality, vulnerability to psychological problems and maladaptive coping styles. See Table 2.3 for a summary of factors.

2.6.1 HIV-related factors

As discussed in Chapter 1, there are two main stages at which psychological problems tend to occur: after notification of a positive HIV test result and later, when symptomatic disease develops. The process of adjusting to a positive result may be a difficult one, and the circumstances in which the test is performed, whether consent was given, the way the news is broken, and the nature of any subsequent counselling will all be important in influencing the person's response (Pierce, 1987; Ostrow et al, 1989a, b; Perry et al, 1990b; Pace et al, 1990; Beevor and Catalán, 1993; Pergami et al, 1994a, b).

Asymptomatic disease may sometimes be associated with the development of psychological problems, and when this happens it is likely that other important factors are contributing (Kessler et al, 1988) (see below). One example of psychological distress in an otherwise well HIV person may be the case of someone whose laboratory investigations suggest the development of progressive immune suppression (declining CD4 count) and who is offered anti-retroviral treatment or prophylaxis for *Pneumocystis carinii* pneumia (PCP). In this situation, the person may become anxious about impending illness, with a reawakening of fears of disease and death. However, this is not an inevitable outcome, some finding hope in the offer of treatments with the potential of preventing disease progression (Hedge et al, 1991).

It is in the symptomatic stages that psychological morbidity is more likely, as shown by research surveys (Tross et al, 1987; Atkinson et al, 1988; Schneider et al, 1991a, b; Lovejoy et al, 1991; Viney et al, 1989; Bialer, 1992; Dening et al, 1992; Catalán et al, 1992a and 1992b; Franke et al, 1992; Hoover et al, 1993; Fell et al, 1993) and by clinical reports of people with HIV infection referred to the mental health services (Perry and Tross, 1984; Dilley et al, 1985; Buhrich and Cooper, 1987; Baer, 1989; Lyons et al, 1989; Ayuso-Mateos et al, 1989; Sno et al, 1989; Seth et al, 1991; Douzenis et al, 1991). Disease stage can be associated with the development of psychological problems in several ways. The presence of physical symptoms such as persistent diarrhoea, tiredness, or shortness of breath is likely to have an effect on the person's quality of life (Burgess et al, 1993). More disturbing psychological impact may follow the onset of severe visual problems resulting from cytomegalovirus (CMV) retinitis, disfiguring conditions like Kaposi's sarcoma involving the face or other visible parts of the body, marked weight loss, or neurological disorders resulting in reduced mobility and independence. Side-effects of medication can also cause psychological symptoms either as a direct pharmacological result or indirectly because of the malaise and short-term symptoms they can produce, as in the case of chemotherapy or radiotherapy.

Psychological distress may follow the doctor's offer of prophylactic interventions by highlighting the person's vulnerability to further complications. Particularly significant in its symbolic and practical implications is the presence of an AIDS-defining illness, even when the physical symptoms are not very marked. For somebody who has worked hard at keeping healthy and maintaining a positive and constructive attitude to the infection, receiving a diagnosis of AIDS can have very significant impact, by seemingly undermining the person's sense of control over the infection. The recently revised classification of HIV infection adopted by the Centers for Disease Control from January 1993 which can lead to a diagnosis of AIDS on the basis of a low CD4 count and in the absence of one of the traditional AIDS-defining illness is an example of the kind of clinical situation that can have profound psychological effects on people with HIV.

Reporting of positive symptoms may itself be an indication of the presence of psychological morbidity. People complaining of symptoms suggestive of cognitive impairment, such as memory problems or difficulty with thinking are usually found to neuropsychologically intact, but suffering from anxiety or depression (Wilkins et al, 1991; Riccio et al, 1993).

2.6.2 Past psychiatric history

As mentioned in Chapter 1, in developed countries, a history of psychiatric treatment before HIV infection is not uncommon, and there is evidence that those with a past history of psychiatric problems are more likely to experience further problems in relation to HIV infection. The contribution of a past psychiatric history (history of in-patient or out-patient care or a history of deliberate self-harm) to the presence of current psychological morbidity has been reported in several studies involving gay men (Catalán et al, 1992a; Fell et al, 1993; Riccio et al, 1993) and men with haemophilia (Dew et al, 1990; Catalán et al, 1992b). Interestingly, in these studies the effect of a past psychiatric history was stronger than the HIV status of the subjects, suggesting that it is not the infection itself that leads to psychological problems, but other pre-existing factors. This finding is consistent with that of Perry et al (1993), who found levels of psychological distress at the time of HIV testing to be the best predictor of psychological morbidity a year later, regardless of serostatus. The presence of personality disorder, whether associated to a past psychiatric history or not, also increases the risk of developing psychological problems (Perkins et al, 1993a).

2.6.3 Social supports

Community studies and surveys of psychiatric populations have confirmed that the presence of social supports is associated with greater psychological well-being, even if the mechanisms by which social supports reduce distress and the contribution of other variables are unclear (Cohen and Wills, 1985; Monroe et al, 1986; George et al, 1989; Goldberg et al, 1990). Similar results have been reported in people with HIV infection, although the relationship between social support, perceived threat and psychological stress is a complex one (Britton et al, 1993).

In cross-sectional studies, Blaney et al (1991) found social supports to be associated with less distress in people with early HIV infection, and Hays et al (1990a) found depression levels in people with AIDS to be strongly correlated with having fewer close relationships, while psychological well-being was correlated with greater support levels and with the quality of close relationships, as was also reported by Wolcott et al, 1986a). In people with AIDS, depression was associated to reduced supports and to dependence on health care professionals (Noh et al, 1990). Depressed people with HIV infection report significantly poorer quality of social supports (Murphy et al, 1991; Kelly et al, 1993a), and women with HIV showing psychological distress tended to be isolated and dissatisfied with their social supports according to Franke et al (1992). HIV asymptomatic gay men with good social supports who were facing the threat of progressing to symptomatic disease showed more adaptive coping responses than those without community involvement (Leserman et al, 1992).

These findings have been confirmed in a handful of prospective studies. Loneliness and fewer close supports at baseline were some of the variables associated with greater levels of depression two years later in a cohort of San Francisco gay/bisexual men (Castro et al, 1989). Poor quality of social support in men with haemophilia and HIV was found to predict psychological morbidity one year later, two factors: low 'social belonging' and 'social guidance', accounting for 35 per cent of the variance (Catalán 1991b). Social supports also predicted psychological functioning at four months in the study by Lamping et al (1992). In a study involving a five-year follow-up, subjective perception of social support was found to contribute to depression ratings during this period (Lackner et al, 1993). Unstructured support groups have been shown to contribute to a reduction in distress, in particular for those with higher distress levels (DiPasquale, 1990), thus confirming the importance of interpersonal supports. It has to be stressed that the relationship between perceived social supports and psychological health is a complex one, and that there are difficult methodological issues involved (Monroe et al, 1986; Britton et al, 1993).

2.6.4 Coping style

The way we cope with specific stresses, whether they involve perceived threat, loss or challenge, is to some extent influenced by long-standing personality traits (Deary and Matthews, 1993), and both personality and coping style contribute to psychological well-being (McCrae and Costa, 1986). For example, problem-focused coping, such as using rational action and seeking help, and emotional-focused coping, such as expressing feelings, are generally effective in reducing distress. Other usually effective coping methods are humour, regarding difficulties as opportunities for learning, and religion. On the other hand, hostility, self-blame, indecisiveness, wishful thinking and avoidance are usually ineffective in reducing distress (McCrae and Costa, 1986). There is some evidence from work with people with cancer that 'hopeless–helpless' coping is associated with psychological morbidity (Burgess et al, 1988) and that coping mechanisms change over time with the specific circumstances of hospitalization, treatment modality, and with stages of disease progression like remission, relapse and terminal phases (Heim et al, 1993). One important methodological problem with many of these studies is the possible effect of low mood on the person's rating of coping styles, which may result in spurious results. This problem is particularly relevant to cross-sectional studies.

Studies of people with HIV infection have given results consistent with the literature reviewed above. Cross-sectional studies of gay/bisexual men have showed that psychological morbidity is associated with the use of an avoidance coping style (Kurdek and Siesky, 1990); the use of mental and behavioural disengagement from the stressful situation, rather than with active coping or planning (Lovett et al, 1993); and with helplessness, and with a lesser use of fighting spirit, more denial and less positive reframing of experiences (Leserman et al, 1992). AIDS long-term survivors have been reported to use a wide range of coping strategies involving active coping, taking control of their health, and pursuing pleasurable activities in addition to making good use of social supports, and having internal or chance health locus of control (Remien et al, 1992) (see Chapter 6 for further discussion of long-term surviving in HIV infection).

Study of health beliefs regarding locus of control indicate that having less internal locus of control is associated with distress (Lovejoy et al, 1991) and severe depression (Murphy et al, 1991) in gay men, and with greater psychological morbidity in women (Pergami et al, 1993), although there may be some circularity about these cross-sectional findings.

2.6.5 Life events and losses due to AIDS

The role of stressful life events, in particular those involving loss or threat, in the development of psychological problems such as depression and anxiety, is well established (Uhlenhuth and Paykel, 1973; Harris and Brown, 1989). There is some evidence that life events can contribute to psychological morbidity in people with HIV infection (Lovett et al, 1993). However, a particular phenomenon characteristic of the epidemic and one that has significant psychological implications is the way individuals with HIV infection and those involved in their care are exposed to multiple AIDS-related deaths. In developed countries, the provision of adequate psychological and social care for people with HIV infection would not have been possible without the presence of voluntary community organizations, in particular those involving gay/bisexual men. One inevitable negative consequence of such community structures has been the concentration of individuals with HIV infection, and thus of individuals at risk of becoming ill and dying, with the subsequent impact on survivors in the organization, who will then be exposed to the repeated experience of HIV-related deaths.

The process of grieving the loss of a person dying of AIDS is often complicated: stigma, possible lack of support, fears of contagion, young age of the person involved and the course and pattern of illness, involving disfigurement, neurological disorders and blindness can add to the difficulties (Klein and Fletcher 1987; Worden 1991). Studies of gay men have shown that those involved in caring for someone dying of AIDS experience greater psychological distress, especially when social supports are limited (Lennon et al, 1990). About a third of gay men in a New York community sample had experienced the loss of a lover or close friend to AIDS, one-third of whom had experienced multiple losses, and an association was found between the number of bereavements and psychological distress levels (Martin, 1991), while other authors reported an association between the number of losses and the pattern of grief (Neugebauer et al, 1992). Loss of a loved one was found to be a predictor of subsequent depression in a prospective two-year follow-up study (Castro et al, 1989). Gay men who have suffered greater exposure to AIDS deaths show higher anxiety and anger levels (Viney et al, 1992). Amongst HIV infected people, mostly gay men, referred by their physicians for psychological help Sherr et al (1992) found 43 per cent to have experienced bereavement, with an average of nearly 13 deaths per person. Depression, guilt, and anger were the most commonly reported emotions. HIV infected people tend to experience greater distress following the death of their partners, while discordant couples may suffer other difficulties (see Bor, 1992). In addition to the feelings of anxiety and anger described above, some people report disturbing feelings of numbness in the face of yet another death and funeral, and others suffer distress at their own survival, while everyone else seems to be dying. Not surprisingly for some, avoidance of and withdrawal from gay community organizations may seem an attractive escape.

2.6.6 Demographic factors

There is no clear evidence that age is associated with the development of psychological problems, although it is not uncommon for people at the extremes of the age range to experience difficulties, in particular adolescents or people over 55. Older persons appear to have worse clinical outcome and a greater risk of HIV-encephalopathy (Ship et al, 1991; Ferro and Salit 1992) and it is therefore likely some will also experience important psychological problems related to the speed of progression, brain effects and possible lack of the kind of social supports to which younger people would have access.

In developed countries, women with HIV seem to have worse access to medical services than men, and this may contribute to differences in survival and physical morbidity (Hankins and Handley, 1992), and in turn to their greater psychological morbidity reported in some studies (see Catalán and Riccio, 1990a). Other factors, such a history of injecting drug use, may also be relevant (see below).

Ethnicity has been found to be a contributor to psychological problems in a number of studies from developed countries. Hispanic gay men reported greater distress related to their sexual orientation than other HIV infected white gay men (Ceballos-Capitaine et al, 1990). Black and Hispanic US men have been found to experience greater distress than white men (see Catalán and Riccio, 1990a), and Black men with HIV infection appear to have poorer social supports than white men, and a culturally different pattern of family relations (Mays and Cochran, 1987; Ostrow et al, 1991). As in the case of gender, ethnic and cultural factors are closely related to important social and political issues such as restricted access to medical care, discrimination, and economic adversity, which will play a significant part in the risk of developing psychological problems.

HIV transmission category is also of relevance. Injecting drug users of either sex have been found to suffer greater psychological morbidity than other transmission groups (Gala et al, 1993), a finding not altogether surprising, as many injecting drug users will have experienced psychological and social difficulties prior to HIV infection which will have worsened as a result of it. Unfortunately, in spite of their increased risk of psychological problems, injecting drug users are less likely than other groups to make use of mental health services designed to help them cope with HIV infection (Gala et al, 1992b).

2.7 Summary

In addition to the common psychological reactions seen in people with HIV infection, a proportion of individuals can develop major psychiatric syndromes requiring intensive and specialized care. Suicidal behaviour is a particularly important area of concern. Suicidal ideas are common in people with HIV infection and among those seeking testing. The risk of suicide has been reported to be increased in people with HIV infection, figures ranging from 7 to 36 the rate of suicide compared with sex- and age-matched control populations. There are, however, methodological problems in this area of research that make it difficult to know for certain whether suicide risk is increased in HIV and, if so, to what degree. Deliberate self-harm not leading to death has also being reported in people with HIV infection.

Psychotic disorders are often seen in people with HIV infection, although their exact prevalence is not clear. Many factors can contribute to the development of such disorders, including pre-existing psychotic illness, substance misuse, psychogenic reactions, side-effects of medical treatments, and possibly HIV related brain disease. New-onset psychotic disorders in HIV patients are indicative of poor HIV prognosis.

Sexual dysfunction problems are common in HIV, and they can result from psychological reactions to the infection, pre-existing difficulties, HIV-related organic factors, and treatment side-effects. Other conditions and problems which can be seen in people with HIV infection include: personality problems, feigned HIV infection, eating disorders, sexual identity disorder, and learning difficulties. There is also an association between sexual offences and sexual abuse and HIV.

The factors associated with the development of psychological problems in HIV disease include those that are known to be important in general such as past psychiatric history, lack of social supports, coping style, life events, and demographic characteristics. There are also risk factors which are specific to HIV infection and these include multiple losses of friends and partners, the development of illness and the stigma associated with the disease.

3 HIV and the brain

3.1 Introduction

The initial recognition of AIDS in Los Angeles and New York in 1981 was prompted by the identification of an abnormally high incidence of two rare diseases (*Pneumocystis carinii* pneumonia and Kaposi's sarcoma) in a group of young men. It was not until some time later that it was realised that many people with AIDS also suffered from neurological disease. In an early report, Snider et al (1983) found that half of all people with AIDS suffered neurological complications and later post-mortem studies have suggested that nearly all those who die with AIDS have significant cerebral pathology.

In many cases, central nervous system (CNS) disease is secondary to the immunosuppression caused by HIV. McArthur (1987) described a series of 186 HIV seropositive patients who had been referred for neurological examination. Of these, more than half (n = 101; 54 per cent) had a significant CNS complication including 71 (38 per cent) with a neurological disease secondary to HIV infection. The most frequent of these were viral infections (n = 26; 14 per cent), intracranial mass lesions (n = 29; 16 per cent) and bacterial infections (n = 12; 6 per cent). The single most common neurological complication, however, seen in 16 per cent of the patients (n = 30), was a progressive dementia associated with the HIV infection thought to be caused by the direct effect of HIV on the brain.

This chapter includes a clinical description of the dementia sometimes seen in people with AIDS, and the terminological difficulties, the epidemiology and the prognosis of this disease are also addressed. The nature and type of cognitive difficulties seen in advanced HIV disease, which do not amount to a full clinical dementia, are also described. Whether there is any cognitive impairment in the asymptomatic stage of infection remains controversial and the evidence for and against early impairment will be discussed. Finally, the neuropathological, neuroradiological and psychophysiological changes seen in association with the cognitive changes in HIV disease are described.

3.2 HIV-1 associated dementia

Clinical characteristics

The first detailed descriptions of the dementia seen in AIDS were reported by Navia et al (1986a, b). They presented detailed clinical and neuropathological data on a series of patients who had died of AIDS. Of their 121 patients, more than 40 per cent had some degree of cognitive impairment caused by CNS disease secondary to their HIV infection. In addition, more than a third of this group showed some cognitive or behavioural changes for which, at that time, there was no explanation. From the medical records of this group, Navia et al (1986a, b) were able to describe a triad of clinical features which they later labelled the AIDS Dementia Complex (ADC). The triad consisted of *cognitive impairment* (including forgetfulness, loss of concentration, confusion and slowness of thought), *motor dysfunction* (including loss of balance, leg weakness, deterioration in handwriting) and *behavioural changes* (including apathy, social withdrawal, organic psychosis and regressed behaviour). Most of the patients with ADC had a pre-existing diagnosis of AIDS ($n = 29$) but in 17 cases, ADC had developed in people who were otherwise well. Although there have been many reports of dementia being the first manifestation of AIDS (Navia and Price 1987) this is relatively uncommon (McArthur et al, 1993). The Centers for Disease Control (CDC) criteria for a diagnosis of AIDS now include dementia as an AIDS defining syndrome (CDC group IV; see Table 9.2). This means that, by definition, it is no longer possible for a person with asymptomatic disease to be demented.

Terminology and concepts

The concept of the 'AIDS dementia complex' (ADC) has been developed by Price and Brew (1988) to include a clinical rating scale that has been widely used in research studies. The ADC scale allows individuals to be rated on one of 6 levels from Normal (Stage 0) through equivocal (Stage 0.5) to end stage dementia (Stage 4). Ratings are made by comparing a patient's clinical presentation with descriptive exemplars (Table 3.1). Navia et al's (1986a) clinical description of the cognitive and behavioural changes seen in advanced HIV disease has been widely accepted. The use of the term 'ADC', however, has been more controversial. One of the major criticisms of the ADC is that the term 'complex' suggests that the triad of features of cognitive impairment, motor dysfunction and behavioural change necessarily go together. From Navia et al's (1986a) report, it was clear that some individuals displayed evidence of either motor or cognitive impairment without the other features of the ADC triad. The use of the term 'dementia' has also been challenged. Under existing diagnostic schemes such as DSM-III-R and ICD-10, the term 'dementia' applies only in cases of profound, dense amnesia. Under the ADC terminology, the term 'dementia' can apply to people whose cognitive deficits are mild and would not have warranted that diagnosis under existing diagnostic schemes (e.g. Catalán, 1991c).

ADC has been one of the more widely used diagnostic categories to describe the cognitive and behavioural changes sometimes seen in AIDS. As Catalán (1991c) points out, however, at least 12 other different labels have been used to describe a variety of broadly similar clinical presentations. In an attempt to rationalize this terminological confusion, the WHO (1990b) recommended the adoption a new diagnosis, 'HIV-1 associated dementia', based on operationally defined criteria adapted from the ICD-10 diagnosis of dementia (Table 3.2). To achieve a diagnosis of HIV-1 associated dementia the ICD-10 criteria for dementia

Table 3.1 The AIDS dementia rating scale. (From Price and Brew (1988), reproduced with permission.)

STAGE 0 (normal)	Normal mental and motor function.
STAGE 0.5 (equivocal/ subclinical)	Absent, minimal or equivocal symptoms without impairment of work or capacity to perform activities of daily living (ADL). Mild signs (snout response, slowed ocular or extremity movements) may be present. Gait and strength are normal
STAGE 1 (mild)	Able to perform all but the more demanding aspects of work or ADL but with unequivocal evidence (signs or symptoms that may include performance on neuropsychological testing) of functional intellectual or motor impairment. Can walk without assistance.
STAGE 2 (moderate)	Able to perform basic activities of self-care but cannot work or maintain the more demanding aspects of daily life. Ambulatory, but may require a single prop.
STAGE 3 (severe)	Major intellectual incapacity (cannot follow news or personal events, cannot sustain complex conversation, considerable slowing of all output or motor disability (cannot walk unassisted, requiring walker or personal support, usually with slowing and clumsiness of arms as well).
STAGE 4 (end stage)	Nearly negative. Intellectual and social comprehension and output are at a rudimentary level. Nearly or absolutely mute. Paraparetic or paraplegic with urinary and faecal incontinence.

must be met with the following modifications: (i) the decline in memory may not be severe enough to impair activities of daily living; (ii) motor dysfunction may be present; (iii) aphasia, agnosia and apraxia are uncommon; and (iv) the symptoms should have lasted for at least one month. Further, the patient must be HIV seropositive and other possible aetiologies should be excluded.

The WHO diagnostic system has several advantages. First, it re-aligns the use of the term 'dementia' with its use in other diseases such as Alzheimer's. Second, it reduces the importance of the non-cognitive and motor aspects of the disorder which although common are not always seen. Third, it emphasizes the importance of excluding other causes of cognitive impairment that may occur in AIDS. This last point is of great clinical importance as some CNS diseases are treatable (e.g. toxoplasmosis) whereas a diagnosis of dementia is often taken to suggest that nothing can be done.

A parallel attempt to rationalize the terminology in this area has been presented by the American Academy of Neurology AIDS Task Forces (AAN, 1991). The AAN nomenclature is consistent with the WHO definition of HIV-1 associated dementia, although not identical with it. The major difference is that the dementia, called HIV-1 associated cognitive motor complex, is divided into two main categories which specify whether the dementia has a primarily

Table 3.2 World Health Organization definition of HIV-1 associated dementia. (From WHO, 1990b, reproduced with permission.)

A	Evidence of a dementia, of a specified level of severity, based on the presence of each of the following:
(i)	A decline in memory which may not be severe enough to cause impaired functioning in daily living. The decline should be objectively verifiable and not based on subjective complaint. The level of severity should be assessed as follows: Mild impairment: A degree of memory loss sufficient to interfere with everyday activities, though not so severe as to be incompatible with independent living. The main function affected is the learning of new material. Moderate impairment: A more severe degree of memory loss. Only highly learned or familiar material is retained. This degree of memory impairment is a serious handicap to independent living. Severe impairment: Severe memory loss with only fragments of previously learned material remaining. The individual is not able to function in the community without close supervision.
(ii)	A decline in intellectual abilities characterized by deterioration in thinking and processing of information of a degree leading to impaired functioning in daily living. The level of intellectual impairment should be assessed as follows: Mild impairment: The decline in intellectual abilities causes impaired performance in daily living, but not to a degree making the individual dependent on others. Moderate impairment: The decline in intellectual abilities makes the individual unable to function without the assistance of another in activities of daily living. Severe impairment: The decline precludes not only independence from the assistance of others, but is characterized by an absence, or virtual absence of intelligible ideation.
(iii)	Decline in motor function may be present.
(iv)	Aphasia, agnosia and apraxia are unusual.
(v)	Symptoms should be present for at least one month.
B	Absence of clouding of consciousness.
C	A deterioration in emotional control or social behaviour.
D	Laboratory evidence of systemic HIV-1 infection.
E	No evidence of another aetiology.

cognitive or motor component: HIV-1 associated dementia complex and HIV-1 associated myelopathy.

In recognition that cognitive impairment is frequently seen in people with AIDS that does not amount to a dementia, the WHO have also proposed an additional diagnosis of 'HIV-1 associated minor cognitive/motor disorder'

(WHO 1990b). The AAN term is 'HIV-1 associated minor cognitive/motor disorder'.

Whilst other diagnostic terms, particularly the AAN nomenclature, will continue to be used, it is recommended that the WHO advice is followed and the term HIV-1 associated dementia should be used where appropriate.

Epidemiology

Good estimates of the prevalence of dementia in people with AIDS have only recently been available. Early prevalence figures were based upon unrepresentative samples of patients attending specialist neurological centres (e.g. Navia et al, 1986a; McArthur, 1987). In addition, relatively liberal definitions of dementia were sometimes used. As a consequence, some estimates suggested that up to 40 per cent of people with AIDS would develop dementia. Such high prevalence figures raised the spectre of potentially overwhelming demands on the limited medical resources available from large numbers of otherwise healthy people dementing in their youth. Fortunately, later studies of more representative samples of people with AIDS have suggested that the prevalence of HIV-1 associated dementia is very much lower than was at first feared. The WHO Consultation Meeting (1990b) concluded that the point prevalence of dementia in AIDS to be between 8 and 16 per cent. Even this figure may be too high. A detailed retrospective examination of all reported AIDS cases in a single health district in the UK in a single year (n = 662) found 75 (11 per cent) with a substantial clinically identified cognitive impairment. In most cases, this was associated with either a pre-existing impairment or the secondary effects of HIV infection (Meadows et al, 1993d). In this sample, only 17 (2.6 per cent) met the WHO definition of HIV-1 associated dementia.

Estimates of the annual incidence of dementia in people with AIDS are now available. A review of all AIDS cases reported to the Centres for Diseases Control in the US between 1987 and 1988 estimated the incidence of dementia to be 7.3 per cent (Janssen et al, 1990). One of the most detailed reports on this issue has come from the Multicenter AIDS Cohort Study (MACS) (McArthur et al, 1993). The MACS study is a large prospective study of people with HIV infection in the US which includes a broad range of health evaluations including regular neuropsychological assessment. In the MACS cohort, the annual incidence of dementia, using AAN criteria, in people with AIDS was 7 per cent, confirming Janssen et al's (1990) findings. Of those people in the MACS cohort who were followed through to death, 15 per cent demented. In addition, the MACS report identified several risk factors that were present before the first AIDS diagnosis that were associated with an increased risk of dementing. These were low body mass index, low haemoglobin, more constitutional symptoms and older age.

These studies, summarized in Table 3.3, give widely varying estimates of the prevalence not only because of differences in subject populations and diagnostic criteria, but also because the true prevalence of dementia may have been changing. There are several possible reasons for this. First, one risk factor for the development of dementia may be the length of time that a patient has been

Table 3.3 Operational criteria for the American Academy of Neurology diagnosis of HIV-1 associated cognitive/motor complex. (Adapted by McArthur et al, 1993, with permission.)

Possible HIV-1 dementia	
	One or more of the following
1. History	Third party report of progressive cognitive/ behavioural deterioration with clear consciousness, sufficient to interfere with social or work activities.
2. Neurologic assessment	Deterioration in cognition from pre-morbid level with either normal examination or diffuse CNS signs.
3. Neurophsychological testing	Two or more measures ≤ 2 sd below age/ education mean or a decline of ≥ 1 sd below previous neuropsychological test in at least two independent measures or one global measure of intellectual function.
Probable HIV-1 dementia	
	History, neuropsychological testing and neurological assessment as above.
	and all of the following
Psychiatric disease	No active thought disorder; stable psychiatric medication regime.
Confounding medical conditions	No metabolic derangements, e.g. uraemia, sepsis, hepatic failure or intoxication.
Opportunistic processes and neurosyphillis	imaging studies, serum fluorescent treponemal antibody, CSF analysis, autopsy, or prolonged survival without empiric treatment.

carrying the virus. This means that after entry into a population, the prevalence of HIV should be expected to rise for many years before levelling off. Second, the use of zidovudine appears to have reduced the risk of developing dementia and may partially ameliorate the cognitive impairment, at least in the short term (see Chapter 5). Third, the changing pattern of medical treatment and the emergence of resistance to existing therapies may result in the fluctuations in the incidence of dementia in the future.

Most of the data on the prevalence of HIV-1 associated dementia has been based on samples of well-educated gay/bisexual men from Western Europe and North America. Given that only 15 per cent of people living with HIV infection live in the Western world and that 75 per cent of HIV infections are transmitted via heterosexual contact (Mann et al, 1992), this is a serious limitation. Some estimates of the prevalence of HIV-1 associated dementia in the developing world are available although they vary widely. Belec et al (1989) found a 3 per cent prevalence rate in the Central African Republic, compared with 9 per cent

Table 3.4 Epidemiology of dementia in AIDS

Authors	Country	Patient source	Prevalence (%)
Navia et al, 1986a,b	US	Post-mortem study. Diagnosis of dementia based on retrospective analysis of medical records using ADC criteria.	38
McArthur, 1987	US	Consecutive series of patients with AIDS referred for neurological assessment using ADC criteria.	16
Janssen et al, 1990	US	All patients with AIDS reported to the CDC 1987–8. Diagnostic criterion *cognitive and/or motor dysfunction interfering with occupation or activities of daily living*	Incidence 7
Meadows et al, 1993	UK	Retrospective study of all registered patients with AIDS in a single health district in 1990. Diagnosis made from medical notes and interviews with clinical staff according to DMS-III-R criteria.	Possible dementia 11 Probable dementia 3
Belec et al, 1989	Central African Republic	Consecutive series of in-patients with AIDS. Diagnostic criteria not specified.	Dementia 3 Neuropsychiatric complications 16
Howlett et al, 1989	Tanzania	Consecutive series of patients with AIDS. Dementia defined as *a decline of memory and other cognitive functions in comparison with the patient's previous level of function.*	
Perriens et al, 1992	Zaïre	Consecutive HIV+ in-patients. Structured interview giving diagnosis based on DMS-III-R and ICD-10 criteria.	
McArthur et al, 1993	US	Patients enrolled in the Multicenter AIDS Cohort Study. Diagnosis based on AAN definition of dementia.	Probable dementia 6 Possible & probable 15 Incidence 7
WHO Study Maj et al, 1994b	Brazil Germany Kenya Thailand Zaïre	Representative selection of AIDS patients attentind out-patient clinics. DSM-II-R and ICD-10 diagnoses used.	6.5 5.4 6.9 0 5.9

in Zaïre (Perriens et al, 1992) and an alarmingly high 54 per cent reported by Howlett et al (1989) from Tanzania, although the last used a very liberal definition of dementia.

Recently, more representative estimates of the prevalence of HIV-1 associated dementia have been reported by the WHO Cross-cultural study on the neuropsychiatric consequences of HIV infection (Maj et al. 1991, 1994a, b). In this study, subjects were selected from five centres around the world (Bangkok, Thailand; Kinshasa, Zaïre; Munich, Germany; Nairobi, Kenya; and São Paulo, Brazil) selected to represent the four different epidemiological patterns of HIV infection identified by the WHO. Subjects were recruited sequentially from patients with HIV infection who presented themselves at out-patient clinics and the resulting samples were an accurate reflection of the local HIV seropositive population in terms of age, sex, education level, disease stage, and probable route of infection. As part of a more detailed neuropsychiatric evaluation, subjects were also assessed to see whether they met the ICD-10 or DSM-III-R criteria for dementia. The prevalence rates for dementia did not differ substantially between DSM-III-R and ICD-10 nor between four of the five recruitment centres where the rate was 4.4–6.9 per cent of people living with AIDS. In one centre, Bangkok, no cases of HIV-1 associated dementia were recorded. This probably reflects the more recent entry of HIV into the population where no cases of HIV had been identified prior to 1987. In none of the centres did any people who were otherwise asymptomatic meet the criteria for HIV-1 associated dementia. The WHO cross-cultural study gives the best indication of the prevalence of HIV-1 associated dementia based on a more representative sample of persons infected with HIV than has been available to date. The major limitation of the study is that the sample is based upon patients attending out-patient clinics and may, therefore, exclude the most seriously ill patients who have the highest risk of developing dementia. At present, it is not known whether the extremely poor prognosis for those with HIV-1 associated dementia reported by Navia et al (1986a, b) is reflected in this wider population, but this will be answered by in the future by the longitudinal phase of the WHO cross-cultural study.

Course and Prognosis

Navia et al (1986a, b) found that in most cases, the onset of dementia was insidious but in some case an abrupt onset was seen, usually associated with a serious systemic illness. More recent reports from longitudinal neuropsychological studies have suggested that dementia typically develops over a relatively short period of time and is not necessarily preceded by any significant cognitive difficulties. Selnes et al (1991) described 12 gay men who had enrolled in a prospective longitudinal study for whom neuropsychological data was available *before* the onset of dementia. In each case, secondary causes of dementia, such as cerebral infections and neoplasms, had been excluded by magnetic resonance imaging (MRI) and laboratory studies. In all but one case, the changes in cognitive performance were precipitous, occurring within a 6 month period, and were *not* preceded by an insidious decline. The only change that preceded the onset of dementia was some slowing in fine motor speed (Grooved Pegboard). Other cognitive changes developed later. Whilst the numbers are small, Selnes et al (1991) have produced clear evidence that even those individuals who go on to develop HIV-1 associated dementia, may be cognitively unimpaired during the asymptomatic stages of the disease.

For those who develop dementia, the prognosis is extremely poor. More than half of the patients with ADC from Navia et al's (1986a, b) cohort went on to develop a severe global impairment within 2 months and died on average 1.8 months later (range 1–6 months). It is now believed that the prognosis for those who develop dementia may be slightly better than Navia et al's (1986a, b) study initially suggested. The MACS study found that median life expectancy from the time of a diagnosis of dementia was 6 months (McArthur et al, 1993). This means that dementia has a far poorer prognosis than most other AIDS diagnoses. In a retrospective study, Meadows et al (1993d) found that the time from the first diagnosis of AIDS to death was significantly shorter for those who developed dementia than for people with other AIDS diagnoses. For those with HIV-1 dementia, the median life span was only 16 months from the date of first AIDS diagnosis, less than half that of those who did not develop dementia. Mayeux et al (1993) found that people living with HIV infection who showed mild to moderate degrees of cognitive impairment were four times more likely to die over the 36-month period of follow-up than those with no impairment regardless of whether they had symptomatic disease or not. Similar prognostic value has been reported for MRI and computed tomography (CT) scans (Mundinger et al, 1991). They found that the life expectancy of people with AIDS who had normal neuroradiological images was twice that of those with atrophy and nearly nine times as long as those with focal lesions.

3.3 Neuropsychology of HIV infection

3.3.1 Neuropsychology of advanced HIV disease

Although a frank clinical dementia is relatively uncommon in people with AIDS, significant degrees of cognitive impairment are more frequently seen. In some cases, cognitive impairment will be due to opportunistic infections in the brain or cerebral neoplasms, but even in those with no secondary cerebral involvement, some impairment will often been seen. Grant et al (1987) reported that people with AIDS tended to show poorer memory (Prose Recall) and attention (Digit Span), were slower at information processing (Paced Auditory Serial Addition Test) and had difficulty with abstract thinking (Category Test). Ayers et al (1987), using the Luria–Nebraska Neuropsychological Battery (LNNB), found that a third of their subjects with AIDS were impaired on three or more of the LNNB scales. The scales most frequently impaired were Writing, Memory, Tactile, and Intellectual functions.

Perhaps the most detailed of the early studies was that by Tross et al. (1988) who compared the neuropsychological performance of a group of seronegative gay men (n = 20) with an asymptomatic seropositive group (n = 16), and two AIDS groups. The first group of people with AIDS included those who had been newly diagnosed (early AIDS; n = 44) and the second, those who had been referred for neurological examination (late AIDS; n = 40). The neuropsychological battery was made up of well established clinical tests and assessed language, memory, visuo-spatial performance, attention, speed of information processing and motor control. Tross et al (1988) found no difference between any of the groups in terms of their performance on the language, memory tasks or attention. Both AIDS groups, however, had significantly impaired fine motor speed (Grooved Pegboard), psychomotor speed (Trail Making Test, WAIS-R Digit Symbol) and visuo-spatial ability (WAIS-R Block Design). Further, on most of these tasks, the late AIDS group performed more poorly than the early AIDS group with over 60 per cent of the late AIDS rated as 'impaired' compared with only 5 per cent in the early AIDS group.

Other researchers have generally confirmed Tross et al's (1988) findings although there has been some variation in the types of deficits seen (e.g. Ayers et al, 1987; Grant et al, 1987; Rubinow et al, 1988; Van Gorp et al, 1989; Derix et al, 1990; Krikorian and Wrobel, 1991). In addition to motor speed, language, memory and executive functions are frequently found to be impaired as well. A similar, though less marked pattern of cognitive deficits has been seen in patients with symptomatic disease (Janssen et al, 1989; Perdices and Cooper, 1990).

In summary, the most frequently seen deficits are in fine motor control (e.g. Grooved Pegboard; Matthews and Klove, 1964) and psychomotor speed (e.g. Trail Making Test; Reitan, 1958; Digit Symbol; Wechsler, 1981). Memory and language impairments are often reported, though they are typically less prominent than in cortical dementias (e.g. Alzheimer's disease) and are most common in the final stages of the disease. Other cortical dysfunctions such as the agnosias and apraxias are only rarely seen unless there is some other cerebral pathology.

Deficits in executive functions, which involve planning, problem solving, sequencing and concept formation have also been reported (e.g. Category Test, Grant et al, 1987; the Stroop Test, Perdices and Cooper, 1990; the Odd Man Out Test; Stern et al, 1991), though these have been investigated less often than other functions. Deficits in executive functions are typically ascribed to the frontal lobes (Walsh, 1987) or subcortical grey matter structures, particularly the basal ganglia (Flowers and Robertson 1987). As would be expected from the neuropathology of HIV-1 associated dementia (pp. 77–8), which predominantly, though not exclusively, involves subcortical structures (Price et al, 1988), the pattern of cognitive deficits resembles that of a subcortical dementia and involves '. . . psychomotor slowing, memory impairment, affective and emotional disorders and difficulties with strategy formation and problem solving' (Cummings 1986).

Pattern of neuropsychological decline

The question arises as to when do the cognitive deficits seen in advanced HIV disease first become apparent. Perdices et al (1991) found no evidence of cognitive deterioration as individuals progressed from a diagnosis of asymptomatic to symptomatic disease suggesting that the first development of symptoms is not usually associated with cognitive impairment. Although cognitive impairment or dementia may be the first presenting sign of AIDS (e.g. Navia and Price 1987) this is usually only seen in the context of other AIDS-defining illnesses (McArthur et a. 1993). Nor is a diagnosis of AIDS necessarily associated with the development of cognitive dysfunction. Dunbar et al (1991) described a prospective longitudinal study in which a group of patients with symptomatic disease who progressed to AIDS were compared with a group who remained clinically stable. They found no significant cognitive associated with progression to AIDS, although both groups did show a decline in performance over time and both performed at a lower level than a matched control group.

Biological markers of neuropsychological performance

Although changes in neuropsychological performance are not strongly linked to changes in CDC stage, it is undoubtedly true that cognitive impairment is more common in advanced disease stages. For this reason, many researchers have attempted to identify biological markers that link cognitive changes with some measure of disease stage. The most obvious measure to use is CD4 count. There is, however, little evidence of a correlation between neuropsychological performance and CD4 count despite many attempts to show one. Particularly for CD4 counts above 400 (e.g. McArthur et al, 1989; Perry et al, 1989) there is almost no association with cognitive performance. For CD4 counts below 200, there have been some reports of increased probability of cognitive impairment (Mitchell et al, 1989) but the association is still not strong. Bornstein et al (1991) have suggested that it is the change in CD4 count rather than the absolute level that is related to cognitive performance, but this result has yet to be replicated.

In addition to CD4 count, a number of other biological markers of HIV-1 associated dementia have been proposed including cerebrospinal fluid (CSF) levels of quinolinic acid, interleukin, p24 antigen (Wiley et al, 1992), beta-2 microglobulin (McArthur et al, 1992), macrophage-tropic viruses (Brew et al, 1991), dopamine (Levin et al, 1991), gp120 (Trujillo et al, 1991) and vitamin B_{12} (Robertson et al, 1993). At present, the biological markers that have been identified are non-specific and correlations with cognitive and clinical measures are modest.

3.3.2 Neuropsychology in asymptomatic HIV infection

Whilst some degree of cognitive impairment is a common feature of advanced HIV disease, there is considerable doubt as to whether people with HIV infection, but who are otherwise well, show any cognitive deficits. Grant et al. (1987), in an influential paper reported that 44 per cent of their sample of gay/bisexual men with who did not meet the criteria for AIDS or ARC were cognitively impaired. The impact of this paper was enormous both in terms of changes in social policy (including the introduction of mandatory HIV testing for US service personnel) and in the initiation of numerous research projects into the neuropsychology of early HIV disease around the world. Subsequent studies have mostly been less pessimistic about the prevalence of cognitive impairment in asymptomatic HIV disease and many have found no evidence of impairment at all. Burgess and Riccio (1992) identified 56 studies which had been published or presented at symposia that reported neuropsychological data on people with asymptomatic HIV infection, including follow-up reports of earlier studies. Of these, 30 reported that people with asymptomatic HIV infection do show some degree of cognitive impairment compared with seronegative controls and 26 studies reported no difference. A simple tally of the studies gives a rather misleading picture. On the whole, the larger better designed studies have failed to find any impairment with asymptomatich HIV infection though there have been some notable exceptions (e.g. Stern et al, 1991; Burgess et al, 1994).

Methodological difficulties

There are many possible reasons for the differing conclusions between the studies reported to date. Many of the studies were quite small and lacked the statistical power to detect minor cognitive changes. Other differences may have been due to variations in the methods of data analysis and in the definitions of impairment used. Particularly with smaller studies, it is difficult to control adequately other factors that might cause neuropsychological impairment such as alcohol and drug usage, pre-existing neurological disease and psychiatric illness (including subclinical variations in mood and psychological distress). In some studies the groups have not always been well matched for pre-morbid IQ, years of education or age. Wilkins et al (1990) have argued strongly that much of the controversy over the presence or absence of cognitive impairment stems from failure in many studies to control properly for such confounding factors. In their study, out of a sample of 40 HIV seropositive gay men at different stages of disease, only 10 were free from confounding factors altogether. In addition, there was a strong association between the presence and severity of confounding factors and neuropsychological performance.

Aside from narrow statistical concerns, some studies assessed only a limited range of neuropsychological functions and did not include tests sensitive to the types of deficits seen in HIV infection. Many of the clinical neuropsychological tests used were originally developed to identify cortical deficits. Many of these are not sensitive to the types of deficits seen in what is predominantly a subcortical disorder. For this reason, it is not surprising that there has been a tendency for abnormal performance amongst asymptomatic HIV seropositive individuals to be detected on non-clinical tests using highly sensitive paradigms such as reaction time measures (e.g. Wilkie et al, 1990b).

In is also worth noting that asymptomatic HIV infection includes an heterogenous selection of persons and may include some people who are very well, others with lymphadenopathy and yet others in the early stages of immunosuppression who are without clinical presentation of disease. The selection of subjects may also be important. Self-selected patients presenting at tertiary medical facilities may provide a misleading selection of the wider HIV seropositive population.

In some transmission groups, the situation is further confounded by the fact that the risk of infection may be associated with an increase risk of neuropsychological impairment. The risk of infection for men with haemophilia was greatest for those with the most severe disease who required most blood-clotting factor VIII. More severe haemophilia increases the risks of cerebral bleeds and a consequent risk of cognitive impairment. The frequency of injecting drugs with shared needles increases both the risk or HIV infection and drug-related cognitive impairment. Similarly, children infected by vertical transmission will frequently have been exposed *in utero* to drugs injected by the mother or to heavy alcohol usage, and the severity of the mother's drug habit will increase both the risk of infection and the probability of developmental delays in the child. Further, children born to drug using mothers will typically have received low levels of prenatal care, have low birth weight, be born into socioeconomically impoverished and receive erratic care giving: all factors associated with an increased risk of developmental delay.

Neuropsychology of HIV infection in gay/bisexual men

Most of the studies that have investigated the neuropsychological consequences of HIV infection during the asymptomatic stage of disease have used cohorts of gay/bisexual men. The reasons for this are that in the much of the Western world, gay/bisexual men make up the largest single group of HIV infected individuals. The main alternative group in Western countries are injecting drug users, who are typically less willing to endure prolonged neuropsychological testing and may have pre-existing cognitive impairments due to their drug usage.

The largest prospective longitudinal study of the neuropsychological consequences of asymptomatic HIV infection to date is from the Multicenter AIDS Cohort Study (MACS). The MACS sample was made up of 463 gay/bisexual men with asymptomatic HIV infection recruited from four centres in the US: Baltimore, Chicago, Los Angeles, and Pittsburgh. The first report of MACS study (McArthur et al, 1989) found nearly half of their 463 volunteers (226 out of 463; 49 per cent) showed some degree of abnormality on a brief neuropsychological screening battery. Of these, only 24 (5 per cent) were found to be impaired on a more detailed neuropsychological assessment. In most cases, the neuropsychological impairment was associated with another identifiable aetiology (e.g. alcohol use, anxiety/depression or low pre-morbid IQ) and was *not* related to HIV serostatus. Miller et al (1990) reported the neuropsychological results from the MACS study in more detail, including additional recruits giving a total sample of over 1500 subjects. Again, they found no evidence of neuropsychological impairment amongst people in the asymptomatic stages of disease when compared to HIV seronegative controls.

Although the MACS study is the largest to date, its main limitation is that only a relatively limited neuropsychological battery was used. Other relatively large, well-designed studies using more detailed neuropsychological batteries have confirmed the MACS findings (Goethe et al, 1989; Janssen et al, 1989; Riccio et al, 1993; Clifford et al, 1990; McAllister et al, 1992). There have been some notable exceptions. Stern et al (1991) reported that asymptomatic seropositive subjects performed more poorly than HIV seronegative controls on tests of memory (Selective Reminding Test), language (Controlled Oral Word Association), attention (Digit Span) and executive function (Odd Man Out Test). This study has been criticized on the grounds that the asymptomatic group had very low CD4 counts and included large numbers of people whose first language was not English (Miller et al, 1992). Stern et al (1992) have shown that the differences are still seen when these effects are taken into account. Nor are Stern et al (1991) alone in finding neuropsychological impairment amongst those with asymptomatic HIV infection. Fitzgibbon et al (1989) reported motor slowing in a group of gay/bisexual men with asymptomatic infection and Lunn et al (1991) have also found differences in both memory (Word Pair Learning) and psychomotor speed (Trail Making Test).

To date, few longitudinal studies have been reported. The MACS cohort has now been followed up for several years. Selnes et al. (1990) has reported on the follow-up assessments of 132 asymptomatic HIV seropositive gay/bisexual men form the MACS cohort compared with a matched HIV seronegative control group. Over the course of the follow-up period (average time 18 months) there were no differences between the HIV seropositive and seronegative groups, nor was HIV status a significant predictor of neuropsychological performance. Only two longitudinal studies have found impairment in people with asymptomatic disease. In the first of these (Sinforiani et al, 1991), the sample size was small ($n = 30$), the differences seen were small and had not increased at follow-up 18 months later. The stability of the differences between these groups suggests that they are due to pre-existing differences groups rather than to the progressive effects of HIV. This cohort has now been followed for over three years with no evidence of any significant cognitive changes in those individuals who remain well (Mauri et al, 1993). The second study reported neuropsychological follow-up over four years in a group of injecting drug users (Silberstein et al, 1994). They found that there were small, but statistically significant deteriorations on motor and psychomotor speed tasks, but that the changes were slow to develop and generally paralleled changes in immunological function. Other longitudinal studies have failed to find any differences in terms of mean scores on neuropsychological tests between HIV seropositive subjected and seronegative control (Selnes et al, 1990; Saykin et al, 1992; Burgess et al, 1994). There is some evidence that people with asymptomatic HIV infection do perform marginally poorer on neuropsychological tasks than might be expected. Bornstein et al (1993) found a higher proportion of people with asymptomatic infection developed neuropsychological abnormalities than matched controls. Similarly, Burgess et al (1994) predicted neuropsychological performance at follow-up from baseline performance and a range of medical and psychosocial variables for groups of asymptomatic HIV seropositive individuals and seronegative controls. They found that there was a small but significant tendency for those with asymptomatic disease to perform at a lower level than predicted. Even in this case, however, the effect of HIV was very small and was not sufficient to have a significant impact on any individual's everyday life.

For the most part, the studies have used well-established neuropsychological tests which are commonly used for clinical assessment though recently, there has been a trend towards using reaction time (RT) measures adapted from experimental psychology paradigms. The majority of studies using simple or choice RTs have not found any impairment of asymptomatic HIV seropositive men (Perdices and Cooper, 1989; Miller et al, 1991a; Stern et al, 1991; Dunlop et al, 1992), though as usual, there have been some exceptions (Karlsen et al, 1992; Martin et al, 1992). More complex RT's appear to be more sensitive. Dunlop et al (1992) found that asymptomatic HIV seropositive subjects were slower at a RT task which involved judging distances between objects presented on a computer screen. Similarly, Wilkie et al (1990b) reported that asymptomatic HIV seropositive gay/bisexual men showed poorer performance on both the Posner (Posner and Mitchell, 1967) and Sternberg tasks (Sternberg, 1969). The use of RT measures appears promising as a means of detecting early cognitive changes in HIV infection. They also possess the advantages that the administration can be automated and they are suitable for repeated measurements. It should be stressed, however, that most of the studies reporting the efficacy of RT measures in early HIV infection have been with relatively small samples and few RT trials and it would be premature to select RT measures as the sole or primary measures of cognitive function in future studies.

Neuropsychology of men with haemophilia

Most of the studies that have reported on the neuropsychology of HIV infection have involved gay/bisexual men. Several studies have reported on the adult men with haemophilia and in each case the conclusion was that there was no measurable impact of HIV on cognitive performance during the asymptomatic stages of disease (Catalán and Klimes, 1991; Klimes et al, 1990; Turnbull et al, 1990; Reidel et al, 1991). This pattern holds even over follow-up periods of more than a year (Klimes et al, 1991).

Neuropsychology of injecting drug users

The effect of HIV on cognition in injecting drug users (IDU) is less clear. In an early study, Silberstein et al (1987) found that asymptomatic HIV seropositive IDUs were impaired compared with seronegative controls and this finding has been confirmed (McKegney et al, 1990). Other studies, however, have found no effect of HIV in the asymptomatic stages of disease (Selnes et al, 1992). One problem in evaluating cognitive performance in those who inject drugs is that some degree of cognitive impairment is quite common although this is probably unrelated to HIV serostatus (Egan et al, 1990; Royal et al, 1991; Grassi et al, 1993). Certainly no follow-up study with injecting drug users has yet reported any progressive cognitive changes which would be expected if HIV had any serious impact on the brain during the asymptomatic stages of disease (Selnes et al, 1992; Egan et al, 1992).

Neuropsychology of children

The impact of HIV infection on the neurological development of children depends upon the mode of transmission. The prognosis is poorest in those children infected in the first days or months of life whether by vertical transmission (i.e. from the mother *in utero*, during labour or, more rarely, via breast milk). In cases of vertical transmission, one-third will develop AIDS, serious symptomatic disease or die in the first year of life (Gibb, 1991). Estimates of the prevalence of neurodevelopmental abnormalities in HIV infected children vary considerably but most studies suggest that the majority of children with AIDS or ARC show some impairment or developmental delay (e.g. Epstein et al, 1986; Belman et al, 1985; Diamond et al, 1987). The pattern of deficits seen parallels that seen in adults. As well as delays in developmental milestones, there are particular deficits in areas of psychomotor skills, visuo-motor integration, visuo-spatial perception (Belman et al, 1988; Diamond et al, 1987; Epstein et al, 1986), often leading to regression (Epstein et al, 1988).

Relatively few studies have investigated children with asymptomatic HIV infection, but of those that have, some developmental delay is usually seen compared with children from similar social and family situations (Epstein et al, 1988; Cohen et al, 1991). Most reports from European centres have tended to be more optimistic. The European Collaborative Study investigating neurological abnormalities in children with HIV infection (European Collaborative Study, 1990) found that 31 per cent of the children in their sample with ARC or AIDS showed some neurological abnormality but no abnormalities were seen amongst those children who remained asymptomatic. Differences between the European and American studies have been consistently reported. This is probably due to differences in the assessment procedures (no neuropsychological assessment was included in the European study) though other social and health care factors or differences in viral strain and infectious co-factors cannot be excluded.

Compared with adults, however, children infected by vertical transmission appear to have a very much higher rate of neuropsychological abnormality than adults, even in the early stages of disease. In a recent study, Aylward et al (1992) examined the neurodevelopmental performance of a small group, of HIV seropositive children between the ages of 5 and 24 months of age using the Bayley Scales of Infant Development. They found that the HIV seropositive children showed significant developmental delays compared with matched controls. This was true even though most of the children were in the early stages of disease. Cohen et al (1991) reported a study looking at a sample of children who had been infected with HIV through contaminated blood transfusions, mainly in the first few weeks of life. They assessed these children between 4 and 8 years after infection and found only minor differences in terms of neuropsychological performance between the HIV seropositive group and a matched seronegative control sample. Whilst there were no differences in overall IQ, the HIV seropositive children did less well on tests of motor speed (Finger Tapping) and mental flexibility (Colour Form Test). In addition, they were slightly poorer at reading and arithmetic and had poorer ratings from their teachers.

Children infected later in life (e.g. children with haemophilia and survivors of sexual abuse) may be less severely affected, at least in the asymptomatic stages of disease. Whitt et al (1993) found no evidence of neuropsychological impairment in HIV seropositive boys with haemophilia over a 7 year follow-up period. Tennison et al (1992) reporting on the same cohort, found no evidence of abnormality on neurological examination, magnetic resonance imaging (MRI), electroencephalogram (EEG) or event-related potentials (ERP). Overall, the impact of HIV on older children seems less severe than on those infected by vertical transmission and appears to follow a pattern comparable to HIV infected adults.

Neuropsychology of HIV infection cross-culturally

In addition to determining the prevalence of dementia in five centres around the world (Munich, São Paulo, Kinshasa, Nairobi, and Bangkok), the WHO cross-cultural study investigated the neuropsychological performance of its recruits at each stage of disease (Maj et al, 1994a, b). Cross-cultural comparisons of neuropsychological performance are notoriously difficult and overcoming the worst of the problems involved the development of new testing instruments that, as far as possible, were 'culture-free'. As well as established neuropsychological tasks (Timed Gait, Digit Symbol, Block Design, Grooved Pegboard, Trails A and Verbal Fluency) the battery included tests of memory (WHO Auditory Verbal Learning Test: WHOAVLT and the WHO Picture Memory Test: WHOPLT) and an adaptation of Trails B (The WHO Colour Trails).

Comparing the asymptomatic HIV seropositive and HIV seronegative groups revealed few differences on the neuropsychological tests and there was no consistent pattern between recruitment centre. The HIV asymptomatic group performed more poorly on the WHOAVLT in Munich, on Block Design in Kinshasa and on the Grooved Pegboard in Bangkok. No differences were seen in São Paulo and Nairobi. The higher incidence of neuropsychological impairment seen in these two centres was only found in those with low levels of education and there was a trend in all centres for those with poor educational background to be neuropsychologically impaired. An analysis of the data from all centres together suggested that there was a significant interaction between low educational level and HIV serostatus such that the impact of HIV on neuropsychological performance was much more marked in those with poorer education.

The importance of level of education has been interpreted in the light of the 'cerebral reserve theory' (Grady et al 1988; Satz, 1993). This theory suggests that vulnerability to cerebral insult is determined, in part, by the degree of redundancy and efficiency of neuronal networks in the brain. People who have lost brain tissue (e.g. head injuries) or have not developed efficient neural systems because of poor psychosocial conditions (e.g. lack of education, unstimulating environment or malnutrition) will be more vulnerable to the impact of cerebral pathology, however caused. On the basis of this theory, it would be expected that those people recruited in the developing world would, on average, have less 'cerebral reserve' (due to lower educational levels and poorer social conditions) and would, therefore, be more vulnerable to the impact of HIV infection. The results of the WHO cross-cultural study are consistent with the cerebral reserve theory but it remains unclear whether the effect of educational level is a direct one or simply a reflection of fact that those who receive little education typically suffer the worst social and environmental conditions.

Neuropsychology of HIV infection: summary

Although the controversy over the neuropsychological effects of HIV in asymptomatic HIV disease continues, there seems little doubt that HIV has minimal impact on day to day cognitive performance. Certainly, the effect of HIV is often dwarfed by the effect of other factors on neuropsychological performance such as poor education, drug and alcohol usage, psychiatric illness and other neurological disease (Wilkins et al, 1990). It would be unwise to conclude that the relatively silent effect of HIV on the brain in asymptomatic disease is the same for all. Children, at least those infected by vertical transmission, seem to be particularly vulnerable and there is some evidence to suggest that older people are more susceptible. Similarly, those people from educationally and socioeconomically deprived backgrounds or those who have been infected over longer periods of time may also be at particular risk (Maj et al. 1994a, b). Overall, whilst the impact of HIV on the brain during asymptomatic infection is often minimal, there is a disproportionate effect on those who are very young, very old or socially disadvantaged.

3.4 Neuropathology

Given that some degree of cognitive impairment is common in advanced HIV disease, it is not surprising that neuropathological studies have found a high frequency of cerebral pathology in those who die with AIDS. Petito et al (1986) in a retrospective study found that over 80 per cent of their sample displayed neuropathological abnormalities. Similarly, Budka et al (1987) found abnormalities in 95 per cent of their cases and Lantos et al (1989) in 88 per cent. The most common abnormalities seen were opportunistic viral infections (e.g. cytomegalovirus: CMV, herpes simplex virus: HSV, varicella-zoster and progressive multifocal leucoencephalopathy), fungal infections (e.g. cryptococcus and candida), parasitic infections (e.g. toxoplasmosis), neoplasms (e.g. primary non-Hodgkin's lymphoma) and cerebrovascular lesions.

In addition to neuropathological abnormalities caused by secondary processes, such as opportunistic infections and neoplasms, there are the direct effects of HIV on the brain. These primary HIV-induced brain lesions come in several different identifiable forms (Budka et al, 1991) of which the most important are HIV encephalitis and HIV leucoencephalopathy. HIV encephalitis involves multiple foci of inflammatory cells (microglia, macrophages and multinucleated giant cells) distributed predominantly in the white matter, basal ganglia, brainstem, and cortex. HIV leucoencephalopathy results in diffuse damage to the white matter of the cerebral hemispheres and cerebellum caused by myelin loss and astrocytosis. Whilst HIV encephalitis and HIV leucoencephalopathy have been recognized as separate pathologies, they have similar features (Everall and Lantos 1991) and frequently coexist (Budka et al, 1991). It is of interest that the correspondence between the presence of these neuropathological markers and clinical dementia is surprisngly poor. Although multinucleated giant cells or diffuse myelin pallor are found only in those with a clinical history of dementia, there is no evidence of either of these features in up to half of all patients with dementia (Glass et al, 1993). This suggests that other neuropathological changes, as yet unknown, must also exist.

HIV enters the brain within the first few months of infection (Ho et al, 1985) and there is some evidence that it may do so even earlier. Davis et al (1992) have reported a tragic case study in which HIV was isolated from the brain of a man who died of hepatorenal syndrome within days of his having been accidentally infected with HIV during his medical care. Blood cultures were seropositive for HIV 14 days after the initial infection, despite having been treated with anti-retroviral medication (zidovudine and dideoxyinosine) and HIV was isolated from his brain at post-mortem the next day.

The method of entry of HIV into the brain is disputed, but the most likely route is via HIV-infected microglia and macrophages: the so-called 'Trojan Horse' theory. Once in the brain, HIV infects monocytes, microglia, and macrophages, though other cell types may also be targeted. The most distinctive histological marker of HIV in the brain are multinucleated giant cells which are derived from the fusion of numerous HIV infected macrophages.

Although there is no evidence that HIV infects neurones, it is now known that substantial neuronal loss is a common consequence of HIV infection (Ketzler et al, 1990). In a careful quantitative analysis, Everall et al (1991) found between 35 and 38 per cent fewer neurones in the frontal cortex in a sample of people who died with AIDS compared to age- and sex-matched controls. Similarly, Wiley et al (1991) have reported a 30–50 per cent loss of neurones form the frontal, temporal and parietal lobes of the brains of people who died of AIDS. This neuronal loss is found not only in the absence of any opportunistic infection or neoplasm, but also in people who showed little evidence of encephalitis (Everall et al, 1991, 1993).

Although the occurrence of neuronal loss in people who die of AIDS is now well established, the mechanisms by which this occurs are not clear. A number of mechanisms have been suggested including coexisting opportunistic infections (e.g. CMV, HSV), excess cytokine production (e.g. α-tumour necrosis factor), changes in brain metabolism (possibly related to vitamin B_{12} deficiency) and the neurotoxic effects of HIV products (e.g. the HIV envelope glycoprotein gp120). In addition, neuronal death may be a secondary consequence of HIV infection of other cells, particularly microglia which result in demyelination and changed neuronal metabolism.

The question as to when these neuropathological changes first occur is difficult to answer. The very nature of post-mortem studies of neuropathology mean that most patients examined will have died of AIDS. There are, however, a few studies in which patients with HIV have died through other causes in the asymptomatic stages of infection (Lenhardt et al, 1988; Lantos et al, 1989; Esiri et al, 1990; Gray et al, 1991). In these asymptomatic cases, there was evidence of some non-specific changes, but no sign of HIV encephalitis or HIV leucoencephalopathy, suggesting that the most important neuropathologies occur only in advanced HIV disease.

3.5 Neuroradiology

3.5.1 Computerized tomography (CT) and magnetic resonance imaging (MRI)

Magnetic resonance imaging (MRI) and computerized tomography (CT) typically reveal clear abnormalities in the brains of people with HIV-1 associated dementia. The most common abnormalities are cerebral atrophy, particularly widened sulci (Dal Pan et al, 1992), but also ventricular enlargement and, particularly with MRI, white matter lesions in the subcortical and periventricular regions (Levy et al, 1986; McArthur, 1987; Pederson et al, 1991) and basal ganglia (Aylward et al, 1993). In addition, there is some evidence or more specific lesions. Both Kieburtz et al. (1990) and Broderick et al (1993) have reported lesions in the splenium of the corpus callosum, but only amongst those patients who had been referred because of cognitive difficulties.

Neuroradiological abnormalities are not only seen in people with HIV-1 associated dementia. High rates of cerebral atrophy on CT or MRI scans of greater than 70 per cent have been reported amongst people with AIDS (Grant et al, 1987; Post et al, 1988; Chrysikopoulos et al, 1990; Pederson et al, 1991; Raininko et al, 1992), although other studies have found very much lower rates (Olsen et al, 1988; Post et al, 1991; Levy et al, 1990). Other abnormalities on scans are less common. The prevalence of white matter lesions on MRI is generally thought to be much lower (Pederson et al, 1991; Raininko et al, 1992) though the range varies substantially and in at least one study the proportion of people white matter abnormalities did not differ between people with AIDS and comparable controls (McArthur et al, 1990a). Although much attention has focused on the deep white matter lesions often seen with MRI, there is some doubt as to their clinical significance. Because the most common foci of these lesions are in the subcortical white matter, the area which post-mortem studies haves found is most commonly affected in HIV-1 associated dementia, it has been assumed that the MRI signals correspond to an early manifestation of the dementing process. Recently, some doubt has been cast on this suggestion as high rates of hyper-intense signals have been found in the same regions in the brains of healthy control subjects (McArthur et al, 1990a; Dooneief et al, 1992; McAllister et al, 1992; Collier et al, 1992). Furthermore, there was no correlation between white matter abnormalities and markers of HIV disease state such as CD4 count (McArthur et al, 1990a) or neurologic or neuropsychological performance (Dooneief et al, 1992; McAllister et al, 1992) although some results to the contrary have been reported (Post et al, 1991).

Perhaps the most important use of MRI and CT is in the differential diagnosis of CNS disease in AIDS. Lesions caused by opportunistic infections and neoplasms will often show up clearly on scans, particularly MRI (Whiteman et al, 1993). It should be noted, however, that a normal CT or MRI does not indicate that the brain is unaffected. Several recent studies haves shown that MRI or CT will fail to identify some pathologies (Grafe et al, 1990) or lead to misdiagnosis (Anson et al, 1992).

Recent developments in MRI spectroscopy make it possible to identify the density of specific cell types. This method has been applied by Chong et al (1993) to measure loss of neurones in people with HIV infection. In this study, they reported that there was no evidence of neuronal loss in people with HIV infection who were otherwise well or had a CD4 count greater than 200. More than half their sample of people with symptomatic disease however, showed evidence of neuronal loss. Using a similar technique, Meyerhoff et al (1993) found clear evidence of neuronal loss in a sample of patients with HIV related cognitive impairment even though most showed normal scans using conventional MRI.

Whilst MRI or CT abnormalities are common in people with AIDS, there is little evidence of any difference between people with asymptomatic infection and HIV seronegative controls (McArthur et al, 1990a; Koralnik et al, 1991a, b; Cohen et al, 1992; McAllister et al, 1992; Dooneief et al, 1992; Collier et al, 1992). At least one large study (Raininko et al, 1992) however, has found that people with asymptomatic infection do show greater rates of atrophy, particularly in the frontal lobes and cerebellum) though not of white matter lesions.

Few longitudinal studies have been published in this area although Post et al (1993) have reported on a cohort of 64 people with asymptomatic infection who were followed up over a period of up to 42 months. They found that 13 out of their sample (20 per cent) had abnormal MRI scans at baseline, mainly atrophy and white matter lesions and that only two of these had deteriorated at follow-up. The findings have been confirmed by Manji et al (1994) who found no evidence of developing cerebral atrophy over the course of a year in a sample of gay/bisexual men provided they remained asymptomatic. These studies suggest that abnormal MRI scans are not strongly predictive of further deterioration, at least in people with asymptomatic disease.

The wide variation of findings from both MRI and CT studies reflects a number of methodological weaknesses in the area. Studies differ not only in because of variations in the technical details of the scans and the variations in the samples of HIV subjects investigated, but because of differences in the ratings between radiologists. Ratings of the degree of cortical atrophy vary substantially because the judgement is subjective and will depend not only upon the criteria used but upon the individual rater. Nor are the definitions of normal and abnormal well defined. In one otherwise well-designed study (Dooneief et al, 1992), 97 per cent of the control subjects were rated as having at least mild cerebral atrophy by a single blind rater. Such high rates of 'abnormality' in otherwise healthy individuals raises questions about the usefulness of such criteria and for these reasons, quantitative methods of analysis are to be preferred.

The whole question of how MRI or CT findings relate to clinical and functional performance in people with HIV is uncertain. There is good agreement that most patients defined as neuropsychologically impaired or demented will show MRI abnormalities. Grant et al (1987) found a 74 per cent agreement between individuals defined as abnormal by both methods and Raininko et al (1992) found that all of their subjects with a clinical diagnosis of dementia had significant cerebral atrophy. With less marked cognitive impairments, the agreement is much less good and although some studies have found some correlations between MRI abnormalities and neuropsychological performance (Cohen et al, 1992; Hestad et al, 1993) others have failed to do so (Dooneief et al, 1992; McAllister et al, 1992). The relatively poor correlation between neuroradiological measures and cognitive performance are consistent with the theory of 'cerebral reserve'. A corollary of this theory is that the amount of brain tissue lost is not the only important factor. The efficiency and organization of what tissue remains is important too and this is not measured by structural imaging techniques (3.3 and pp. 79–81).

3.5.2 Single photon emission tomography (SPET) and positron emission tomography (PET)

In addition to structural abnormalities, there is increasing evidence of metabolic abnormalities in the brains of people with AIDS as measured by positron emission tomography (PET) and single photon emission tomography (SPET). Rottenberg et al (1987) reported subcortical *hyper*metabolism (basal ganglia and thalamus) in the early stages of dementia with *hypo*metabolism in the cortical and subcortical grey matter in more advanced disease. Several subsequent studies have confirmed that metabolic abnormalities are common in people with AIDS or HIV-1 associated dementia (Pohl et al, 1988; Ajmanii et al, 1991; Masdeu et al, 1991; Pascal et al, 1991). Although these metabolic changes seem contradictory, they make sense in terms of the brain's response to infection. Hypermetabolism is seen in the early stages of dementia when the brain attempts to compensate for HIV related changes by placing additional demands on those parts which continue to function. In time, the amount of tissue lost is so great that the overall levels of metabolism diminishes.

Few studies have used PET or SPET to examine people with asymptomatic disease. Tran Dinh et al (1990) found abnormalities of cerebral perfusion, mainly in the frontal regions of 16 out their 18 asymptomatic HIV seropositive subjects compared with their control group and Pascal et al (1991) reported a high incidence of metabolic lateral asymmetries. Similar findings have been reported from several uncontrolled studies (La France et al, 1988; Schielke et al, 1990; Rosci et al, 1992). The pattern of perfusion abnormalities that have been reported are not specific to people with HIV infection. Holman et al (1992) found that the SPET images of regular cocaine users were indistinguishable from those of people with HIV-1 associated dementia.

Several studies have compared SPET or PET with other measures of brain function. Most reports have claimed that the metabolic abnormalities seen in the people with AIDS correlate significantly with neuropsychological test scores (Rottenberg et al, 1987; Kuni et al, 1991) and clinical ratings of the severity of dementia (Ajmani et al, 1991). Interestingly, correlations between neuropsychological testing and metabolic abnormalities in the asymptomatic stage of HIV infection have not been found (Rosci et al, 1992).

Most reports have found that both SPET and PET show higher rates of abnormality than either CT, MRI (Rottenberg, 1987; Masdeu et al, 1991; Ajmani et al, 1991; Pascal et al, 1991), EEG (Pohl et al, 1988) or neuropsychological testing (Rosci et al, 1992). Frequently, the higher incidence of abnormality detected by PET or SPECT than by other measures has been interpreted as suggesting the greater sensitivity of metabolic measures, although this is not the only possible explanation. The metric properties of these measures have not been thoroughly reported and it will be necessary to determine the false positive rate, specificity and sensitivity of both SPET and PET before a reasonable judgement can be made. The use of both SPET and PET in clinical studies is a relatively new development and the definition of normal and abnormal is not well defined. In particular, there are large variations in healthy individuals and this makes clinical ratings without control groups effectively uninterpretable (Holman and Johnson, 1991). Certainly quantitative studies, particularly those using relative measures of metabolism, are to be preferred and appropriate control groups should always be used. At present, although PET, and particularly SPET, appear to be promising clinical instruments for the measurement of brain function in HIV disease, their main usefulness in the immediate future, is for research purposes.

3.6 Psychophysiology

Psychophysiological measures including the electroencephalogram (EEG), multimodal evoked potentials (MEP) and event-related potentials (ERPs) have frequently been used to investigate functional changes in the brains of people with HIV infection. The evidence for psychophysiological abnormalities in advanced HIV disease is strong and there is some evidence that psychophysiological measures may reveal abnormalities even in the asymptomatic stages of disease (Baldeweg and Lovett, 1991).

3.6.1 Electroencephalography (EEG)

The earliest reports of EEG abnormalities came from uncontrolled retrospective studies of patients referred for EEG assessment. Parisi et al (1988a), reviewed 101 HIV seropositive patients at different disease stages and found that those with 'sub-acute encephalopathy' showed a pronounced generalized slowing of theta and delta rhythms. Other abnormal signs included slowed frontal theta and delta activity together with less severe generalized slowing. Low amplitude EEG has also been reported in people with AIDS (Harden et al, 1993). Of the 101 patients reported by Parisi et al (1988a), only 37 were classified as having normal EEG. This non-specific pattern of slow wave activity in the frontal areas has been replicated although focal delta and theta abnormalities may also be seen in cases of localized lesions caused by opportunistic infections or neoplasms in the advanced stages of disease (Gabuzda et al, 1988, Parisi et al, 1989; Tinuper et al, 1990).

Parisi et al (1988a) have claimed that abnormal EEG in people with asymptomatic disease is a strong predictor of progression to cerebral disease. They found that 55 per cent of patients with an abnormal EEG who were otherwise asymptomatic went on to develop 'sub-acute encephalitis' 11 months later.

EEG abnormalities have also been reported in asymptomatic HIV infection but, in most cases, the studies have not included an appropriate control group which makes it impossible to determine the significance of these findings (Gabuzda et al, 1988; Parisi et al, 1988a; Parisi et al, 1989; Somma-Mauvais et al, 1990). There are some exceptions. Koralnik et al (1991a) reported the findings of a relatively small but well-designed controlled study. They found that nearly one-third of their asymptomatic patients had EEG abnormalities compared with none in the seronegative control group. These findings have been criticized on methodological and statistical grounds (Nuwer et al, 1991) although the objections have been disputed (Koralnik et al, 1991b). Nor are Koralnik et al (1991a) alone in identifying EEG abnormalities in people with asymptomatic HIV infection. Elovaara et al (1991) found that people with asymptomatic HIV infection showed on average a 12 per cent decrease in EEG amplitude compared with health controls. Jabbari et al (1993) found that none of their 42 asymptomatic patients showed abnormal EEG though three (7 per cent) developed diffuse slow waves at follow-up a year later. Recording EEG in passive conditions may not be the most sensitive method of detecting early abnormalities. Baldeweg et al (1993b) found that although none of their sample of people with asymptomatic infection showed abnormal EEG when at rest, differences did emerge during a motor task. Compared with the baseline condition, people with asymptomatic infection showed less attenuation of delta, theta, and alpha during hand movement than matched controls.

The finding of abnormal EEG in people with asymptomatic HIV infection has not always been found. Nuwer et al (1992) reported on a large sample of 200 gay/bisexual men from the Multicentre AIDS Cohort Study (MACS) and found that there were no differences in the proportion of abnormal EEG traces in the HIV seropositive and HIV seronegative groups (36 per cent and 29 per cent, respectively). Where there were abnormalities, they were frequently associated with neuropsychological impairment. Overall, whilst EEG abnormalities in advanced HIV disease have frequently been reported, abnormalities during asymptomatic disease are not well established.

3.6.2 Multimodal evoked potentials (MEP)

Abnormalities of somatosensory (SEP), visual (VEP) and brainstem auditory evoked potentials (BAEP) have all been reported to show delays in advanced HIV disease (Smith et al, 1988; Jakobsen et al, 1989). Again, it is less clear whether abnormalities in MEPs are seen in people with asymptomatic disease. For example, Koralnik et al (1991a) found that SEPs were delayed in people with asymptomatic HIV infection compared with their seronegative controls, though this finding has failed to be confirmed (McAllister et al, 1992). Generally, there have been few published controlled studies which have measured MEPs in people with asymptomatic infection and for this reason, the values of these techniques in HIV disease is largely unknown.

3.6.3 Event-related potentials (ERP)

Event-related potentials (ERP) include a number of procedures that involve the recording of psychophysiological responses to changes or omissions in a frequently presented stimuli. These methods have been used in the study of memory, attention and other cognitive processes (Donchin et al, 1986). A number of studies have reported an increased latency of the P3 (an ERP thought to relate to attentional processes) in people with AIDS (Ollo et al, 1991; Baldeweg et al, 1993a; Arendt et al, 1990). In people with asymptomatic HIV disease some studies have reported delayed P3 (Goodin et al, 1990; Ollo et al, 1991; Ragazzoni et al, 1993) whilst others have found no such effect (Goodwin et al, 1990, McAllister et al, 1992). Messenheimer et al (1992) have reported results of one of the few longitudinal studies of ERPs in HIV disease. Although they found no difference between P3 latency for the HIV seropositive subjects and their control group at baseline, differences were seen between both the symptomatic and asymptomatic patients and the controls at 18-month follow-up. In contrast, Goodwin et al (1990) only found increased latency amongst those with a CDC IV diagnosis at 12-month follow-up. Overall, whilst there is some evidence of delayed ERPs in asymptomatic HIV disease, this has not always been confirmed.

Although psychophysiological measures, such as the P3, are believed to be manifestations of basic cognitive processes, correlations with neuropsychological performance have proved elusive. Whilst Messenheimer et al (1992) and Baldeweg et al (1993a) have found some such associations for the P3, others have failed to do so (McAllister et al, 1992; Arendt et al, 1990). There is, however, some evidence to suggest that psychophysiological abnormalities may be found in people with HIV who in other respects function normally. Whether such abnormalities are predictive of later cognitive difficulties is less clear. Such a situation makes interpretation of psychophysiological abnormalities in terms of functional performance problematic.

3.7 Summary

Cognitive impairment is a common feature of advanced HIV disease and may be caused by the direct effect of HIV on the brain or by secondary factors (opportunistic infections or neoplasms). In the most severe cases, the result is a frank clinical dementia which may affect 5–6 per cent of people with AIDS. Neuropathological studies show that the most common abnormalities in the brains of people who have died with AIDS are HIV encephalitis involving multiple foci of immflammatory cells in the white matter and subcortical grey matter and HIV leucoencephalopathy which involves diffuse damage to the white matter. In people with AIDS who are not demented, cognitive deficits are common particularly those of fine motor control, psychomotor speed, memory and executive function. Abnormalities are also seen on CT and MRI scans, PET and SPECT and psychophysiological measures (e.g. EEG and ERP). It is uncertain at what stage of disease functional abnormalities of the brain become apparent. Even in those reports of abnormality in the asymptomatic stages of disease, it is clear that for adults, any deficits are mild and not likely to have any noticeable impact on an individuals daily life. For children, particularly those infected *in utero*, developmental deficits may have a more serious impact.

4 Assessment of mental health problems

4.1 Introduction

In earlier chapters we have described the range and extent of the psychological and neuropsychiatric syndromes that can occur in people with HIV infection, and the psychological impact on their partners and relatives. Here we review the process of identification of mental health problems and the detailed assessment of psychological and neuropsychiatric syndromes and other mental health problems. Research evaluations are often undertaken when dealing with HIV problems, partly in response to the need to investigate a new disease process, but also as part of an effort to develop ways of minimizing the psychiatric impact of the disease. Commonly used instruments and techniques are also reviewed here.

Mental health specialists do not work in isolation, but rather, in close contact with physicians and others involved in the medical and nursing care of people with HIV infection. Good collaboration between professional groups is essential to ensure that mental health problems are identified promptly, and that the right help is provided. Prior to considering in detail the assessment of mental health problems, the organization and links of specialist mental health services are discussed.

4.2 Organization of mental health services

The provision of psychological care to people with HIV infection is not limited to mental health specialists. In practice, a variety of individuals working in the statutory and voluntary sectors are involved in providing different levels of expertise in the assessment and management of psychological problems.

4.2.1 Care by statutory services

Primary level of psychological care

Physicians and nurses, usually hospital-based but also those working in primary care, are in a good position to provide front line psychological support for common difficulties, and to carry out an assessment of problems requiring more intensive or specialized interventions.

All patients with HIV infection will at some stage come into contact with medical and nursing teams, and the quality of rapport that develops with patients will be important in helping them cope with the complications of the disease. Patients' satisfaction with the way staff discuss their HIV status or how they are given an AIDS diagnosis is influenced by doctors' attitudes as well as by the quality of information given (Pergami et al, 1994a, c). Doctors and others need to have the skills to listen to patients' concerns and difficulties, answer questions about prognosis and further care, and generally be able to contain distress and cope with situations where there is no favourable or easy solution. While many of these skills are relatively easy to acquire, others may be more difficult to master, and senior medical and nursing staff and mental health care workers can be in a good position to train and support junior staff in the development of these skills.

Family doctors can play an important role in the care of people with HIV infection in the community and their partners and relatives, although it has to be said that general practitioners have not been as involved with patients with HIV infection as with those suffering from other conditions (King, 1989d; Singh et al, 1993), with some notable exceptions (Robertson et al, 1986; Winiarski, 1993). Similarly, family doctors could play an important part in the prevention of the spread of HIV infection, but there is evidence that this opportunity is often missed (Loft et al, 1994).

Secondary level of psychological care

The practical pressures created by the number of patients and the complexity of the clinical problems upon doctors and nurses make it difficult for lengthy or detailed consultations to discuss social and psychological issues to occur regularly. Other staff attached to the medical teams, such as health advisers, midwives or others involved in pre- and post-test counselling, and those with regular contact with patients such as occupational therapists, physiotherapists and drugs counsellors are often in a good position to provide continuing support and counselling about the infection and about family and other problems. Social workers, whether hospital-based or in the community, are an essential element in the provision of social and community care, and in giving advice about welfare benefits and practical help. As in the case of those involved in providing primary levels of care, it is important that staff have the skills to identify problems requiring greater expertise.

Tertiary level of psychological care—mental health teams

Only a minority of people with HIV infection are likely to require this facility. The experience in our centre is that between one-third and one-quarter of patients receiving care for their HIV infection are referred to the specialist mental health team for assessment and management of more severe, urgent or complex problems, such as major depression, suicidal ideas, substance misuse problems, symptomatic treatment of psychotic illnesses or acute brain syndromes, or for neuropsychological assessment. Our experience is comparable to that of other centres (Fernandez et al, 1989b; Ellis et al, 1994) (see Chapters 1 and 2). Care can be provided to medical in-patients, out-patients and in the community. A proportion of patients with HIV infection referred to the mental health services will require psychiatric hospitalization, while the care of those with HIV-associated dementia and those requiring palliative care may need to involve specialist non-psychiatric residential facilities (see Chapter 5).

Ideally, a mental health team should include psychiatrists, psychologists and nurses, each professional group providing unique expertise (detailed neuropsychological assessment and cognitive behavioural interventions in the case of the psychologists; neuropsychiatric evaluation and psychotropic drug prescribing by psychiatrists; awareness of nursing care issues and support of general nurses by psychiatric nurses), while at the same time sharing a range of skills. Many HIV units have some access to psychologists with an interest in the field, while access to psychiatrists is dependent on local interest and the presence of liaison psychiatry services, an area of psychiatric specialization with uneven development (Mayou and Huyse, 1991). Psychiatric liaison nurses are rare. In areas with high prevalence of substance misuse, drug dependency services may be involved (Sherrard et al, 1993). Often, mental health services are not well co-ordinated, being under different management structures and even duplicating facilities in the same locality.

Access to specialist mental health facilities is not uniform within and between countries. In a recent WHO-sponsored European survey of mental health services for people with HIV infection (Catalán, 1993) the lack of emergency mental health facilities was identified as the main area of unmet need, followed by lack of facilities for the care of injecting drug users.

4.2.2 Psychological care by voluntary and non-statutory services

In many developed countries voluntary and non-statutory services for psychological and social support and practical help for people with HIV have become an essential element of their care, so that the extensive and easily accessible range of facilities available would not have been possible with the statutory services alone. Self-help organizations have a long tradition in Anglo-Saxon countries, and the unique combination of a serious illness affecting young people against a background of negative public attitudes and rejection, have contributed to generating a strong positive organizational response, in particular in metropolitan areas. While not all countries have managed to marshal resources and efforts in this way, there are many examples of community organizations, including in those that have sprung up in developing countries (see Chapter 5). Non-statutory services can provide support for people in many groups, such as gay men, women, drug users, and people from ethnic and cultural minorities. Counselling and more formal psychotherapeutic intervention for the newly diagnosed, the bereaved, partners and relatives are available. Palliative and respite care and other forms of residential care may be available (see Chapter 5).

4.2.3 Co-ordinating the provision of mental health care

The existence of a wide range of teams and professionals involved in the psychological and social care of people with HIV infection means there is potential for conflict and confusion: sometimes professionals or teams compete with each other for patients, or struggle to maintain some involvement when other professionals have already become involved; there may be rivalry between professional groups, so that the more specialized professionals resent the involvement of the less experienced, while the latter cling to their patients and are reluctant to ask for an opinion. When conflicts arise, the loser is usually the patient, and it is therefore essential to develop mechanisms to minimize between-team problems, and to involve the patient and relatives in the discussions. Here are some possible actions to prevent difficulties.

1. *Clarification of areas of competence*
   It helps if each team attempts to clarify what its expertise consists of, and what are its in particular by reference to other professionals. There may well be role differences within a particular team, and these will need to be made explicit to those in and outside the team.
2. *Explicit referral process and responsibility*
   How does one professional group refer a patient to another, and who is responsible for the overall care of the individual?
3. *Communication between groups*
   When several professionals are involved, regular communication about the person's contact with the various groups needs to occur, ensuring that the patient's consent has been granted and that information is treated in confidence.
4. *Identification of key worker*
   When several people are involved, it is important to identify professionals in the community and in hospital who can act as key workers, co-ordinating efforts and involving others when required.
5. *Mechanisms to deal with problems*
   Telephone contact will be a minimal requirement, but often case conference-type meetings to evaluate and review progress and iron out difficulties will be necessary. When disagreements occur between people or teams, it is important to provide opportunities for early discussion and exchange of views.
6. *Explicit discharge or change in care plans*
   When a particular professional pulls out others involved need to be aware of the change in circumstances.
7. *Rationalizing care*
   Sometimes several therapists are involved in providing support, including voluntary and statutory professionals. It is important to review whether all should be involved, or whether it would be better to concentrate efforts into a lesser number of helpers. If this is the case, the reasons for the change and the process through which it is to be achieved should be made explicit.
8. *Monitor progress*
   Regular review of needs and plans needs to be built into the care plan to ensure that objectives are met.

4.3 Recognition of mental health problems

Mental health problems, as described in Chapters 1 and 2, are common in people with HIV infection and thus likely to present to doctors and others involved in their care. Recognition of the existence of a substantial degree of psychological morbidity will be an essential first step in the process of clarifying its severity, causes, and treatment. Recognition of mental health disorders in people suffering from a physical disorder, however, is not always an easy matter.

4.3.1 Obstacles to the recognition of mental health problems

The fact that a person with HIV infection may be suffering from a significant somatic illness can cloud the recognition of a psychiatric disorder. This can happen in a variety of ways:

1. Psychological symptoms are perceived by doctors or others as only a manifestation of physical disease, resulting in a desperate search for an organic aetiology. While exclusion of a primary physical cause for mental or behavioural abnormalities is essential (Hall et al, 1978), there are obvious dangers in failing to recognize from the start that psychological and physical factors are always involved, the crucial question being the degree to which they contribute to the clinical syndrome.
2. The psychological syndrome is regarded as normal under the circumstances, and therefore not requiring a psychiatric diagnosis. It is true that it is sometimes difficult to discriminate between normal and pathological reactions to events, but inability to recognize that some psychological responses, no matter how understandable, can benefit from specialist mental health intervention, can only work against the patient's best interests.
3. Attitudes to psychiatry: if mental health specialists are perceived as punitive or controlling, or mental illness is regarded as a sign of moral weakness or personal failure, it is less likely that referral to mental health services will occur. Patients and their doctors may well share these beliefs.
4. Perceived competence in the management of psychological disorder: doctors and others involved in the care of people with HIV may fear identifying distress if they do not feel confident in their ability to support and counsel those experiencing difficulties.
5. Access to mental health specialists: absence of facilities to deal with the more complex problems will discourage the recognition of mental health problems; the converse could conceivably also happen where specialist services are over provided, leading to immediate referral to specialists, and the subsequent loss of skills for the primary care teams.

4.3.2 Psychiatric symptoms as side-effects of medical treatments

Many commonly used drugs to deal with the complications of HIV infection can have adverse side-effects which include symptoms of mental disturbance. When

Table 4.1 Psychiatric manifestations of commonly used treatments in HIV disease

Medicine	Symptoms
Acyclovir	Tremor, lethargy, agitation, confusion, hallucinations, sleeplessness (Ricci et al, 1988; MacDiarmond-Gordon et al, 1992)
Gancyclovir	Nightmares, hallucinations, confusion, seizures (Chen et al, 1992; Davies et al, 1990; Barton et al, 1992)
Cotrimoxazole	Agitation, hallucinations, tremor, panic disorder (McCue and Zandt, 1991; Zealberg et al, 1991)
Ciprofloxacine	Restlessness, insomnia, dizziness, hallucinations, confusion, anxiety, paranoid states (McCue & Zandt, 1991; Reeves, 1992)
Dapsone	Psychotic states (Garrett & Corcos, 1952; Gawkrodger, 1989; Carmichael and Paul, 1989; Daneshmend, 1989)
Anti-TB	Paranoid states, mania, hallucinations (Bernardo et al, 1991; Reboli and Mandler, 1992)
Amphotericin, fluconazol, ketaconazol	Delirium, tremor, confusion (Winn, 1979; Pillans, 1985)
Steroids	Anxiety, depression, euphoria, delirium, hallucinations (Milgrom and Bender, 1993)
Anti-HIV	Mania, insomnia, confusion (see Chapter 2)
Anabolic steroids	Euphoria, increased energy, irritability, aggression, steroids, violence, mood swings, forgetfulness, and confusion (Su et al, 1993)
Interferon	Depression, aggression, forgetfulness, lethargy, confusion (Marimsky et al, 1990; Prasad et al, 1992)

assessing individual cases it is important to consider the possible role of medication in contributing to the psychiatric picture. Some examples of therapeutic agents which have been the subject of reports are listed in Table 4.1.

4.3.3 Diagnosis or problem-orientated formulation?

Psychiatric diagnosis, like those made in general medicine, have several functions: they provide a descriptive label which makes communication easier and can give indications about the aetiology, treatment and prognosis of a condition. While there are dangers in 'medicalizing' human behaviours and experiences, it is clear that conceptualizing some mental states and behaviours as abnormal or pathological has contributed significantly to their amelioration.

Formal psychiatric disorders such as major depression or organic brain disorders can develop in people with primarily physical disease, but other abnormal mental or behavioural states associated with difficulties coping with physical illness may not be so easily labelled: to make a diagnosis at any cost may be a fruitless exercise. In such instances it is usually better to use a problem-orientated formulation, based on the cognitive–behavioural analysis of the person's difficulties, and of the individual's circumstances. One important advantage of a problem-orientated approach is that it can facilitate intervention, by pinpointing and clarifying the problems that require help. It is often possible to use a combined diagnostic and problem-orientated formulation.

4.3.4 Factors associated with the development of psychological disorders

Knowledge about the circumstances and events that can contribute to mental health problems can help doctors and others involved in the care of people with HIV infection recognize their presence. Factors associated with psychological morbidity were discussed in detail in Chapter 2, and here we shall only summarize them.

1. Factors related to HIV infection: symptomatic and, in particular, advanced HIV infection are associated with the development of mental health problems, although notification of a positive test result can also lead to persistent problems.
2. Factors related to the person with the infection: past psychiatric history, gender, ethnic and socioeconomic characteristics, and past or current injecting drug use.
3. Ways of coping: avoidance and hopeless-helpless approach, and persistent denial.
4. Social supports and continuing adverse life events: social isolation and absence of confiding relationships, and accumulation of adverse events such as losses, or financial and employment difficulties.

The assessment of mental health problems will require the clarification of the likely factors that contribute to the problems. It is useful to think in terms of predisposing, precipitating, and maintaining factors. For example, **predisposing or vulnerability factors** will include such things as the existence of a past psychiatric history or a history of difficulties coping with life stresses, parental discord and separation, and a pattern of behavioural problems in childhood and adolescence. **Precipitating factors** will include events chronologically associated with the onset of the difficulties, such as bereavement, notification of an AIDS diagnosis, loss of employment or other practical problems. **Maintaining factors** will be the current stresses or difficulties that keep the problem going, such as lack of supports, maladaptive mental attitudes, social isolation, fears of impending decline in health and relationship problems.

4.3.5 Psychiatric assessment

Formal, standardized assessment of a person's mental state and behaviour and psychiatric history is the principal method of establishing the presence of psychiatric disturbance. Psychiatric assessment is comparable to medical history-taking and examination, although there are differences of content and emphasis. Psychiatrists and other mental health specialists are well trained in this form of clinical evaluation, but health workers in general should be familiar with psychiatric interviewing and with the way the manifestations of mental disorders can be identified. An outline of the contents of the psychiatric interview will be given here, detailed accounts being available in standard textbooks (see Gelder et al, 1989; Rose, 1994).

Psychiatric history-taking

It is important to be familiar with the areas about which information needs to be obtained and to have a structured plan, even if the interview is carried out in a flexible and semi-structured way.

History of current problems leading to referral: what are the reasons for referral, when did the problems started, what are their effects on the person's life, what makes the situation better or worse; if the difficulties are long standing, why is the person referred now?

Family history: information about parents and other siblings, with emphasis on the relationship with the person both currently and in the past. History of mental health problems in relatives.

Personal history: chronological outline of the person's life history, including childhood, schooling and further education, work, sexual experience and attitudes, relationships, marriage and children when appropriate, use of alcohol or illicit substances. Detailed information about past psychiatric and other health problems when relevant.

Usual personality: information about the sort of person the patient was before the current problems began, including interests, relationships, temperament and achievements.

Current social circumstances: living arrangements, financial situation, employment, and social supports, and the presence of difficulties in any of these areas.

Mental state examination

Systematic assessment of the individual's behaviour and mental state at interview involves listening to and observing spontaneous utterances and behaviour, as well as the asking of specific direct questions. Together with the psychiatric history, mental state examination forms the basis of the diagnostic formulation.

Mental state assessment is usually structured under a number of headings covering a wide range of mental manifestations.

Appearance and behaviour: self-neglect and standard of dress, restlessness, psychomotor retardation and appropriateness of behaviour, degree of co-operation, facial appearance indicating sadness or distress.

Mood: in particular the presence of depression and anxiety, their degree and the extent to which they are persistent or variable, feelings of hope for the future, and suicidal ideas and plans; **elated mood** with feelings of overconfidence and happiness out of keeping with the actual circumstances.

Thinking: presence of abnormal beliefs such as **delusions** (false unshakeable beliefs out of keeping with the person's cultural background, and usually involving the person having especial powers or suffering persecution), **ideas of reference** (random events and situations are interpreted as having special personal significance), or **morbid fears** (fear of HIV infection, obsessional thoughts, and phobic anxieties). Thinking may be reported as fast or retarded, or may be observed to be disjointed and incoherent. Thoughts may be described as under the control of external forces or persons.

Perceptions: illusions (misperceptions where the person realises there has been a transient mistake) and hallucinations (the experience has all the qualities of a real perception in the absence of an external stimulus).

Cognitive function: the clinical assessment of the higher mental functions usually involves asking about orientation (in time, place and person), **attention and concentration** (asking to give the months of the year backwards or to subtract 7 from 100 and to keep repeating the calculation with the next figure), **recent memory** (registration is tested by asking to repeat straight away a name and address or series of digits, and recall is assessed by asking again five minutes later), and **remote memory** (asking about well-known historical events or personal history details).

Insight: degree of understanding of the person's predicament, awareness of the presence of psychiatric disturbance and attitudes to receiving help.

By the end of the psychiatric assessment, the interviewer should be in a position to start answering several questions:

1. Is the person suffering from a psychiatric disorder?
2. Whether or not the person has a psychiatric disorder, are there any substantial social or other problems?
3. What are the causes of the psychiatric disorder and/or problems?
4. What further information or investigations are required?
5. Is there a risk of harm to the person or to others as a result of mental illness or other problems?

6. What kind of help does the person want? what kind of help is appropriate and is the person willing to accept it?
7. If the person is not willing to accept help, is intervention against the person's wishes indicated?

4.4 Clinical assessment of specific psychiatric problems

It is beyond the scope of this book to describe in detail the assessment of all possible mental health problems in HIV infection, but a review of some issues and difficulties in the evaluation of common problems will be given, including: depressed mood, suicidal ideas, problems coping with HIV infection, and the possibility of psychotic disorders such as mania and schizophrenia. Organic brain syndromes, whether acute or chronic, are also a common reason for mental health evaluation.

4.4.1 Assessment of depressed mood

Low mood can be a normal reaction to events, and as such part of a normal human response. However, low mood can also be a symptom of a physical or psychiatric disorder, in particular of a depressive illness (or major depressive disorder). While there is a debate about the classification and aetiology of depressive syndromes (see, for example, Taylor et al, 1985; Gelder et al, 1989; Rodin et al, 1991), in practice it is important to identify depressive syndromes, regardless of their aetiology, which are likely to be associated with the risk major problems such as suicidal behaviour, and likely to respond to antidepressant medication.

In major depressive disorders, **low mood** is persistent over several days or weeks rather than hours, and shows minimal response to external events that would be expected to improve it. There may be some variation in the intensity of the depressed mood during the day, with the worst mood in the earlier part of the day. Anhedonia (loss of enjoyment of usually pleasurable activities) is common. **Thought content** is consistent with depressed mood, with marked feelings of hopelessness, guilt and self-reproach. **Suicidal ideas** may be prominent, and suicidal plans made. So-called **somatic** or **biological symptoms** are present: insomnia in the form of either delayed sleep or early waking; loss of appetite and weight; tiredness and lack of energy; retardation in common activities. Concentration, attention and memory can be impaired. In severe forms, **delusional ideas** and **hallucinations** can occur.

When severe physical disease is present, the diagnosis of major depression can be difficult to make, as many of the symptoms listed above, in particular the somatic or biological ones, could be the direct result of physical disease (House, 1988). It is important to focus on the more psychological, as opposed to somatic symptoms associated with low mood to avoid misdiagnosing depression. In a study of general medical patients (not including people with HIV infection) depressed mood and feelings of panic, followed by lack of confidence, social withdrawal, sleep delay, anxiety and anergy were found to be the best predictors of affective disorder (Van Hemert et al, 1993a).

Assessment of depressed mood will also require evaluation of the likely factors contributing to its presence, attempting to formulate the possible mechanisms that contribute to its development. Even in the case of major depression requiring antidepressant medication, personal and social factors will be important in the course and prognosis of the condition, and in their management.

4.4.2 Assessment of suicide risk

As discussed in Chapter 2, suicidal ideas are common in people with HIV infection, and there is strong evidence that they are at an increased risk of suicide. It is therefore important to be able to evaluate suicidal ideas so as to allow people with HIV infection the opportunity to discuss their fears and concerns, and to identify those at risk of suicide, in particular those suffering from psychiatric disorders likely to respond to treatment (Taylor et al, 1985; Hawton and Catalán, 1987; Gelder et al, 1989; Gunnell and Frankel, 1994).

The evaluation of suicidal risk is closely related to the assessment of major depression, as there is a strong association between them. The presence of strong feelings of hopelessness is an important indicator of risk. A history of substance misuse, past psychiatric treatment, and a past history of suicidal behaviour are also indicators of risk. Male sex, middle or old age, and living alone are some of the demographic indicators.

For many people with HIV infection, the opportunity to discuss their suicidal ideas with a sympathetic doctor or nurse will the first step in acknowledging the seriousness of their situation and of their acceptance of their illness. The wish to end one's life may be an initial panic-driven response to the diagnosis, but sensitive questioning and realistic reassurance can help to clarify the person's fears, for example, concerning pain, disfigurement, stigma or rejection. It is not unusual for people with HIV infection to ask their doctors at this stage for help to end their lives. Again, this is often the start of the process of recognizing the seriousness of the situation, and the doctor or nurse is in a good position to clarify the person's fears and concerns, establish the boundaries of professional ethics and responsibility, and stress his or her willingness to help minimize the person's problems (see Chapter 8, for discussion of ethical dilemmas).

4.4.3 Assessment of psychotic disorders

In mania, the main symptoms are: elevated or irritable mood; hyperactivity, including insomnia; increased appetite and sexual interest; and abnormalities of thinking, including pressure of speech and flight of ideas, and delusional ideas often of a grandiose nature. In schizophrenia-like disorders, delusions and hallucinations may be prominent. Visual hallucinations are often associated with organic brain syndromes, while auditory hallucinations are characteristic of schizophrenia and related disorders.

As discussed in Chapter 2, psychotic illnesses in people with HIV may be the result of a variety of factors: pre-existing disorder, illicit drug induced, side-effect of medication, or related to brain disease. Assessment should take into account the careful evaluation of these possible aetiological factors.

4.4.4 Acute organic brain syndromes: delirium

Following the work of Lipowski (1990), delirium is defined as a transient organic mental syndrome of acute onset, characterized by global impairment of cognitive function, reduced level of consciousness, attentional abnormalities, perceptual disorder, abnormal psychomotor activity and disordered wake–sleep cycle.

The precipitant organic factors involved include: primary cerebral disease, either focal or diffuse; systemic disorders with indirect cerebral effects; intoxication and medication side-effect; and withdrawal from substances like alcohol or other addiction-inducing drugs. Older people, and those with pre-existing brain disease, are more likely to develop delirium, and it has been argued that factors such as sleep deprivation, stress, sensory underload or overload, and immobilization could contribute to its development (Lipowski, 1990).

Studies carried out in general medical patients, rather than specifically those with HIV infection, suggest that the development of an acute brain syndrome is a bad prognostic indicator associated with excess mortality (Van Hemert et al, 1993b). Clinical experience indicates that this is likely to apply to people with HIV infection as well. Mental health workers deal with only a minority of cases of delirium occurring in medical patients, the milder and more transient cases seldom requiring specialist intervention.

4.4.5 Chronic organic brain syndromes: dementia

Dementia syndromes are characterized by abnormalities in memory, general intellectual functioning and personality, while level of consciousness is usually unimpaired. The history of the changes in mental functioning and behaviour as given by someone who knows the person well will be an important part of the evaluation (see Chapter 3 for a detailed discussion of HIV associated dementia).

Memory can be tested by asking the person to repeat three items or objects or a name and address (to test registration), and then asking to repeat them once more five minutes later (short-term memory). **Concentration** can be tested by asking the person to subtract 7 serially from a hundred, or to repeat the months of the year backwards, or spell 5 or longer letter words forward and backwards. **Global orientation** is tested by asking about time, place and person. Some idea of the person's **general intellectual functioning** can be obtained from the content and structure of speech, by the general level of information and awareness of current events, in particular when compared with the person's pre-morbid level of education and achievement. Changes in **behaviour** and **personality** may include: slowness, decline in standards of self-care, disorganization, irritability, inability to cope with simple tasks, and uninhibited or anti-social behaviour.

Evaluation of chronic brain disorders will require investigation of possible current focal or diffuse brain disease, systemic disorders, and the exclusion of major psychiatric disease. A past history of head injury, epilepsy, or other conditions likely to have brain consequences, such as substance misuse, may be of relevance. It is important to note that subjective complaints of impaired cognitive function in asymptomatic HIV individuals are seldom indicative of chronic brain disorder, but rather of anxiety or depression (Wilkins et al, 1991; Riccio et al, 1993).

4.4.6 Mental illness or abnormal personality?

Non-psychiatrists are often puzzled by the seemingly unclear and not always helpful distinction favoured by psychiatrists between mental illness and personality disorder, in particular when it comes to considering the use of mental health legislation to deal with undesirable behaviour (for detailed discussion see Gelder et al, 1989). The concept of mental illness implies that the individual has developed a disease after a period of normal health, the disease being the result of the interaction of genetic factors, upbringing and contemporary events. Mental disorders have more or less effective treatments, and at times the severity of the condition is such that the person can be at risk or can put others at risk, as result of the disease: it is in such cases that mental health legislation can be used to detain and treat the person for a specified period of time.

By contrast, personality disorders are regarded as exaggerations of personality traits of such degree, that they are maladaptive and often lead to problems with society. For example, a person may be particularly aggressive, dependent, anti-social or histrionic. The assumption is that such personality traits have been present since childhood or early adolescence, and they are regarded as part of the way the person is, rather than as a disease that affects the individual. It is quite possible for someone with a personality disorder to develop a mental illness, say depression, at some stage. Personality disorders are not regarded as responsive to mental health interventions, although mental health workers are often involved in the care of people described as having a personality disorder. Such individuals are regarded as responsible for their actions, while this is not always the case for those suffering from severe mental disorders, and this is reflected in mental health legislation which is usually not applicable to people with personality disorders.

There is some suggestion that personality disorders are not uncommon in people with HIV infection (see chapter 2), although much depends on the criteria used to define personality disorder. Whether personality disorders are over-represented amongst people with HIV infection or not, in practice those involved in the care of HIV will come across patients who are demanding, dependent, or anti-social, and who will test their ability to set limits, clarify the degree to which the patients' psychological and social needs can be met, and who will put pressure on the teams involved in their care. It is when dealing with people with difficult personalities that it is particularly important to have a co-ordinated provision of care.

4.5 Standardized and research assessments

In a new area of research and clinical work like HIV infection, it is important to ensure that different investigators and clinicians speak a comparable language, hence the value of standardized instruments to assess the nature and severity of problems and to evaluate the outcome of interventions. There are well-validated instruments developed by psychiatric and behavioural researchers to quantify psychological distress and social and other problems (Thompson, 1989), and many of these are easily applicable to HIV infection, while few new instruments have been developed specifically for this condition (Huang et al, 1988).

4.5.1 General and specific psychiatric morbidity

Interview-based measures

Standardized psychiatric interviews based on the systematic evaluation of operationally defined symptoms allow the formulation of diagnosis and the measurement of severity of symptoms and symptom-clusters. Training of the interviewer is essential to ensure adequate validity and reliability. Compared with self-report questionnaires, interview-based measures can be time-consuming, but the interviewer can generate more meaningful information.

Amongst the standardized instruments of value are the Present State Examination (PSE) (Wing et al, 1974); Clinical Interview Schedule (CIS) (Goldberg et al, 1970), the Structured Clinical Interview for DSM-III-R (SCID) (Thompson, 1989) and the Diagnostic Interview Schedule (DIS) (Robins et al, 1981). Maj et al (1994a) reported the use of the Composite International Diagnostic Interview, which is provides psychiatric diagnosis according to the ICD-10-R and DSM-III-R in the WHO multicentre study. In view of the common occurrence of mania in people with HIV, the Mania Rating Scale (MRS) (Young et al, 1978) could help in quantifying its severity and monitoring treatment response. These instruments were not developed specifically for the assessment of psychiatric status in people with physical disorders, and their ratings may well be affected by the presence of physical symptoms unrelated to psychological morbidity.

Self-report questionnaires

There are many questionnaires to assess overall psychological morbidity and specific symptoms, such as anxiety or depression. Questionnaires are easy to use, but the information they provide is more limited than that offered by interview-based measures.

The General Health Questionnaire (GHQ) (Goldberg, 1972) is a good screening instrument, although its sensitivity and specificity can be affected by physical symptoms. The Hospital Anxiety and Depression Scale (HAD) (Zigmond and Snaith, 1983) was developed specifically for the assessment of mood in people with physical disorders, and it avoids the use of questions that might be affected by the presence of physical symptoms. The Profile of Mood States (POMS) (McNair and Lorr, 1964) covers a wide range of feelings from anxiety and depression to anger and fatigue, which can be relevant when dealing with HIV infection.

The Beck Depression Inventory (BDI) (Beck et al, 1961) is a well-known instrument which requires care when using it with physically ill populations. Cavanaugh et al (1983) have shown the value of the cognitive–affective items of the inventory (feeling a failure, loss of interest in people, feeling punished, suicidal ideas, dissatisfaction, difficulty with decisions and crying) in the identification of depression in the physically ill. Two other useful instruments developed by Beck are the Hopelessness Scale (Beck et al, 1974a) and the Suicide Intent Scale (Beck et al, 1974b). The Spielberger State–Trait Anxiety Inventory (Spielberger et al, 1983) has the advantage of assessing separately current anxiety and anxiety as a personality trait.

4.5.2 Neuropsychological assessment

Although gross cognitive impairment of the type seen in HIV-1 associated dementia will be readily identified during a routine mental state examination, the detection of minor cognitive deficits requires a more comprehensive neuropsychological assessment. The selection of appropriate testing instruments should be based on a knowledge of those cognitive functions which are most likely to be compromised. In the case of HIV infection, the major cognitive deficits include psychomotor slowing, memory impairment, affective and emotional disorders, and difficulty with strategy formation and problem solving (see Chapter 3). Adequate evaluation of these functions takes time and cannot be done in a few minutes. In addition, good neuropsychological assessment requires more than a simple knowledge of how to administer tests, and the interpretation of results requires more than an ability to use tables of normative data. A good neuropsychologist will obtain information from both the qualitative aspects of performance during testing and from information obtained during interview.

Perhaps the most common reason for referral for neuropsychological assessment is because of subjective complaints of cognitive, particularly memory, difficulties. In asymptomatic infection, subjective complaints of memory problems are usually more closely associated with anxiety or depression than with objectively verifiable cognitive impairments. In contrast, subjective complaints in more advanced disease stages are more reliably associated with measurable deficits. For this reason, assessment of mental health is a crucial part of neuropsychological assessment in people with HIV infection.

Neuropsychological assessment also requires a detailed knowledge of the patient's state of health. This should include not only broad indices of health such as CDC stage and CD4 count, which may be thought of as indicating the degree of risk of impairment, but also details of specific diseases. Many diseases can result in impaired performance on some neuropsychological tests where there is, in reality, no cognitive impairment. For example, cytomegalovirus retinitis may result in poor visual acuity, and myelopathies and peripheral neuropathies will often result in impaired motor performance. In each case, impaired performance may occur where there is no neuropsychological deficit. The same effect may be seen, more generally, as the consequence of the debilitating effects of illness.

In the early days of HIV infection, little was known about the impact of HIV on cognitive performance and neuropsychologists had little clear idea of which functions were most vulnerable. As more has been learned about the neuropsychological impact of HIV, it has become possible to refine the range of functions assessed and tests used. The National Institutes for Mental Health (NIMH) in the US published the conclusions of the workgroup on neuropsychological issues in HIV infection and AIDS which included recommendations for both a comprehensive and short assessment battery (Butters et al, 1990). The comprehensive battery (Table 4.2) includes assessment of attention, speed of processing, memory, abstraction, language, visuo-perception, constructional abilities, motor abilities, psychiatric assessment and an evaluation of pre-morbid ability. Most of the instruments recommended are well known standardized clinical tests but some are adaptations of tasks used in experimental psychology such as the Sternberg Search Task and the Simple and Choice Reaction Times. The NIMH battery is certainly the most authoritative statement yet published on clinical neuropsychological assessment in HIV infection, but it has the major drawback that completion of the comprehensive battery takes 7–9 hours. Although the NIMH workgroup strongly recommended the use of the comprehensive battery, it was recognized that it might not always be possible to complete this. For this reason, a shorter battery taking 1–2 hours was also proposed which included evaluation of attention, speed of processing, memory, psychiatric state and pre-morbid intelligence.

Similar recommendations for neuropsychological assessment have not been published in other countries, and although the NIMH report may be appropriate for the US, it is not necessarily suitable for the way neuropsychological services are set up in other countries. In the UK, and in many other European countries, neuropsychologists have traditionally avoided using large comprehensive batteries which are administered on a routine basis to most patients. Rather, the emphasis is on shorter assessments where the instruments used are selected according to the strengths and weaknesses revealed during the session. In our Unit of Psychological Medicine, Charing Cross and Westminster Medical School, in London, a core of established clinical tests has been selected for use with people with HIV infection referred for neuropsychological assessment (Table 4.3). Although the Charing Cross and Westminster and NIMH batteries were developed independently, comparison of Tables 4.2 and 4.3 shows there is considerable overlap between the two. At Chelsea and Westminster, most patients will be assessed using these core instruments and additional tests will be selected by the neuropsychologist depending upon the patient's performance. In this way, most patients can be assessed in 2–3 hours.

Other strategies for assessment have focused on tasks designed specifically to be sensitive to the deficits seen in HIV infection. A good example of this is the

Table 4.2 Domains of the National Institutes for Mental Health (NIMH) core neuropsychological battery (Reproduced with permission)

A	Indication of pre-morbid intelligence
	Vocabulary (*WAIS*-R)
	National Adult Reading Test
B	Attention
	Digit Span (WMS-R)
	Visual Span (*WMS-R*)
C	Speed of processing
	Sternberg Search Task
	Simple and Choice Reaction Times
	Paced Authority Serial Addition Test
D	Memory
	California Verbal Learning Test
	Working Memory Test
	Modified Visual Reproduction Test (WMS)
E	Abstraction
	Category Test
	Trail Marking Test, Parts A and B
F	Language
	Boston Naming Test
	Letter and Category Fluency Test
G	Visuo-spatial
	Embedded Figures Test
	Money's Standardized Road-Map Test of Directional Sense
	Digit Symbol Substitution
H	Constructional abilities
	Block Design Test
	Tactual Performance Test
I	Motor abilities
	Grooved Pegboard
	Finger Tapping Test
	Grip Strength
J	Psychiatric assessment
	Diagnostic interview schedule
	Hamilton Depression Scale
	State–Trait Anxiety Scale
	Mini-mental State Examination

Note: *italics* indicate instruments in the abbreviated version of the NIMH neuropsychological battery. WMS-R = The Wechsler Memory Scale – Revised. Wechsler, 1987; WAIS-R = Wechsler Adult Intelligence Scale – Revised. Wechsler, 1981.

Dual Attention Task, a complex computerized test which gives requires accurate tracking, fast reaction times and attention to two different tasks simultaneously (Kocsis et al, 1989). The preliminary results from this task suggest that it is highly sensitive to HIV-related cognitive impairments but details of the specificity of the test have not been published. New HIV-specific neuropsychological tests

Table 4.3 Domains of the Charing Cross and Westminster Unit of Psychological Medicine neuropsychological battery

A	Interview
	educational and occupational background
	health history especially disease of the CNS
	current health status
	handedness
	psychiatric state and history
	drug and alcohol usage
B	Pre-morbid ability
	Vocabulary (WAIS-R)
	National Adult Reading Test
C	Attention
	Digit Span
D	Memory*
	Story Recall (AMIPB)
	Figure Recall (AMIPB)
	List Learning (AMIPB)
	Design Learning (AMIPB)
E	Psychomotor speed
	Digit Symbol (WAIS-R)
	Trail Making Test, Parts A and B
F	Language
	Letter fluency
	Similarities (WAIS-R)
G	Constructional ability
	Block Design
H	Motor ability
	Grooved Pegboard
I	Non-verbal intelligence
	Picture arrangement
J	Psychiatric assessment
	Hospital Anxiety and Depression Scale

Note: *italics* indicate instruments to the core Charing Cross and Westminster neuropsychological battery.
*If recall memory is normal, the learning tasks are omitted.
AMIPB = The Adult Memory and Information Processing Battery, Coughlan and Hollows (1985); WAIS-R = Wechsler Adult Intelligence Scale – Revised. Wechsler, 1981.

may become increasingly important in the future as most established clinical instruments were designed to assess cortical function and are often not particularly sensitive to the types of deficits seen in HIV infection. At present, however, these new instruments are either in the process of development or are not widely available and for these reasons, most neuropsychologists will continue to rely most heavily on traditional clinical tests.

Although a comprehensive neuropsychological battery should assess at least the range of functions listed in Table 4.3 there will be times when circumstances require a briefer assessment. Many screening batteries have been proposed for use in HIV infection, but none has gained widespread acceptance. Inevitably, producing brief assessment batteries involves a trade-off between time on the one hand and specificity and sensitivity on the other. Where the optimum balance between these factors lies will depend upon the purpose of the assessment and the circumstances under which the assessment is made. In many cases, however, the most important functions to assess are psychomotor speed (e.g. Digit Symbol, Trail Making Test), Memory (e.g. List Learning Task, Design Learning Task) and mood state (e.g. the Hospital Anxiety and Depression Scale).

4.5.3 Health-related quality of life

For many diseases, demonstrating the effectiveness of medical interventions is straightforward and in the most dramatic cases, the outcome is that the patient is either dead or alive. In other cases, the patient makes a full recovery and becomes symptom-free or remains permanently unwell. Such clear cut examples are unusual. For most diseases, and HIV disease is a good example, the benefits of medical treatment may be much less obvious. Where clear-cut cures are absent, physicians have traditionally evaluated their interventions by measuring changes in the signs or symptoms of disease. For example, the Concorde study investigated the efficacy of zidovudine (ZVD) asymptomatic HIV infection by looking at how it delayed progression to symptomatic illness and by its impact on CD4 levels. Although CD4 levels and CDC stages are considered important medically, it is not clear how they relate to other aspects of a person's life. For this reason, there has been a growth of interest in evaluating medical interventions in terms of both traditional medical indices and in terms of their wider impact on patients' lives. This broader range of outcome measures has come to be termed 'quality of life' (QoL).

The prospect of evaluating QoL in HIV infection may seem daunting. There is, however, nothing unusual or uncommon about quality of life evaluations in medicine. Making value judgements about a patient's quality of life and deciding whether to give or withhold treatment on the basis of those judgements is an everyday part of medical practice. In some cases, the benefits of treatment may be so marginal, the prospects of improvement so small, and the potential cost in terms of side-effects so great, that a clinician may decide that it is in the patient's interest to withhold treatment even if this decision ultimately results in the patient's death. It is no accident that much of the early research into the quantitative evaluation of QoL related to patients with cancer where such issues are commonplace. For the same reasons, interest in QoL has grown enormously amongst HIV physicians and patients in recent years.

Others have become interested in QoL as a way of rationalizing decisions about the allocation of funds to health services. Increasingly, decisions to treat or not to treat in medicine are not solely determined on the basis of clinical judgement or the patient's wishes. Resource limitations demand that difficult decisions have to be made and in some cases established treatments may be withheld because the necessary funding is no longer available. For these reasons, health economists have devised ways of evaluating health care, not only on the basis of conventional outcome measures, such as survival time or symptom reduction, but also in terms of QoL.

Quality of life in the health care context concerns only those aspects of life that are 'health-sensitive'. Listening to music may add to the quality of life of some people, but it is only a QoL issue if the ability to listen to music is impaired or prevented by illness or disease. For this reason, it is preferable to refer to *health-related quality of life*, acknowledging that such assessments address only part of what makes up any given individual's quality of life.

There is no universally accepted definition of QoL, yet there is considerable agreement as to what may *detract* from good quality of life. For this reason, QoL is most often defined negatively. For example, most people would agree that pain or physical handicap, may have an adverse impact on QoL. There is a surprising degree of consistency in the domains that most researchers have considered important. Whilst different reviewers tend to use slightly different taxonomies, most include the *physical*, the *functional*, the *psychological* and the *social* domains.

The *physical* domain is the most commonly assessed area includes an evaluation of symptoms (e.g. pain or nausea), side-effects and toxicities of treatment. The *functional* domain includes assessment of the patient's mobility, activities of daily living, work performance, and so on. The *psychological* domain typically addresses questions of depression and anxiety, but also other aspects of psychological well-being. Finally, the *social* domain evaluates social and recreational aspects of a person's life including family, peer, and sexual relationships.

The earliest formal measures of QoL, such as the Karnofsky index (Karnofsky and Burchenal, 1949), were simple scales in which the clinician rated the degree of impairment caused by illness. Later researchers, influenced by behavioural psychology, relied on indices that could be objectively measured such as 'How many days has the patient been confined to bed in the last month?' and 'How far can the person walk unaided?'. More recently, the emphasis of QoL measurement has been on the subjective evaluation of quality of life by the patient. Provided that care is taken in the design of measuring instruments, subjective measures may be at least as reliable as many routine clinical judgements.

Although QoL is not tightly defined, it is not difficult in principle to develop appropriate scales using standard psychometric principles. This involves asking a wide range of relevant questions about QoL and then selecting those which show the best reliability and validity. In practice this process will often be unnecessary as there are a large number of measurement scales already available that can be used to assess a wide range of different aspects of QoL. When selecting a QoL measure there are several issues that should be considered.

1. *Psychometric properties* As with any measurement instrument, QoL measures should be both valid and reliable. Unfortunately, many of the scales

that have been used to measure QoL, do not, meet these most basic psychometric criteria.

2. *Practical issues* Selection of a QoL measure requires that the practicalities of the data collection be considered. In some ways interviews have advantages over self-report questionnaires in that a skilled interviewer is more likely to ensure that the patient's views are accurately recorded. Also, more detailed information can be obtained by this means than is typically available from questionnaires. However, interviews are time-consuming and self-report questionnaires will often make acceptable substitutes. This is an important consideration, particularly when the patients may be quite ill and the assessment is to be repeated. In such circumstances a short, user-friendly instrument is a boon. It is often better to have a large number of brief completed assessments than a smaller number of more comprehensive evaluations which fail to be completed.

3. *General versus disease-specific assessment* One of the most basic questions is to ask whether any existing scale measures those aspects of ill health that are relevant to the disease in question, in this case HIV. Many instruments are general in that they aim to be appropriate for any conceivable health condition the Quality of Well Being Scale (Kaplan and Anderson 1988), the Nottingham Health Profile (Hunt et al, 1981), and the Medical Outcomes Studies Short Form (Stewart et al, 1988). Others have been designed for specific diseases. Already there are several scales designed specifically for HIV infection including the HOPES (HIV Overview of Problems Evaluation Systems; Ganz et al, 1993) and the HIV-QAM (HIV Quality Audit Marker; Holzemer et al, 1993). One of the main advantages of using generic measures is that comparisons with other health conditions are possible. In many cases, generic measures will be sufficient, although sometimes more specific instruments will be required. For example, if QoL is measured in an heterogeneous group of people with HIV then a generic measure may be useful. If, however, the investigation focuses on only those people with HIV who also have Karposi's sarcoma skin lesions, a more specific measure which looks at the impact of this condition may also be required. The major disadvantage of using specific measures is that it may be necessary to develop a new scale, a process that can take several years if done properly.

4. *Uni versus multidimensional measures* It is widely agreed that QoL has many dimensions. One of the motivations for measuring QoL, however, is to produce an index that can be used by health economists to compare the cost-effectiveness of different treatments. For this purpose, a multidimensional construct needs to be reduced to a unidimensional index, an example of which is the Quality of Well Being Scale (QWB). The QWB is widely used in the US but, to date, has not been used much elsewhere. It is in two parts; the Functional Classification Scale including scales to measure mobility, physical activity, and social activity and the Symptom/Problem Complex Scale listing 21 different health conditions ordered in severity from no symptoms to death. The ratings

on these two scales are weighted and entered into a standard formula which results in a score between 0 and 1. This score, the QWB index, can then be used to evaluate health care outcome using a system of Quality Adjusted Life Years (QALYs) where the life expectancy following a given treatment is adjusted by the expected quality of life during that time. For example, different treatments may be compared by considering mortality statistics such that a person on treatment A has a life expectancy of 5 years and on treatment B only 4 years. Using conventional mortality statistics, it is clear that treatment A is superior to treatment B. When QoL ratings are used, the situation is rather different. Treatment A has a QWB index of 0.7 and treatment B a QWB index of 0.85. In terms of Quality Adjusted Life Years, the QWB index of 0.7 can be interpreted to mean that each year of life lived by the patient is equivalent to 0.7 years of full quality life. Thus, comparing the treatments again, the QALYs for treatment A is 3.5 (i.e. 5 × 0.70) years and for treatment B, 3.4 (i.e. 4 × 0.85), suggesting an approximate parity between treatments.

The attraction of unidimensional approaches to health care evaluation is that they appear to provide a useful guide to help resolve complex decisions, both clinical and financial. However, the QALY approach has been widely criticized both on methodological grounds and in its application to real health care decisions which may result, if applied uncritically, in counter-intuitive policy decisions. Perhaps the most alarming aspect of measures of this type is that different evaluation systems give rise to different outcomes which raises serious concerns over the validity of this approach. The fact that it is *possible* to produce a single index of quality of life does not mean that it is appropriate to do so and it could be argued that any such approach inevitably oversimplifies a host of complex ethical and practical issues. Whilst the unidimensional approach has a number of attractive features, it should be used with caution. Certainly for most clinical evaluations of QoL, multidimensional measures are generally to be preferred.

Multidimensional scales have the advantage over unidimensional scales in that they provide information, not only about the overall level of quality of life, but also about particular *facets* of quality of life. Clinicians are used to making decisions based on many sources of information and may prefer the detailed information from a multidimensional scale to a single index number.

Some well-established, high-quality multidimensional QoL scales have been used in HIV infection. Perhaps the most best known of these have been derived from the Medical Outcomes Studies Health Ratings (the MOS-HIV and the SF-36). The Medical Outcomes Study was a large research project set up in the US with the aim of improving ways of evaluating health outcomes (Tarlov et al, 1989). One of the most important consequences of this project was the publication of a series of QoL measures, including a 20-item short form, which have subsequently been used extensively around the world. The MOS-HIV is a measure based on tht MOS Short Form with additional scales to cover areas specific to HIV infection (Wu et al, 1989). The final scale is made up of 30 items in 11 subscales measuring Overall Health, Pain, Physical Functioning, Role Functioning, Social Functioning, Mental Health, Energy and Fatigue, Health

Distress, Cognitive Functioning, Overall Quality of Life, and Health Transition. This measure has been shown, both in the US and in the UK, to be reliable, valid and sensitive to change. The MOS-HIV is a self-completion questionnaire which most people can complete unaided in less than five minutes. For these reasons, and because it is already commonly used both in the UK and in the US, the MOS-HIV scale is a good choice to consider when planning QoL investigations in HIV infection (Burgess et al, 1993).

Multidimensional measures are not without problems, however. Very often, the scales have been designed on the basis of face validity (i.e. items are put into the same scales because it seems sensible that they should go together) rather than on some more rigorous basis such as through an exploration of the factor structure of the scale. The result is that the subscale structure of multidimensional scales may at worst be rather arbitrary and with considerable redundancy among the scales used.

The importance of evaluating health care in broader terms than traditional medical measures is now widely recognized. Until recently, however, only a few studies had even attempted to measure QoL in HIV infection. The situation has, however, changed dramatically, and nowadays most treatment evaluations routinely include some QoL measures. Indeed, quality of life issues are not new in medicine. What is new about QoL evaluation is the attempt to make explicit the value judgements that go to make up decisions about quality of life and then measure and evaluate clinical choices in as systematic and as scientific a manner as possible.

4.5.4 Adjustment to illness, coping with stress and social supports

There are many instruments available to assess methods of coping with stressful events. The COPE (Carver et al, 1989) is a self-report instrument that provides information about problem-focused strategies, emotional expression-based methods, and maladaptive techniques such as denial. The Psychosocial Adjustment to Illness Scale (PAIS) (Derogatis, 1986) gives information on its effects on relationships, sex, health care, and psychological distress, amongst other variables.

Substance misuse can worsen as a result of adverse life events, and its evaluation may be desirable when monitoring the effects of psychological and other interventions. Standardized instruments for the assessment of alcohol misuse include questionnaires both for the screening of individuals likely to be drinking excessively, such as the CAGE (Mayfield et al, 1974) and the Michigan Alcoholism Screening Test (MAST) (Selzer, 1971), and for the assessment of severe alcohol misuse, such as the Severity of Alcohol Dependence Questionnaire (SADQ) (Stockwell et al, 1983).

The presence of adequate social supports plays a crucial role in reducing the likelihood of psychological distress when faced with adverse life events and difficulties (Cohen, 1991; O'Brien et al, 1993). The Interpersonal Support Evaluation List (ISEL) (Cohen et al, 1985) is a good instrument which can be used in research in HIV.

4.6 Summary

Practical aspects of the assessment of mental health problems in people with HIV infection are reviewed here. The organization of services, combining the role of statutory bodies and voluntary agencies is discussed, with advice about co-ordination of services.

Obstacles to the recognition of mental health problems in people with HIV are discussed, and the principles of assessment of mental symptoms reviewed, with focus on common disorders, such as major depression, psychotic disorders, acute and chronic brain syndromes, and the assessment of suicide risk. Finally, standardized and research assessment of neuropsychological function, psychological status, mood, quality of life, adjustment to illness, and coping are discussed.

5 Management of mental health problems

5.1 Introduction

In previous chapters we have reviewed the types and nature of psychiatric problems that can occur in association with HIV infection, and described the detailed assessment of mental health problems and difficulties. Here we discuss approaches to intervention to deal with such mental health problems.

As in the case of other situations where mental health problems can develop, there is a wide range of interventions of the kind familiar to psychiatrists, psychologists, and psychiatric nurses, and they include, amongst others: psychological therapies, psychopharmacological interventions, and treatment in residential settings. In addition, the social impact of HIV infection has led to the development of novel approaches to the delivery of care, involving voluntary, non-governmental organizations, of an extent that the statutory services would not have been able to provide on their own.

While a good deal of descriptive work illustrating treatments to minimize the psychiatric consequences of HIV infection has been published, there is a dearth of research to evaluate the efficacy of psychiatric interventions, traditional or novel, when applied to problems associated with HIV infection. Whenever possible, the results of outcome research studies are summarized.

Mental health interventions are usually provided in combination, but for the sake of clarity they are discussed here under several categories: (1) psychological; (2) psychopharmacological; (3) residential care; (4) care provided by community organizations; and (5) complementary therapies. Sometimes the same therapist will be involved in providing several forms of care, although usually different team members with individual skills will be responsible for specific interventions.

5.2 Psychological interventions

Psychological treatments well known to mental health workers, such as cognitive behaviour therapy, brief focal psychotherapy, crisis intervention or psychodynamic therapies, can be employed to deal with the problems associated to HIV infection.

The term *counselling* is much used in the context of HIV infection, but unfortunately often in a vague and all-inclusive way, which makes it difficult to understand what it actually involves. There are at least three kind of activities covered by the term counselling:

(a) counselling about the significance and consequences of testing for HIV antibodies;
(b) counselling about HIV risk reduction; and
(c) counselling to deal with the psychological and social consequences of HIV infection.

Clearly the knowledge and skills needed for each of these forms of counselling are different, and it can not be assumed that a given 'AIDS counsellor' will be equally at home in the three modalities. Detailed discussion of theoretical and practical aspects of counselling are provided by Green and McCreaner (1989) and Bor et al (1992).

5.2.1 Psychological interventions at the time of HIV testing

Pre-test counselling about the significance of HIV testing

There is evidence that individuals who regard themselves as being at risk of HIV infection and who seek testing have higher than expected rates of lifetime psychopathology, in particular mood disorders and substance misuse problems (see Chapter 1). A substantial proportion report suicidal ideas (Perry et al, 1990b) and anecdotal reports have documented the occurrence of completed suicide following notification of a positive HIV test result (Pierce, 1987). The presence of such psychological vulnerability in people coming forward for testing highlights the need to make sure that a careful evaluation takes place of the reasons for seeking testing, risk perception, and in particular assessment of how the person is likely to cope with the result of the test. The World Health Organization (1993) has stressed the need for informed consent in HIV testing and has rejected mandatory testing programmes.

Counselling before HIV testing should contain an explanation of the significance of the test, including likelihood of progression to symptomatic disease, and the possible advantages of knowing the result (e.g. access to early treatment to prevent progression or ability to make a decision about continuation of pregnancy), as well as its disadvantages (Miller and Pinching, 1989; Dent, 1989; Catalán and Riccio, 1990b; Bor et al, 1991; Meadows et al, 1993b).

Establishing the likelihood of the person having HIV infection will require enquiring about behaviours associated with high risk: history of unprotected anal or vaginal intercourse, sharing of injecting drug using equipment, such as needles and syringes, blood transfusion or use of blood products. Focusing on behaviours is preferable to thinking about membership of so-called 'risk groups', which may not only tend to stigmatize those thought to belong to such groups but, more importantly may lead to failure to identify those who are really at risk because of their behaviour but do not belong to recognized 'at risk' groups (Catalán, 1990b). Issues concerning confidentiality, and the likely personal and social reactions to a positive result need to be explored (Perry and Markowitz,

1988). For example, there are real concerns about the chances of obtaining life insurance after undergoing HIV testing, even when the results are negative.

Pre-test counselling is sometimes regarded as a complex and highly skilled procedure which requires a good deal of time. In practice, most individuals considering HIV testing will not need intense and lengthy counselling, although some will need more careful and detailed before they make up their mind (Miller and Bor, 1992).

Post-test counselling about the implications of test result

Counselling following HIV testing may require more time than pre-test counselling, in particular when the person is found to be HIV seropositive. Post-test counselling will include notification of the result, some help to reduce stress, discussion of how to prevent spread of infection, consideration of the practical implications, including to whom to tell the result, and an offer of further opportunities for discussion (Perry and Markowitz, 1988; Sonnex et al, 1989).

These commendable goals are not always met, however. Retrospective investigations have suggested that only a minority of individuals are satisfied with how they were told their HIV positive status (McCann and Wadsworth, 1991; Pergami et al, 1994a). The attitude of the person breaking the news and the quality of the information given were regarded in the latter study as the main determinants of satisfaction with the consultation.

Perry et al (1991) compared three different interventions to reduce distress after HIV testing in a study involving 1307 individuals. All participants received standard pre- and post-test counselling, and after notification of the results, they were randomly allocated to one of the following:

(a) six weekly individual 'stress prevention training' sessions;

(b) three-weekly 'interactive video programme' sessions; and

(c) standard post-test counselling alone.

Three months later significant reductions in levels of distress were seen in the three conditions for both HIV seropositive and seronegative individuals, although those with HIV infection who had received stress prevention training showed greater reductions in psychological distress.

Risk reduction counselling

Counselling to modify sexual and drug using behaviours in the direction of lowering the risk of acquiring or transmitting HIV infection is often provided at the time when individuals consider HIV testing, although it can be provided in other situations. Counselling will involve information about risky behaviours, assessment of the person's risk perception and obstacles to risk reduction, as well as provision of practical help in the form of condoms, needles and syringes, and access to cleaning materials and exchange of injecting equipment. The results of such counselling are not always effective or persistent: a study of childbearing women in Kinshasa, Zaïre, showed that while a majority of women intended to use condoms after notification of the test result, only a minority were using condoms a year later (Heyward et al, 1993) (see Chapter 6).

It is often wrongly assumed that risk reduction counselling is only necessary when a person is found to be HIV seropositive. However, people who are found to be seronegative, in particular after practising risky behaviours, may become overconfident as a result of a negative test and thus fail to alter their behaviour. There is disturbing empirical evidence to indicate that in the six months following HIV testing and post-test counselling, those individuals who turn out to be uninfected increase their rates of sexually transmitted disease, while those who are HIV seropositive experience a reduction (Otten et al, 1993). One possible reason for the increase in risky sexual behaviour in those found to be seronegative may be their falsely increased sense of confidence in their ability to avoid HIV infection in spite of having taken risks. By contrast, those found to be seropositive, as a group, may be initially too distressed and shocked to engage in sexual activity of any kind, let alone unprotected sex.

Risk reduction counselling can be associated with favourable changes regardless of testing, although the results vary considerably with the population counselled and the behaviours considered (Higgins et al, 1991; Perkins et al, 1993b; Simpson et al, 1993; Thornton and Catalán, 1993). Encouraging results have been published about the value of counselling to prevent HIV transmission in heterosexual couples where one of the partners is infected (Padian et al, 1993) (see Chapter 6 for further discussion of risk reduction interventions).

Abnormal beliefs in people seeking HIV testing

As discussed in Chapter 1, amongst people seeking HIV testing, some present with persistent concerns about being infected, often in spite of repeated negative tests. Reassurance and basic counselling provide minimal relief, the individual soon returning to a state of distress about HIV infection. Many different terms have been used to describe these individuals or the syndromes they suffer, often adding to the confusion, rather than helping to clarify the problem. A good example is provided by the unfortunate term 'the worried well', which was originally introduced before HIV testing was available to refer to a mixed group of individuals including some who had been sexual partners of people with AIDS, but who had no symptoms at the time and had no way of knowing if they were likely to develop AIDS, as well as others with hypochondriacal preoccupations (Forstein, 1984; Morin et al, 1984). What at the time was a good attempt at dealing with a new problem, is now an unhelpful label with derogatory connotations.

Worrying beliefs about HIV infection which do not subside after a negative test result and appropriate counselling about its significance should be regarded as a *symptom* rather than a diagnosis (see chapter 1). For example, they may be part of an adjustment reaction, obsessional disorder, somatization disorder, or hypochondriasis; they may be delusional and occur in the context of an affective disorder or schizophrenic illness; or they may present in someone with a personality disorder. People with hypochondriasis have received a good deal of attention in the HIV literature (Davey and Green, 1991) compared with those with delusional or other disorders, perhaps reflecting the prevalence of syndromes.

Psychological interventions will clearly depend on the nature of the principal diagnosis, cognitive behavioural approaches being the treatment of choice in hypochondriasis and obsessional or phobic disorders (Salkovskis and Warwick, 1986; Miller et al, 1988; Logsdail et al, 1991; Stern and Fernandez, 1991; Sharpe et al, 1992), while explanation and change in misguided attitudes may be all is needed in less complex cases (Bor et al, 1989). Delusional beliefs secondary to major depression or to a schizophrenic disorder will require appropriate pharmacological treatment.

HIV testing in psychiatric settings

The association between HIV infection and psychiatric disorder means that HIV infected individuals will present in psychiatric settings, regardless of whether their HIV status is known to them or their carers. Studies in the US and Europe show that over 6 per cent of acute psychiatric admissions are HIV seropositive, the majority remaining undetected (Cournos et al, 1991; Sacks et al, 1992; Empfield et al, 1993; Ayuso-Mateos et al, 1994). In a New York City shelter for homeless male psychiatric patients 13 per cent were known to be HIV seropositive (Susser et al, 1993). HIV-related risk behaviours are common in acute and chronic psychiatric patients (Baker and Mossman, 1991; Kelly et al, 1992a; DiClemente and Ponton, 1993; Cournos et al, 1994; Kalichman et al, 1994; Avins et al, 1994).

Psychiatrists and other mental health workers will be faced with a series of questions in relation to the possibility HIV infection in their patients (Binder, 1987; Catalán, 1990b):

(a) when to think of the **possibility** of HIV-related psychiatric disorders: history of behaviours with risk of HIV infection; type of psychiatric syndrome; patient's characteristics; suggestive physical symptoms; and known HIV seropositive status;

(b) how to proceed when it is **probable** that the patients has HIV infection: would knowledge of the patient's HIV status affect assessment and treatment?; if establishing a patient's HIV status is thought to be desirable, how should this be done?; how should patients be managed if they refuse HIV testing?; in what circumstances would it be permissible to test psychiatric patients without their consent?;

(c) how to manage **individuals known to be HIV seropositive**: assessment and management of the psychiatric disorder; who should be informed of the patient's status; measures to prevent infection of other patient or staff.

Testing psychiatric patients for HIV infection, as in any other case, should include the need for explicit consent, and provision of pre post-test counselling, as outlined in official documents (see: General Medical Council, 1988; Royal College of Psychiatrists, Catalán et al, 1989; American Psychiatric Association, 1988a, b, 1992a, b); WHO, 1993; Eickhoff, 1994).

Testing without the patient's explicit consent would only be justified in very rare cases, whether in psychiatric settings or in other situations. In psychiatry the question may arise when someone with a psychiatric disorder is unwilling (e.g. in the case of a manic patient) or unable (as in the case of someone with marked cognitive impairment) to give consent. Faced with such situations, psychiatrists should attempt to clarify to what extent the patient's immediate treatment would be influenced by knowledge of HIV status, the degree to which HIV testing would be in the patient's interest, and whether knowing the HIV status would make any difference to the safety of staff or other patients.

The answers to these questions are not always obvious, and discussion with the rest of the clinical team and with a physician with experience in the management of HIV infection with be important. If a decision to test without consent is made, careful documentation of the decision-making process and consultation with a legal adviser would be highly desirable (Catalán, 1990b).

5.2.2 *Clinical management of psychological problems in HIV infection*

The care of psychological problems in HIV infection should be part of the overall clinical management of the condition, and thus involve professionals and volunteers working both in the community and in hospitals.

Doctors and nurses involved in providing day to day care will be in a good position to identify and deal with common psychological and social problems in patients and their relatives (Cline, 1990), and refer on those patients needing more intensive or specialized help. It is a matter of regret that **primary care doctors and their teams**, who are usually well placed to provide long-term care to patients and families, have only had a limited role in the management of people with HIV infection, although there are encouraging changes taking place (King, 1988, 1989c; Kochen et al, 1991; Mansfield and Singh, 1989, 1993).

Social workers, health advisers and a variety of other hospital- and community-based professionals form a second level of intervention, dealing with psychological and social problems requiring more time and skills, and working in close collaboration with the primary medical and nursing teams.

Specialized mental health workers can provide assessment and care of more severe or complex problems, as well as be available to help other professionals. Mental health interventions for people with HIV infection will depend upon the nature of the psychiatric problem and the causal factors involved. As discussed above, a variety of factors contribute to psychiatric morbidity in people with HIV infection, some related to the disease itself, some to the individual's own vulnerability, and some to the social consequences and correlates of the disease. Provision of specialized psychiatric care is not always accessible. A WHO survey of European professionals involved in the care of people with HIV infection has highlighted the inadequacies in the provision of specialist mental health interventions, in particular in emergencies, when dealing with injecting drug users (Catalán, 1993).

In common with other potentially serious and fatal conditions, such as cancer, the physical consequences of the disease and its treatment will be a fundamental element in the development of problems. Those involved in providing psychological care to people with HIV infection will need to become familiar with the specific medical complications and treatments of the condition, as well as with the medical terminology generated by the disease. Unfortunately, standard medical textbooks are usually out of date in relation to HIV and its treatment, and those outside treatment centres may have difficulty keeping up with the literature. Lack of such knowledge will not only make it difficult to understand the patients' predicament, but it will do little to enhance the therapist's credibility in the patient's eyes (see Chapter 9).

5.2.3 General psychological interventions

Psychoeducational interventions

Discussion of the implications of having HIV infection or explaining the nature of treatments, likely complications and their effects may be more complex than expected. While many people with HIV infection are well informed about such matters, misguided media reporting and negative social attitudes may have led some to hold inaccurate beliefs. Methods of transmission and acquisition of HIV infection, and possible concerns about infection to social contacts will need to be addressed. Discussion of risks to unborn children and family planning advice may be necessary.

Clinicians are well placed to provide accurate information and to encourage patients to maintain control over their lives. Advice about keeping healthy, including diet, exercise (Antoni, 1991; Calabrese and LaPerriere, 1993), and minimization of the effects of substance misuse should be included (see below). Much of the advice given by professionals and by voluntary organizations regarding lifestyle changes is generally sensible and may help the person acquire a greater sense of mastery over his or her life, but it has to be stressed that it is not clear that such changes will have significant effect in preventing disease progression (see Chapter 6).

Allowing the expression of painful emotions in the context of a safe therapeutic interview can help patients develop effective ways of dealing with their feelings. Some individuals will have known others who have died as a result of HIV infection, and their fears will need to be noted, including concerns about developing dementia. Partners and relatives may need to be involved in the discussions (Perry, 1993). Psychoeducational interventions have been used with HIV seropositive psychiatric in-patients (Lauer-Listhaus and Watterson, 1988).

Problem-solving interventions

HIV infection is characterized by the seemingly inevitable development of health-related problems leading to gradual or sudden changes in personal autonomy, work, social life, and income, to name a few possible problems. A problem-solving approach of the type that has been shown to be effective in general practice and other settings (Green and McCreaner, 1989; Hawton and Kirk, 1989; Catalán et al, 1991) could help the person develop strategies to cope with a range of moving targets at different stages of disease. For example, in the early stages individuals often feel overwhelmed by multiple concerns about how long they have been infected, who was responsible for their infection, how long they are going to live, who should be told about their status, how parents will respond, or about what they should do with their remaining years. The role of the therapist here would be to help patients identify their concerns, prioritize them in terms of urgency, and then take each one at a time and consider possible solutions. By breaking the problems down into manageable tasks, the person can gain a sense of control and mastery which will allow him or her tackle the more difficult issues that will arise as the disease progresses.

Fawzy et al (1989) have shown the value of a 10-week structured group intervention using problem-solving techniques as a key ingredient of the sessions in reducing distress and improving coping skills in people with AIDS.

Cognitive behaviour therapy

The efficacy of cognitive behavioural therapy for depression (Blackburn et al, 1981) and for a range of other psychiatric disorders is well established (Hawton et al, 1989). Emotional disturbance in people with physical disorders is usually associated with dysfunctional cognitions, and cognitive therapy is therefore an appropriate one to consider (Sensky, 1990). Individual cognitive behavioural techniques have also been shown to be effective in reducing psychological morbidity in patients with cancer (Greer et al, 1992).

There is good evidence for the value of cognitive behavioural therapy for people with HIV infection. Comparison of group behavioural intervention with a waiting list control condition showed significant advantages for the experimental treatment (Auerbach et al, 1992). Group cognitive behaviour therapy and support group brief therapy for depressed individuals with HIV infection have been found to be superior to a non-treatment control condition in improving psychological functioning (Kelly et al, 1993b), although, interestingly, the social support intervention was somewhat more effective. A third controlled study comparing individual cognitive behavioural therapy with a waiting list control condition reinforced the value of this form of therapy in reducing stress and improving quality of life in people with HIV infection (Lamping et al, 1993).

Counselling and supportive therapy

Lack of social supports is an important contributor to psychiatric morbidity (see Chapter 2), and possibly even to physical morbidity (Rosengren et al, 1993). Not surprisingly, access to a confiding relationship, whether with professionals or with others with HIV infection, individually or in groups, can be very effective in reducing distress (Hockings, 1989; Mulleady et al, 1989; Viney et al, 1991; Kelly et al, 1993b). Sometimes, long term contact with a counsellor will be all that is required, but in the case of vulnerable individuals with limited coping resources more skilled help may be needed at times of crisis (Hedge et al, 1992).

In a UK national survey of counselling in HIV infection (Bond, 1991) the themes most often raised by asymptomatic individuals during counselling sessions included: concerns about relationships; avoidance of transmission; death and dying; disease progression; coping with distressing feelings; and fears about stigma, isolation and prejudice. Symptomatic disease tended to add urgency to these themes, with the emphasis on questions related to disease progression an treatment, and the practical implications of declining health.

Brief psychotherapy

Brief focused psychodynamic psychotherapy is sometimes used for people with HIV infection, both in hospital-based services and, possibly more, in non-profit AIDS organizations. While there has been no research of the kind carried out in other physical disorders (Guthrie et al, 1993), clinical experience suggests that brief psychodynamic psychotherapy can be of value in some cases (Ratigan, 1993).

5.2.4 *Specific psychological interventions*

Particular problems related to the disease or its consequences may need specific attention. Some examples are considered below.

Breaking bad news

As with other serious conditions, particular sensitivity will be needed when discussing the implications of an AIDS diagnosis, preparing patients for the possibility of future problems, or when attempting to answer the patient's questions about life expectancy or further treatments.

Empirical research has shown that a substantial proportion of patients are dissatisfied with the way they were given a diagnosis of AIDS (Pergami et al, 1994c), satisfaction being related to the perceived quality of the information given and attitude of the person giving the diagnosis. Doctors and others involved in breaking bad news often fear their own and their patients reactions. Buckman (1984) has discussed some of these fears: being blamed by the patient; unleashing a 'bad reaction'; expressing emotion; not knowing all the answers; one's own fears about illness and death.

Discussing the breaking of bad news in palliative care, Buckman (1993) has summarized the steps involved: (a) ensuring the right setting for the interview, without likely interruptions; (b) finding out how much the person suspects or already knows; (c) finding out how much the person wants to know; (d) sharing medical information; (e) responding to the person's feelings; and (f) planning what to do next. There is always danger of the therapist providing false reassurance to minimize the impact of bad news, or colluding with the patient to avoid facing the unwelcome information. The opposite mistake, to give information in a blunt and insensitive should also be avoided. Information should be given ensuring that there is privacy and sufficient time to answer questions and allow expression of feelings, showing empathy but also with sufficient detachment to be able to contain the patient's distress, and provide some measure of hope (Bor et al, 1993b).

The significance of laboratory tests indicating decline in health

Progress in our understanding of HIV infection has led to identifying predictors of progression before a clinical decline in health, and notification of such changes may have important psychological results (Miller et al, 1991b). For some people, being told that early treatment is available may increase the sense of hope in the chances of remaining well for longer, while others may see it as a sign of impending disease, and this may lead to psychological distress. As when giving bad news, especial care will be needed to allow time to answer questions and provide space for the expression of feelings.

Kaposi's sarcoma and other disfiguring conditions

Skin cancer, in particular when it affects visible parts of the body, severe scarring, or weight loss can lead to dramatic lowering of self-esteem, avoidance of social situations and depression. Intensive help may be needed to help patients mobilize resources and face feared situations, as well as practical cosmetic advice (Bor, 1993).

HIV-associated cognitive impairment

Fear of developing dementia is common among people with HIV infection and their relatives, although the prevalence of severe cognitive impairment is far less common than it was originally feared (Catalán and Thornton, 1993) (see Chapter 3). Providing accurate information about the risk of dementia will be an important part of counselling.

It is not always easy to establish whether someone has cognitive impairment, or when cognitive impairtment is present whether it is due to HIV infection or to other factors (see Chapters 3 and 4). Clear and sensitively given counselling will be needed in those cases where cognitive impairment occurs, in particular in the early stages, when the person may be very aware of what is happening. As when discussing bad news, it is best to be frank and to ensure that explanations are given at a level which the patient understands, and to ensure that sufficient time is allowed to answer questions and permit expression of feelings. Practical concerns about future care and sources of help will need to be addressed. Issues concerning residential and home care of people with HIV-associated dementia are discussed below. Relatives and carers will need to be involved in counselling (Green and Kocsis, 1988; Kocsis, 1989).

Psychological interventions with users of illegal drugs

Drug users with HIV infection may have to deal with many of the problems discussed here, but they also have to face unique difficulties related to their drug taking. HIV infection has led to a major reappraisal of the care and management of people with substance misuse problems, with important initiatives in education and prevention, and the practical care of drug takers (Strang and Stimson, 1990).

Efforts to promote behaviour change in injecting drug users have focused on harm minimization (activities aimed at lowering the severity of the undesirable consequences of injecting drugs), and risk reduction (activities to reduce the risk of transmission of HIV through drug use or sexual behaviour). Counselling should include behavioural assessment and provision of advice about safer injecting behaviours and techniques of injection, syringe cleaning and disposal, and disinfection. Treatment regimes should provide access to the prescription of substitute drugs for people using opiates, such as methadone, although it is true to say that there is still a debate about their value and practice (Strang and Stimson, 1990; Mulleady, 1992; Ward et al, 1992).

Overall, there is research evidence from many countries showing that there has been change in injecting behaviours (Nicolosi et al, 1991) but results concerning sexual behaviour change are disappointing (Martin et al, 1990; Stimson, 1991). Drug users in contact with treatment show evidence of risk reduction, and there is good evidence for the value of syringe exchange schemes and decontamination (Stimson, 1991; Heimer et al, 1993; Keene et al, 1993). It is generally accepted that harm reduction strategies should include outreach health education and counselling for users not in contact with treatment facilities, and access to needle and equipment exchange together with oral substitute prescribing and treatment options for those in contact with services (Brettle, 1991).

Drug users with HIV infection or at risk of acquiring it have an increased prevalence of psychological morbidity, in comparison with other groups (see Chapters 1 and 2), often prior to HIV testing. Paradoxically, drug users are less likely to make use of counselling facilities after notification of a positive test result (Gala et al, 1992b). Furthermore, there social circumstances and legal problems are likely to increase their difficulties (Chiswick et al, 1992). Counselling on pregnancy-related questions (contraception and HIV risk, drug use and pregnancy, abortion, or infant drug withdrawal) may be needed for women users and for couples (Mulleady, 1992).

Collaboration between agencies providing medical care, those involved in treating drug-related problems and the mental health specialists will be essential to ensure adequate care to drug users with HIV (Catalán and Riccio, 1990b; Catalán and Goos, 1991).

Psychological interventions for couples

As discussed in chapter 1, HIV infection has effects beyond the affected person, and his or her partner is also likely to be faced with significant problems. The problems and dynamics will vary depending on whether one or both partners are infected, but in all cases the relationship and HIV, rather than each individual partner, are likely to become the focus of intervention.

There has been limited published research on psychological interventions for couples, although mental health workers and others working with people with HIV infection often see partners of affected individuals. George (1990) illustrated some of the sexual and general relationship difficulties experienced by men and women with the infection, and their successful resolution using cognitive behavioural techniques, and Ussher (1990) described the value of cognitive behavioural intervention in 10 gay couples with relationship problems. Couple counselling and social support have been shown to be both acceptable and effective at preventing heterosexual HIV transmission in couples where one partner was infected, as a result of changes in sexual behaviour in the direction of lower risk activities (Padian et al, 1993).

Interventions with couples usually include as their goals: improvement in communication; development of skills to deal with conflict and disagreement, such as the use of problem-solving techniques; help to balance the relationship, so that the needs of the non-affected individual are also noted; reduction of risk of HIV transmission; dealing with uncomfortable emotions, like guilt and anger; improvement in sexual function; anticipating the problems associated with health decline of the affected partner; and developing supports for the surviving partner.

Psychological interventions for families

Psychological interventions with families tend to occur in the context of heterosexual transmission, and in particular when children are affected, either directly as a result of their own infection, or indirectly when one or both parents are affected (see Chapter 1).

Lippmann et al (1993) have stressed the need to ensure that the integrity and supportiveness of the family are maintained. Education about the risks of infection to other family members and time to answer questions about HIV will be the first step in helping many families. The opportunity to express painful emotions within the family can then lead to finding effective ways of dealing with the difficulties both for the family as a whole, and for its individual members. Fears about breach of confidentiality and isolation from potential sources of support can be explored.

Families with haemophilia and HIV infection face particular problems compounded by the presence of two major health problems (Miller et al, 1989). In the case of children and adolescents 'family secrets' (e.g. parents desire not to inform the child about his HIV status) may have to be tackled firmly but sensitively, especially when the adolescent is likely to commence sexual activity or when treatment for his HIV condition is indicated (Brown and DeMaio, 1992). Greenblat et al (1989) have developed a programme of active intervention for families and individuals with haemophilia and HIV infection, including role play and psychoeducational interventions. In counselling families Tsiantis and Meyer (1992) stress the importance of strengthening the couple and maintaining the family routine, avoidance of secrecy about HIV within the family, avoidance of unnecessary publicity and isolation, and facilitation of mourning.

Counselling about pregnancy in couples where the man has haemophilia and HIV infection will need sensitive and skilled intervention. Goldman et al (1992) counselled 26 such couples, of whom 14 decided against having children, and 12 decided to have a family. Advice was given about methods to reduce risk of infection. A total of 14 children were born, all seronegative. One of the women was HIV seropositive, but the timing and route of infection were not known. The authors made the point that none of the couples regretted their decision.

Further detailed information on interventions with children and their families is available in Claxton and Harrison (1991) and Sherr (1991).

Psychological interventions in prisons

Incarcerated individuals with HIV infection and those at risk of infection face especial difficulties as a result of prison conditions, pre-existing difficulties and legislation. Counselling and testing raise problems of lack of confidentiality and of management of the prisoner as a especial case, and risk reduction strategies can be restricted by prison regulations (Curran et al, 1989). Prisons are an important link in the transmission of the infection, both through injecting drug use and sexual behaviour (Bird et al, 1993), and the care of HIV infected prisoners should be co-ordinated with access to care in general hospitals, including availability of mental health services (Strang and Stimson, 1990; Dixon et al, 1993). The World Health Organization has stressed the need to ensure that drug users in prison have access to treatment for their drug dependence as well as care for HIV-related problems, including the prevention of suicidal behaviour (WHO, 1990a).

5.2.5 Palliative care and bereavement

The final stages of caring for people with advanced HIV infection require attention to the physical and psychological needs when curative interventions are no longer appropriate, and the provision of care for bereaved partners and relatives.

Palliative care

The medical specialty of palliative medicine, less than 30 years old, has led to the development of models of care for those in the final stages of illness, when curative interventions are no longer effective and death is likely in the near future (Hillier, 1988), and its lessons have been applied to the care of people dying as a result of HIV infection (Morissette, 1990; Maddocks, 1990; Cole, 1991; Mansfield et al, 1992). While in curative interventions the main objective is to ensure survival and remission, even at the cost of undesirable treatment side-effects, in palliative care improvement in quality of life, increase in comfort and symptom relief are the principal objectives (Ashby and Stoffell, 1991).

Where does palliative care take place?

The setting where death occurs can be the result of individual choice, but it is likely to be influenced by the existing local resources. **Acute medical facilities** are seldom geared to the provision of comprehensive palliative care, but the fact that acute medical care may be necessary to minimize painful conditions or those that can reduce quality of life means that people with AIDS die in such settings (George, 1991; Mansfield et al, 1992). Many people would choose to die at **home**, provided adequate supports are available. Although there have been important developments in home care provision for people dying with AIDS, it is clear that there is a long way to go before such facilities are the norm (Goldstone, 1992; Higginson, 1993). **Hospice care** is the third alternative, and there are good examples of hospices developed in response to HIV infection, such as the London Lighthouse (Cantacuzino, 1993) and Mildmay Mission Hospital (Moss, 1988). Sadly, not all hospices are prepared to accept people dying with HIV infection (Higginson, 1993), showing that discrimination can occur even when dying. Another form of residential facility, which has developed as a result of HIV, is aimed at caring for with HIV-associated dementia or other major HIV-brain related disorders, often until death. Patrick House in London and the Care Unit, St. Mary's Hospital and Medical Center in San Francisco are two examples of services to deal with this distressing problem.

Interventions in palliative care

Wherever death occurs, in hospital, at home or in a hospice, coordination of medical, nursing, psychological and social care will be required (Sims and Moss, 1991). Common medical problems requiring intervention are: the management of pain, including the use of opiates and other analgesics together with explanation, relaxation and support; treatment of nausea and vomiting; and management of loss of appetite and weight (Moss, 1990) (for detailed review see Sims and Moss, 1991).

Psychological interventions tend to be focused on current difficulties, and will cover the range of approaches used for people with HIV infection (Welsby and Richardson, 1993). Encouraging communication, provision of accurate information in a sensitive manner, exploration of fears and concerns, help to make sense of one's predicament and to complete any unfinished business can occur in the context of a safe, confiding therapeutic relationship (Stedeford, 1984; Sims and Moss, 1991). Fears of dying may be focused on the anticipation of pain or discomfort; separation from loved ones; fear of loss of control and dependence on others; or concerns about after life. Anger and distress may alternate with denial of the consequences of the condition. Concerns for relatives or partners may become prominent.

One situation that can sometimes cause difficulties for those caring for someone receiving palliative care is the presence of persistent denial of the severity of the person's condition. While there are many ways of coping with impending death, denial is sometimes seen as less satisfactory than other forms of coping, in particular if it means that unrealistic plans are being made or that personal affairs are not being dealt with. It is important to try to assess the reasons for the denial: it may well be part of a long-standing way of coping and, thus, not so easy to alter at this stage, but it may still be useful to provide the opportunity for the person to explore his or her fears and concerns. Psychiatric disorders need to be excluded, such as mania or cognitive impairment which prevent accurate perception of the situation (Vachon, 1993).

There is some empirical evidence that some mental strategies used by terminally ill people can help maintain a sense of hope in the face of death. Herth (1990) identified several hope-fostering attributes: presence of meaningful shared relationship with another person; directing efforts to some goal; having spiritual beliefs; perceiving oneself as determined and courageous; being able to maintain a sense of lightheartedness; recalling uplifting memories and events; and feeling accepted and valued by those around them. By contrast, feeling abandoned or isolated; suffering uncontrollable pain; and feeling unwanted or uncared for, all contributed to the loss of hope. Although these experiences may not be universal, they provide practical guidelines for those involved in helping people facing death.

Palliative care raises potentially difficult ethical problems in relation to discontinuation of care, advanced directives and euthanasia (George, 1991; Mansfield et al, 1992) some of which are considered in Chapter 8.

Grief and its management

Grief is a universal human experience but its manifestations are influenced by many factors, such as the circumstances of the death, the nature of the relationship between the bereaved and the dead person, the personality and other characteristics of the bereaved, and the social, cultural and interpersonal circumstances of the survivor.

The majority of bereaved individuals experience a pattern of psychological distress which is within the culturally sanctioned range of responses, while a substantial minority suffer more significant and severe disruption of their psychological and social functioning. It is in such cases that the term **pathological grief** is used (Engel, 1961). While there is a risk of medicalizing grief, as in the case of other human experiences like birth and death, it has to be recognized that for some individuals, grief can reach an intensity or duration of such degree that it interferes significantly with the person's life. Furthermore, individuals experiencing pathological grief can benefit from specific psychological and social interventions.

Normal grief

The psychological, biological and social consequences of loss and bereavement have been the subject of a variety of descriptive studies (see amongst them Lindeman, 1944; Parkes, 1972). Kubler-Ross (1970) thinks of mourning as evolving through a number of **stages**: denial and isolation; anger; bargaining; depression; and acceptance, while stressing that these are not inevitable or fixed in their occurrence. Others like Parkes (1970, 1972) and Bowlby (1980) view grief as involving **phases**: numbness; yearning and anger; disorganization and despair; and reorganization. Worden (1992) uses the concept of **tasks of mourning**: acceptance of the reality of the loss; working through the pain of grief; adjustment to an environment without the deceased person; and emotional relocation of the dead person. It has been argued that the idea of tasks add a sense of activity and working through on the part of the bereaved and the opportunity to focus on specific aspects of the process to achieve completion of the process (Worden, 1992).

Factors associated with the manifestations of grief

Not everyone responds to loss in the same way, and it is clear that descriptions of the process of normal grief provide only an idealized model. In practice, a variety of psychological and social factors will contribute to modulate the expression of grief. Worden (1992) has summarized its most important determinants: who the person was (partner as opposed to distant relative); the nature of the relationship (its strength, security, ambivalence, and conflicts); mode of death (expected, suicidal, or in tragic circumstances); past experience of losses; personality of the bereaved; social variables and supports; and the existence of concurrent stresses.

HIV infection provides a fertile ground for the development of pathological grief. The stigma associated with the disease can lead to reduced social supports and rejection by others, fears of contagion may affect partners and relatives, exposure to multiple losses is likely to lead to increased difficulty accepting the reality of the loss and the expression of affect, death of young individuals does increase the sense of waste and sadness, and the presence of painful and disfiguring complications can add to the persistence of disturbing memories for the bereaved. Child death followed by parental death can lead to problems for the surviving children. Often, relatives have been kept in the dark about the disease until rather late in the condition, curtailing the length of time that they can devote to caring for the sick person.

Pathological grief

As with normal grief, there have been many attempts to develop a conceptual understanding of pathological grief (Freud, 1917; Deutsch, 1937; Lindeman, 1944; Bowlby, 1980) and to obtain empirical evidence for its characteristics and course (Parkes, 1970; Clayton ,1990; Jacobs et al, 1989, 1990). By comparison with uncomplicated grief, pathological grief will be characterized by marked differences in its intensity, specific manifestations, and evolution over time. While it is not always easy to differentiate normal and abnormal grief, there have been useful attempts to provide operational definitions (see Jacobs, 1993). In some cases, grief can lead to clear-cut and well-recognized psychiatric syndromes, such as major depression or anxiety disorders, where the bereavement has acted as a precipitant for the psychiatric disorder.

Lazare (1979) has suggested a number of useful clues to identify pathological grief: the person cannot talk about the deceased without experiencing fresh grief; minor events trigger off an intense grief response; loss is often a topic of conversation; reluctance to move the deceased's belongings; the bereaved reports physical symptoms similar to those of the dead person; radical and sudden lifestyle changes following the loss; or the presence of death or illness fears and phobias. The frequency with which pathological grief occurs will depend to some extent on the criteria used to define it, but a commonly mentioned figure is that quoted by Jacobs (1993), who states that about 20 per cent of bereaved individuals experience pathological grief.

(a) Absent or delayed grief In this form of pathological grief there is absence or delay of the manifestations of numbness and disbelief, separation distress and subsequent features usually associated with normal grief, for a period of at least two weeks. In some cases, the delay may be a matter of months or even years.

Not infrequently, further losses or seemingly less significant experiences of sadness may act as triggers for the onset of obvious grief.

Absent or delayed grief should not be confused with the presence of mild manifestations of mourning in someone who has experienced grief prior to the actual loss, as for example in the case of a person nursing and looking after a loved one during terminal illness. The term **anticipatory grief** (Lindeman, 1944) has been used to describe this form of normal grief.

(b) Chronic grief In normal grief there is a good deal of variation in the duration of the manifestations of mourning, although it is usually assumed that it is within the first year that most of the distressing features occur. Anniversary reactions are regarded as normal even many years after the loss. In chronic grief there is not only persistence over time in the intensity of thoughts and emotions associated to the deceased, but there is also a subjective sense of not being able to return to normal living and of not having worked through the process of mourning. In the terminology of Worden (1992), the tasks of mourning have not been completed, so that the reality of the loss may not have been accepted, adjustment to an environment without the deceased has not begun to happen, or the dead person has not been emotionally relocated by the bereaved. Preoccupation with the grave, either resulting in avoidance of visits, or very frequent visiting is not uncommon. Sometimes the room and possessions of the deceased are left unchanged, as if waiting for the person to return. The bereaved person's life remains dominated by the deceased, without returning to a normal life, and leading to the exclusion of other relationships.

(c) Inhibited or distorted grief Instead of the usual phases or tasks seen in normal mourning, an erratic pattern of emotional responses and thoughts is present, without a clear evolutionary progress. Complaints of somatic symptoms (headaches, palpitations), anxiety or depression, or behavioural manifestations such as hostility, displaced anger, overidentification with the deceased, may become more prominent than the usual features of grief. As in chronic grief, the person may be aware of not working through the loss.

(d) Severe grief The difference between normal and severe grief is only one of degree, with marked separation distress, crying, yearning, somatic manifestations and perceptual and cognitive disturbances. The severity of the early features of grief may be a predictor of chronic grief.

(e) Grief associated with psychiatric disorder Whatever the pattern of the grief reaction, some individuals may develop frank psychiatric syndromes in association with the loss. In some cases, the person may have experienced similar problems in response to other undesirable life events, suggesting the presence of vulnerability or predisposition to psychiatric disorders. When grief is associated with significant psychiatric disturbance, it is legitimate to assess and manage the problem taking into account both the precipitant (the loss) and the characteristics of the specific syndrome, so as to provide effective help. The most

frequently seen psychiatric syndromes are post traumatic stress disorders, depressive disorders and anxiety disorders (see below).

Management of grief

Worden (1992) has made a useful distinction between **grief counselling**: help to facilitate normal, uncomplicated grief, and **grief therapy**: interventions to help resolve pathological grief. In practice, most people faced with uncomplicated grief seldom come into contact with professionals with particular expertise in the field, although they may well come into contact with health and social workers who are in a good position to facilitate or hinder their mourning.

(a) Facilitating normal grief As described above, mourning is an active process which involves tasks, stages or phases, and the role of facilitating normal grief involves working with the bereaved person to work through and complete this process. Few people experiencing grief will seek professional help, the majority being supported by friends and relatives. Some, however, will come into contact with statutory or independent sources of help. In most instances, the person providing help will take a rather non-interventionist role, encouraging and giving permission for the person to explore and experience feelings and thoughts, rather than prescribing a particular kind of mourning. While there are different techniques and approaches to grief counselling, in practice there are some shared themes. Worden (1992) has described ten principles to help the bereaved person work through grief:

1. Help to actualize the loss, for example, by encouraging description of the death, its circumstances and aftermath.
2. Help to identify and express feelings, in particular anger and guilt, which may be regarded as unacceptable.
3. Help to start living without the dead person, which may involve making decisions and changes without being frozen by the need to guess what the dead person might have done or expected.
4. Help to relocate the dead person emotionally, in particular regarding establishing new relationships.
5. Allow time to grieve, recognizing that the whole process does take time, and giving the bereaved permission to do it at their own pace.
6. Reassure the bereaved about the normality of their feelings, so that they do not fear losing their mind as a result of the experience.
7. Allow for individual differences, once more providing reassurance about the range of responses and ways of coping.
8. Give access to longer term, non-intensive support.
9. Explore coping styles, in particular the use of potentially maladaptive methods such as alcohol misuse.
10. Identify unresolved grief and take steps to provide further help when necessary.

In the context of AIDS, reading material prepared by those with practical experience in dealing with the consequences of the infection can help to anticipate problems and to reduce the sense of isolation. Martelli et al (1987), Sims and Moss (1991), and Kirkpatrick (1993) are examples of books with useful practical information which can help prevent problems.

Psychotropic medication is usually not indicated in the majority of cases of uncomplicated grief. However, short-term use of hypnotics to allow the grieving person to have the chance to rest at night, and so have the opportunity to continue adapting to the loss, may be of value if there is severe and persistent insomnia.

(b) Grief therapy The variety of pathological grief reactions and the range of personal and cultural differences that exist suggest that there is no simple, universal approach to dealing successfully with pathological grief, and that it will be important to tailor the intervention to the specific problems and needs of each particular bereaved person. Psychological interventions will sometimes need to be complemented by the use of psychopharmacological approaches, in particular when grief is associated with psychiatric disorders.

1. *Psychological interventions* The majority of specific interventions that have been the subject of outcome research are of relatively brief duration, usually around three or four months. This does not mean that in all cases, psychological intervention is effective in such rapid way. In practice, grief therapy can be a lengthy procedure, requiring a range of therapeutic skills and approaches.

Individual crisis intervention approaches, focusing on the expression of grief, have been shown to be effective for people at risk of complicated grief (Raphael, 1975, 1977a, b), while family-based crisis intervention has not been shown to be effective (Williams and Polak, 1979).

Behavioural therapies, such as guided mourning (Mawson et al, 1981) are effective in dealing with the features of unresolved grief, in particular its avoidant behavioural aspects.

Brief psychodynamic individual psychotherapy (Marmar et al, 1988) has been shown to be as effective as peer-support groups, but the study did not include a no or minimal treatment group.

When pathological grief is associated with psychiatric syndromes, such as PTSD, depression or anxiety disorders, specific psychological interventions for these disorders will be required (Gelder et al, 1989).

2. *Psychopharmacological interventions* There has been no systematic research about the use of psychopharmacological treatments for pathological grief, and what knowledge there is rests basically on clinical experience and is essentially symptomatic: hypnotic medication for insomnia, antidepressants for severe depressive disorders, and sedative for short periods when severe distress and anxiety becoming disabling.

3. *Other psychiatric interventions* Pathological grief associated with psychiatric disorders may sometimes require the use of approaches familiar to

psychiatrists, such as hospitalization or the use of other physical methods of treatment, such as ECT for severe depression. Clearly, what is being treated in such cases is not so much the pathological grief, but its psychiatric manifestations.

4. *Peer or mutual support interventions* Community-based mutual support groups have been an important feature of the HIV epidemic in developing countries, and it is fair to say that the range of services provided by such supports groups could not have been matched by professional statutory agencies (Arno, 1986; Williams, 1988). Bereavement counselling services for people affected by HIV infection have been an integral part of such services, often working in collaboration with professional and statutory services (Sims and Moss, 1991; Kirkpatrick, 1993).

5.3 Psychopharmacological interventions

Here we shall review physical methods of treatment for two groups of conditions: psychiatric problems associated with HIV infection, and HIV-related neuropsychiatric disorders.

5.3.1 Treatment of HIV-related psychiatric disorders

Psychopharmacological and other physical methods of treatment, such as electroconvulsive therapy (ECT), can be very useful in the management of psychiatric disorders associated with HIV infection. As in all cases of psychiatric disorder associated with physical disease (Taylor et al, 1985; Gelder et al, 1989; Lloyd, 1991), it is important to make sure that an accurate assessment of the indications for the use of medication is made before using drugs; that the right preparation and dosage are selected; and that the possibility of interaction with other preparations is considered, including complementary treatments and recreational drugs (Greenblatt et al, 1991; Barton et al, 1994).

It is desirable to select medication with minimal side-effects, such as anticholinergic, sedating or extrapyramidal drugs, as their presence may add to the discomfort of people already suffering from symptoms related to their HIV infection, and in turn affect compliance with treatment. It is often argued on the basis of clinical experience that people with HIV infection, in particular those with advanced disease, are more sensitive to the therapeutic and undesirable side-effects of psychotropic medication, and so particular care is needed when choosing preparations and dosages (Ostrow et al, 1988; Ostrow, 1990; Fernandez and Levy, 1990; Ayuso-Mateos, 1994).

Antidepressants

Antidepressants are the treatment of choice in major depression and in less severe depressive syndromes unresponsive to psychological and social intervention. Phobic and obsessive–compulsive disorders may also respond to treatment with antidepressants (Taylor et al, 1985; Gelder et al, 1989).

Tricyclic antidepressants (imipramine, desipramine and amitriptyline) have been shown to be effective in treating depressed patients with HIV infection in both controlled (Fernandez et al, 1989c; Manning et al, 1990; Rabkin et al, 1994) and open trials (Rabkin and Harrison, 1990) using standard doses (see review by Markowitz et al, 1994). They are thought to be particularly effective in asymptomatic individuals (Fernandez and Levy, 1990). It has been suggested that stimulant antidepressants such as imipramine may be more appropriate in HIV patients in view of the lack of energy associated with depression in many cases (Perry, 1993). There is some evidence from studies not involving HIV patients that dothiepin can be associated with greater toxicity (Buckley et al, 1994) and this should be balanced against its possible advantages.

The new **selective serotonin re-uptake inhibitor (SSRI)** antidepressants appear to be of comparable efficacy to the older preparations and have possibly a better side-effect profile, although they are at present more costly (Song et al, 1993). Their use in people with HIV infection has only being subject to open trials which show encouraging results (Singh and Catalán, 1993; Singh et al, 1994) (see Markowitz et al, 1994 for review).

There are no published reports about the use of monoamine oxidase inhibitors (MAOI) in HIV, although clinical use suggests they can be of value, although it is important to consider the possibility of drug interactions (Ostrow et al, 1988).

Sedatives and major tranquillizers

Sedatives and major tranquillizers are indicated in case of acute brain disorders (delirium) and in HIV-associated psychotic conditions such as mania and schizophrenia-like disorders.

High potency neuroleptics such as haloperidol are commonly used in the treatment of delirium and psychotic disorders in the general hospital, sometimes in combination with diazepam (Lipowski, 1990; Pilowsky et al, 1992). They have been recommended in people with HIV infection, regardless of disease stage (Ostrow et al, 1988; Fernandez et al, 1989b; Ostrow, 1990).

There is concern, however, about the risk of development of extrapyramidal syndromes in people with HIV infection when using high potency dopamine-blocking agents, such as haloperidol and chlorpromazine, in particular in advanced stages of disease when some degree of HIV associated encephalopathy likely to include subtantia nigra abnormalities may be present (Hriso et al, 1991; Reyes et al, 1991). It is recommended to start with relatively low doses, possibly in combination with benzodiazepines, or alternatively to use lower potency neuroleptics. The new atypical antipsychotics, with their selective dopamine D_2 receptor blocking effects and absence of striatal action may well be preferable to the classical antipsychotics (Kerwin, 1994). although reports on their use in people with HIV infection are few. Remoxipride, a selective dopamine D_2 antagonist has been used in the treatment of HIV-associated mania with good results, but in view of its possible contribution to aplastic anaemia, remoxipride should be used with caution (Scurlock et al, 1994).

Anxiolytics and hypnotics

Psychological interventions are the treatment of choice for anxiety disorders and insomnia (see above), and the use of long-term anxiolytic medication should not be encouraged (Livingstone, 1994), although 'psychopharmacological Calvinism', the belief that using mind-altering drugs is bad for one's moral character and therefore should be avoided at all costs, is probably out of place when dealing with people with advanced HIV infection facing major health problems: the efficacy of the drug rather than its ideological connotations should be given priority. In general, it is best to prescribe anxiolytics for a limited period of time, while other psychological and social interventions are also introduced. Benzodiazepines are the drugs of choice, and it is best to avoid the longer-acting ones which are likely to lead to oversedation. Antidepressant drugs can also be used to treat anxiety disorders, in particular those with phobic or obsessional symptoms (Taylor et al, 1985; Gelder et al, 1989).

Psychostimulants

Stimulants, such as methylphenidate and dextroamphetamine, can improve mood and attention and lead to increase in energy, and they have been used in the treatment of psychiatric disorders and in medically ill patients (Chiarello and Cole, 1987).

There are no controlled investigations of the value of psychostimulants in HIV infection, although uncontrolled studies in depressed people with HIV infection who had not responded to tricyclic antidepressants or with some degree of cognitive impairment have shown improvement in mood and cognitive functioning (Fernandez et al, 1988; Holmes et al, 1989; Fernandez and Levy, 1990; Ostrow, 1990). Psychostimulants tend to be used for short periods of time, often during the terminal phase of the illness (Ostrow et al, 1988). The lack of controlled studies and their possible side-effects (agitation, elated mood, restlessness, anorexia, and weight loss, paranoid syndromes, and risk of misuse) means that if they are to be prescribed, it should be under close monitoring and evaluation.

Other physical methods of treatment

Electroconvulsive therapy has been used successfully in people with HIV infection with major depression and delusions, even in the presence of some degree of diffuse cortical atrophy identified by MRI (Schaerf et al, 1989). Careful evaluation of the physical status of the patient will be required.

Lithium preparations are effective in the prevention of bipolar affective disorders, as well as in the treatment of mania and resistant depression (Gelder et al, 1989; Goodwin, 1994).

Anticonvulsants can be used in the treatment of mania (Goodwin, 1994) and they have been reported to be an effective alternative to lithium and neuroleptics in the treatment of HIV-associated mania (Halman et al, 1993).

Appetite stimulants to prevent loss of or to increase body weight are being used in patients with HIV infection. Directly or indirectly these drugs are thought to have some effect on overall well-being. Megestrol, a progestogen, and cyproheptadine appear to be of some value in leading to weight gain, but the former is associated with the development of sexual dysfunctions in men (Summerbell et al, 1992). Anabolic steroids have acquired a certain popularity in recent years, and while uncontrolled studies indicate that they are effective in increasing lean body mass (Jekot and Purdy, 1993), there is concern about possible side-effects (mood elevation, irritability, mood swings and cognitive impairment) and their effects on immune function (Su et al, 1993).

5.3.2 Treatment of HIV-related neuropsychiatric disorders

Zidovudine (ZDV)

Despite the great progress that has been made in treating many of the diseases associated with AIDS and symptomatic HIV infection, there are few available treatments for HIV associated dementia. Indeed, the only well-established treatment is zidovudine (ZDV). The effectiveness of ZDV in prolonging life in people with AIDS and symptomatic HIV infection is now almost universally accepted (Fischl et al, 1987) and there is also a quite substantial body of evidence that ZDV has a beneficial effect on cognitive function in people with HIV-1 associated dementia. The evidence for this comes from several different sources: circumstantial evidence, uncontrolled trials, natural experiments and a few controlled trials.

The **circumstantial evidence** for the efficacy of ZDV comes from retrospective analyses of changes in both the prevalence of dementia and a reduction in the neuropathological markers associated with dementia that were noted at about the time ZDV was introduced. Portegies et al (1989) reported that before the introduction of ZDV to The Netherlands in 1987, as many as 53 per cent of patients with AIDS attending their clinic were diagnosed with AIDS dementia complex. By 1988, the prevalence had fallen to 3 per cent of all AIDS patients and similar changes have been reported from other countries (Vago et al, 1993). On first inspection, the evidence from these studies appears compelling, but some caution is in order. Simply showing that changes in the incidence of dementia or of neuropathological markers occurred at the same time as the introduction of ZDV does not mean that the two events are linked. Changes in the diagnostic and pathological procedures which began during the same period of time could account for the association, although this seems improbable. It is more likely that changes in the incidence of dementia were due to the effects of other treatments, many of which were introduced at around the same time as ZDV. There is some evidence that this might be the case. Maehlen et al (1993) reported that multinucleated giant cells were found in the brains of 50 per cent of their patients who died with AIDS before the introduction of ZDV compared with only 20 per cent afterwards. What is interesting about this finding is that the reduction occurred in both the ZDV treated and untreated patients.

Further evidence for the efficacy of ZDV in the amelioration of HIV-1 associated cognitive deficits comes from a large number of **single case studies and uncontrolled trials**. There are now well over 50 such studies that have been reported at conferences although only a few have been published. These reports consistently show that ZDV can ameliorate or even partially reverse the cognitive impairment that is often seen in people with AIDS (Yarchoan et al, 1987, 1988) or symptomatic disease (Riccio et al, 1990). Although most research has focused on the efficacy of ZDV in adults, some reports have shown quite striking improvements in the cognitive performance of children (Pizzo et al, 1988; Brouwers et al, 1990). In most studies, the effect of ZDV has been assessed using neuropsychological tests but other measures of cerebral function have given similar results. Studies using electroencephalography (Parisi et al, 1988b), single photon emission tomography (Masdeu et al, 1991) and positron emission tomography (Brunetti et al, 1989; Pizzo et al, 1988) have concluded that ZDV can partially reverse the functional cerebral abnormalities in some people with AIDS although the numbers reported so far have been small. There is also evidence of structural improvements in the brains of people who have been on ZDV. Tozzi et al (1993), using magnetic resonance imaging, found a reduction in the number of white matter lesions in some patients following treatment with ZDV compared with their scans 12 months earlier.

There have been several reports on the efficacy of ZDV which may be thought of as **natural experiments**. In these studies the impact of ZDV was examined retrospectively by comparing patients who were treated with ZDV with those who were not. The two largest neuropsychological studies of this type have found that ZDV has a beneficial impact on cognitive function although this benefit is transient and probably lasts little more than 6 months (McArthur et al, 1990b; Baldeweg et al, in press a). Similar findings have been reported from neuropathological studies where those treated with ZDV had a lower incidence of HIV encephalitis, HIV leucoencephalopathy and multinucleated giant cells than those who had never been treated (Gray et al, 1994). Although the neuropathological markers of dementia are usually less common in those treated with ZDV, other opportunistic infections appear to be more frequent (Davies et al, 1993). The most probable explanation of this is that the longer survival time associated with ZDV increases the opportunity for the development of secondary infections in the brain. Although the evidence from these natural experiments is encouraging, since the patients were not matched or randomly allocated to treatment groups, the differences seen may not be due to ZDV, but may reflect other pre-existing differences between the groups.

To date, only two **double blind placebo controlled trials** of the efficacy of ZDV on cognitive performance in people with symptomatic HIV infection and AIDS have been reported (Schmitt et al, 1988; Sidtis et al, 1993). In each case, the follow up periods were short, but those on ZDV showed significant improvement in their cognitive performance compared with controls. It may be, however, that the cognitive benefits were an indirect consequence of the improvement in physical health resulting from ZDV rather than a direct effect of the drug on the brain. As the efficacy of ZDV is now well established, it is no longer ethical to compare ZDV with placebo in controlled trials for patients with symptomatic disease. For this reason, no further double blind placebo controlled studies examining the effects of ZDV on cognition in AIDS and symptomatic disease can be expected.

Two studies are under way which seek to determine whether ZDV given in asymptomatic infection will prevent or reduce the risk of the development of cognitive impairment as the disease progresses (Grunseit et al, 1991; Baldeweg et al, in press, b). Neither study found any clear benefit from taking ZDV, but this is unsurprising as HIV has minimal impact on cognitive function in the asymptomatic stage of disease. The important question is whether early treatment with ZDV prevents the development of impairments later on. Unfortunately, the studies reported so far will not be able to answer this question for some years. In the Baldeweg et al (in press b) study, which analysed a sample of patients from the Concorde study, even over the follow-up period of three years, few patients developed symptomatic disease or AIDS. As cognitive impairment is either rare or minor before the development of symptomatic disease, the chance of detecting differences between the treated and untreated groups was not good. There were, however, subclinical differences between the groups in their EEGs such that the untreated group showed a small increase in slow waves compared with the treated group. It is of note that these changes are of the same type as those reported in HIV-1 associated dementia, albeit of lower magnitude, and it is tempting to interpret them as the precursors of dementia. As these changes occurred only in the untreated group, the implication is that ZDV may provide protection against the earliest signs of dementia. Such a conclusion would, however, be premature at this stage, and will only be confirmed by follow-up over a longer period. Indeed, other evidence suggests that taking ZDV before the development of symptomatic disease has no effect on the risk of developing HIV-1 associated dementia. In a retrospective study of nearly 500 gay men, the risk of developing dementia was found to be associated with several factors including haemoglobin levels and body mass index, but was not associated with ZDV use (McArthur et al, 1993).

Overall, the balance of evidence suggests that ZDV has a beneficial effect on cognitive functioning in advanced HIV disease although the effect is short-lived and probably lasts about six months. In practice, most people who present with HIV-1 associated dementia will either be taking ZDV already or will be intolerant to it which leaves the physician with very limited treatment options. Many of the studies on the cerebral effects of ZDV have used 1000 mg daily, much higher than the usual dosage of 250 mg twice a day. For this reason, one commonly used therapeutic option is to raise the dosage to 500 mg twice a day or higher, but there is no good evidence of improved efficacy with this dose. Another option is to administer ZDV intrathecally and the few reports that have described doing so report that ZDV is well tolerated and effective (Routy et al, 1990). As time goes by, however, the development of ZDV resistant variants of HIV-1, which have already been reported in the brain (Di Stefano et al, 1993) will make even these options ineffective.

Other anti-retroviral medication

ZDV is no longer the only anti-retroviral therapy available but the efficacy of new agents in the treatment of HIV-1 associated dementia remains to be established (e.g. dideoxyinosine, ddI; and dideoxycytosine, ddC). There are some preliminary reports of treatment of dementia using ddI (Wolters et al, 1991), but ddC is unlikely to be effective as it does not cross the blood–brain barrier.

Other pharmacological treatments

Anti-retroviral therapies are no longer the only therapeutic agents available. **Vitamin B_{12}** deficiency is a well-known cause of neurological and neuropsychiatric disease, and abnormalities of vitamin B_{12} metabolism, leading to deficiency, are commonly seen in people with AIDS (Remacha et al, 1991). For these reasons, it has been suggested that vitamin B_{12} deficiency may be a contributory factor in the development of HIV-1 associated dementia. If this were the case, treatment would be straightforward and there is at least one case report of an apparently successful treatment of HIV-1 associated dementia through the administration of vitamin B_{12} (Herzlich and Schiano 1993). The association between vitamin B_{12} deficiency and HIV-1 associated dementia is unclear, however, with some studies finding an association (Kieburtz et al, 1991a; Beach et al, 1992) whilst others find no such link (Robertson et al, 1993). Even if it were found that vitamin B_{12} deficiency is associated with HIV-1 associated dementia, it might not be the case that the two are aetiologically linked. Another explanation would be that both B_{12} deficiency and dementia tend to be seen together because both are most commonly seen only in advanced AIDS. Despite this uncertainty, because treatment is easy and safe, it is advisable to check B_{12} levels in those who present with HIV-1 associated dementia and prescribe accordingly.

Another treatment of HIV-1 associated dementia that has been reported is **peptide T**. It is known that gp120, the HIV envelope protein causes neuronal death *in vitro* and is found in neurotoxic levels in the cerebrospinal fluid of patients in the early stages of HIV infection. It has also been established that peptide T blocks the neurotoxic effects of gp120 (Buzy et al, 1992). In addition there have been reports showing that peptide T is effective in reversing the cognitive deficits in people with AIDS (Bridge et al, 1989) although this is not a treatment that has been used widely.

As more is understood about the ways in which HIV attacks the brain, new medications may become available. Recently, Ca^{2+} has been implicated in neuronal death (Lipton, 1992) which suggests a possible role for calcium channel blockers in treatment, though the widespread physiological importance of Ca^{2+} presents considerable difficulties. Similarly, **quinolinic acid** may play an important role in the destruction of neuronal tissue and strategies that reduce the metabolism of this neurotoxin may prove helpful (Heyes et al, 1991). Such treatments lie in the future, but as our understanding of the effects of HIV on the brain at the cellular and biochemical level improves the prospect of developing new and more effective treatments looks increasingly promising.

5.4 Psychiatric hospitalization and residential care

5.4.1 In-patient psychiatric care

As discussed in Chapters 1 and 2, a small proportion of people with HIV infection referred to mental health specialists requires in-patient psychiatric care.

This group tends to include patients suffering from the more severe psychiatric disorders, such as major depression, mania and schizophrenia-like disorders, and suicidal individuals. It also includes people with a principal diagnosis of personality disorder, who experience persistent difficulties coping with the stresses associated with HIV infection.

Patients with HIV-related brain impairment may require psychiatric hospitalization, especially if they also manifest severe behavioural problems that are difficult to manage in the community or in a medical in-patient unit (Baer, 1989). The experience of a dedicated HIV dementia unit in San Francisco suggest that patients can benefit from rehabilitation and medical care, a proportion being discharged and returning to home care (Ostrow et al, 1992; Esterson, et al, 1992). Early fears about the risk of an epidemic of HIV-related dementia and the need to develop extensive inpatient psychiatric facilities (Tannock and Collier, 1989) have not materialized (Catalán and Riccio, 1990c).

The clinical management of psychiatric in-patients with HIV infection is driven by their principal diagnosis and problems, as in the case of any other in-patient, but there are special issues that need attention. Baer (1989) has described his experiences in an in-patient psychiatric unit in San Francisco, where some beds had been allocated to the care of patients with HIV. Over a period of 18 months they admitted 36 patients with advanced HIV disease suffering from severe psychiatric problems. Prior to the start of the service and at regular intervals a programme of staff training was implemented, and nursing staff were given the opportunity of transferring to another department. Baer identified a range of problems during the study period. Staff were unused to caring for terminally ill people and overidentification with patients and distress required the setting up of supervision and support, individually and in groups. Other patients found young AIDS patients with dementia difficult to cope with, and fears of contagion and feelings of rejection led to the setting up of a weekly educational health group for all patients. Infection control guidelines were made available to all. Diagnostic dilemmas were common, in particular concerning depression and dementia. Development of severe side-effects from medication, neuroleptics in particular, led to greater care with use of medication. Ethical issues were often discussed (Binder, 1987), and also the needs of friends and relatives who might have been unaware of the person's HIV infection.

Other problems in psychiatric units include the need to ensure a very close collaboration with medical colleagues and access to diagnostic and treatment facilities to maintain good standards of care, and the ethical and practical problems involved in managing HIV risky behaviours (Carlson et al, 1989; Cournos et al, 1990). There is evidence for the feasibility and effectiveness of HIV risk reduction education for psychiatric patients (Lauer-Listhaus and Watterson, 1988; Sladyk, 1989).

In addition to the situations described above where the patients' HIV status was known to their professional carers, there is increasing evidence that a small but important proportion of acute and chronic psychiatric patients are HIV seropositive without their serostatus having been identified during their hospitalization. The practical and ethical problems raised are discussed in Chapter 8.

5.4.2 Non-psychiatric residential care

The needs of people with HIV infection and their families has led to the development of residential facilities to deal with some of the problems occurring in advanced disease. These new initiatives have usually been the result of non-statutory agencies that have attempted to fill the gaps left by the statutory health and social services. In practice, residential models of care have complemented care provided in hospitals, which tends to focus on the active treatment of acute problems, rather than longer-term social and palliative care (Singh et al, 1991).

Respite and palliative care services

Using the model of the hospice as its starting point, but usually including also educational, community and pastoral activities, HIV-dedicated facilities have been developed to provide people with advanced HIV disease with non-hospital residential care with access to medical and nursing expertise, and with a strong emphasis on the psychological and social needs. Palliative care facilities are usually combined with access to convalescent care following discharge from hospital and day care. Some centres include facilities for children and families. Good examples of such services are the London Lighthouse, a unique centre for care of people living with HIV infection (Cantacuzino, 1993) and Mildmay Mission Hospital (Sims and Moss, 1991) in London, and Noah's Ark–Red Cross Foundation in Stockholm (Florence, 1994).

Residential care for people with HIV-related brain disorder

The majority of people who develop severe HIV-related brain disease do so in the advanced stages of the disease, when other major HIV-related complications may necessitate acute medical care, respite care and home support. While this range of services is usually adequate for many such patients, there remains a small but important group of patients whose needs cannot easily be met by the combined efforts of the hospital and community services (Boccellari et al, 1991). These patients tend to have more severe behavioural problems, limited social and family supports, and may remain relatively well, without acute medical problems for periods of weeks or months. Some may benefit from in-patient psychiatric care (Ostrow et al, 1992; Esterson et al, 1992). Residential care tailored to their needs may be the best option. Patrick House in London is a good example of one such facility for people with brain-related impairment who are no longer able to live alone and whose carers cannot cope with their difficulties. Patrick House is a family-style home with four double-sized bedrooms and space for personal carers, with a multidisciplinary team providing 24 hour a day care.

Residential services for injecting drug users

The unique problems faced by injecting drug users with HIV infection has led to the development of residential services for their care. The Griffin Project in London is a good example of a continuing care unit for people with HIV infection who are also drug users. A multidisciplinary team offers nursing, medical, and social care, so that convalescent, respite and palliative care are available, together with access to drug stabilization, maintenance and detoxification programmes.

5.5 Community organizations and peer supports

People with HIV infection spend most of their time at home or in community settings, rather than in hospital, and it is therefore logical that the provision of supports for people to cope adequately in the community should be paramount, concentrating on those not requiring acute medical or psychiatric care, but still in need of access to a range of sources of help to prevent or delay their deterioration and to support relatives. Community care interventions need to address the social, psychological and medical needs of those with the infection and their partners and relatives (Wolcott et al, 1986b; Mail and Matheny, 1989; Beedham and Wilson-Barnett, 1993).

Financial and accommodation problems, inability to cope with everyday activities such as cooking, shopping, access to hospital clinics and other practical difficulties, as well as need for emotional support are common (Marazzi et al, 1994). There are, however, barriers to the provision of care outside hospital, and Widman et al (1994) in a study from the US found wide variations in the range of community resources planned for patients after hospitalization. In addition, doctors were less likely to plan further community care than social workers or nurses, and delay in service provision was more likely for white patients, the majority of whom were gay and perhaps perceived as more affluent and therefore less in need of statutory help.

Family doctors play an important part in the care of chronic disorders, both from a medical and psychological point of view, but general practitioners do not appear to have had the same degree of involvement with people with HIV infection as with other patient groups (Singh et al, 1993), with notable exceptions (Robertson et al, 1986). The attitudes and fears of both patients and doctors seem to have been responsible (King, 1988, 1989c, d; Mansfield and Singh, 1989), but there are examples of innovative projects to increase the involvement of family doctors in HIV care, as in the case of the St. Mary's Home Support Team in central London (Butters et al, 1991) and general practice facilitators (Saunders, 1994).

In developing countries. the pressures created by the numbers of people with HIV infection and the limited resources available have made home care programmes essential. The WHO has reported on six home-based models in Uganda and Zambia serving both rural and urban populations (Victor, 1989), providing access to medical and nursing care, palliative care, counselling and education, and practical help. The training of families to care for people at home has been shown to be feasible in developing countries with high HIV prevalence, such as Rwanda (Schietinger et al, 1993).

Many of the developing countries home care programmes mentioned were developed by non-governmental organizations (NGOs), a fact reflected in the services that have developed in the US and other countries (Arno, 1986; Williams, 1988; King, 1993b). Non-profit-making organizations have provided much invaluable support and care which statutory bodies would not have found possible to deliver alone. The Shanti Project in San Francisco, the Terrence Higgins Trust in London, and the Ankali Project in Sydney are examples of organizations offering emotional and practical support and counselling in the community for people with the infection and their families. The model of care developed in relation to HIV infection could well be applied to other severe disorders (McCullum et al, 1989).

5.6 Complementary interventions

Complementary or alternative medicine is not new, and there is a long tradition of tension between traditional or orthodox medicine, based on scientific principles, and a whole variety of other approaches based on different models and belief systems, often with strong philosophical or religious basis (British Medical Association, 1993). The term 'holistic health movement' is sometimes used to refer to this mixed group of interventions (Kopelman and Moskop, 1981). The degree to which these techniques are eventually incorporated into the mainstream therapies is variable, and probably depends on their empirical efficacy, as in the case of acupuncture, as well as changes in public and professional attitudes.

Diseases with an uncertain or chronic course, or those where scientific medical treatments are of limited value are much more likely to lead to the use of alternative or complementary therapies: not only can they reawaken the individual's sense of hope when all other approaches have failed, but they sometimes incorporate beliefs which help to give some meaning to the person's efforts. The practitioner involved in the provision of complementary therapies is usually warm and sympathetic and shows concern for the person's overall well-being, and not just the symptoms of disease, contributing to the person's feeling of being taken seriously. On the other hand, the need to find an effective cure makes the person vulnerable to the possibility of exploitation and abuse by unscrupulous individuals.

Acupuncture, massage, visualization, Chinese herbs, reflexology, aromatherapy, and homeopathy are some of the complementary therapies used in HIV. Exercise is often included amongst them (Calabrese and LaPerriere, 1993). Barton et al (1994) found that 44 per cent of HIV out-patients at a central

London service were using complementary therapies. In the UK, The National AIDS Manual has published an informative and useful *Directory of complementary and alternative treatments in HIV/AIDS* (Alcorn, 1994) to assist potential users. A comparable example is provided by the New York-based *Gay Men's Health Crisis* (GMHC, 1993/1994), a newsletter devoted to alternative therapies.

While there is minimal research evidence for their value, complementary therapies are popular amongst people living with HIV infection, indicating that they are perceived as beneficial. Apart from any specific properties that each of these techniques may have leading to, say, analgesia or anxiety reduction, they all share a number of non-specific factors of potentially beneficial psychological effects, comparable to those found in the psychotherapies. In discussing the therapeutic components of different forms of psychotherapy, Frank (1986) has summarized the factors that combat demoralization, regardless of the approach used: (a) the existence of a confiding relationship based on the patient's trust in the therapist's competence and goodwill; (b) a healing setting which is also perceived as a place of safety; (c) a rationale shared between therapist and patient that explains the symptoms and the role of the treatment; and (d) a set of procedures which require active participation by therapist and patient. Complementary therapies share these characteristics, and some of their beneficial effects can be attributed to these non-specific factors.

While, in general, complementary approaches are reported to have positive effects, it is possible that some may have harmful consequences (Atherton, 1994), especially when they are regarded as the alternative to orthodox medicine, leading to failure to use well tried and effective therapies, or as a result of interaction with other substances (Barton et al, 1994).

The study of the potential value of complementary therapies has been rather neglected by those with a scientific view of the world. Investigation of this area should provide fruitful insights not just into the specific value of these techniques, but also into what influences individuals' coping with major illness and satisfaction with treatment.

5.7 Summary

A wide range of interventions to minimize mental health problems associated with HIV infection have been discussed in this chapter. Psychological interventions at the time of HIV testing; general and specific interventions for people living with HIV; and therapies for the palliative stage of care and for bereaved individuals are discussed. The use of psychotropic medication for the treatment of psychiatric disorders, including antidepressants, major tranquillizers and anxiolytic medication is reviewed. The value of medication in the treatment of brain-related problems and, in particular, the role of zidovudine in the treatment of HIV associated dementia and in the prevention of cognitive impairment are considered. Residential treatments, both those involving psychiatric and non-psychiatric settings, are examined. Finally, the role of community organizations and complementary therapies is discussed.

6 Psychological factors in the prevention of HIV transmission and the delay of disease progression

6.1 Introduction

Pharmacological treatments against HIV and its complications have met with limited success, and progress in vaccine development is slow. For these reasons, preventive strategies to reduce the risk of acquiring or transmitting the infection remain paramount in the containment of HIV infection. Prevention of HIV spread depends on a reduction in the behaviours associated with the risk of infection, in particular sexual and injecting drug use behaviour. Such behaviours are notoriously difficult to change, not just because of the reinforcement created by the pleasure they produce in the short term, but also because of the social, economic and political factors which contribute to their development and maintenance (Mann et al, 1992). Here we review the behaviours associated with the risk of HIV infection, examine the personal and social determinants of risk behaviours, and summarize research into effective intervention to prevent the spread of the infection.

Psychological and behavioural factors may also have an effect on HIV infection by influencing the rate of disease progression. There is much interest in this area of potential psychological intervention, although hard facts are few, and research evidence limited. In the second half of the chapter, the effects of psychological factors on immune function are reviewed, with emphasis on methodological issues and published research evidence.

6.2 Transmission of HIV infection

6.2.1 Behaviours associated with the risk of HIV transmission

Sexual behaviour is the most important mode of HIV transmission with most infections resulting from heterosexual intercourse world-wide although homosexual transmission is more common in developed countries (Piot et al, 1990; Mann et al, 1992). Transmission through injecting drug use is an important mode of transmission in parts of Europe, in Asia and the Pacific region (Mann et al, 1992). In spite the global attention given to HIV, and to the changes that have taken place in recent years (Wielandt, 1993; Melnick et al, 1993), risk behaviours remain common.

Surveys of sexual behaviour from the US show that a majority of young adults have multiple, serial sexual partners, that heterosexual anal intercourse is not uncommon, and that unprotected sexual activity is prevalent amongst heterosexual individuals, both in developed and developing countries (Catania et al, 1992b; Gwede and McDermott, 1992; Campostrini and McQueen, 1993; Fennema et al, 1993; Ku et al, 1993; Leighton et al, 1993; Tessier et al, 1993; Seidman and Rieder, 1994; Wawer et al, 1994; Kassler et al, 1994). Women are at particular risk of infection and reports from the US show that rates of HIV infection among young women are increasing rapidly (Centers for Disease Control, 1994c). In spite of some degree of behaviour change, many women remain at risk of infection (Campbell and Baldwin, 1991; Sherr and Strong, 1992), even in areas of relatively low rates of heterosexually acquired infection (Hudson, 1992; Ades et al, 1993; Johnstone et al, 1994; Nicoll et al, 1994). Reported sexual behaviour among gay/bisexual men has also changed in the direction of lower risk, with reductions in multiple casual partners and unprotected anal intercourse (Centers for Disease Control, 1991a; Lau et al, 1992; Hunt et al, 1993), although there is no room for complacence (Catania et al, 1992b; Kelly et al, 1992b; Gruer and Ssembatya, 1993b).

Injecting drug users have also shown changes in drug use-related risk behaviours (Stimson, 1991; Frischer et al, 1992; Nicolosi et al, 1992; Des Jarlais et al, 1994), although the world picture is uneven, with social and political factors contributing to the variation (Des Jarlais, 1994). In spite of these changes, drug use-related risk remains a major mode of transmission in many regions of the world (Mann et al, 1992).

6.2.2 Factors associated with HIV risk behaviours

Identification of the determinants of behaviours that carry an increased risk of acquiring or transmitting HIV infection is an important step in the planning of intervention strategies and one that should help in the monitoring, evaluation and modification of intervention programmes. There are, however, methodological difficulties in the study of factors associated with unsafe acts, and together with the many cultural differences, individual and social diversity, and sampling problems, the resulting findings can at times be contradictory or inconclusive. Nevertheless, some general impressions can be drawn about the determinants of unsafe behaviour. These include demographic and cultural factors, social norms, type of relationship, use of mood-altering substances, communication and sexual negotiation skills, amongst others.

Determinants of unsafe sexual behaviour

Most of the published work on factors associated with unsafe sexual behaviour concerns gay/bisexual men, although other groups have also been studied, and the relevant research findings will be mentioned when appropriate. A wide variety of factors have been considered, and a summary is presented here. While many of the factors identified are clearly interrelated, in other cases their interactions are unclear (for review see Thornton and Catalán, 1993).

1. Knowledge about HIV and risk perception. Many studies involving gay/bisexual men and heterosexual men and women, including partners of men with haemophilia and HIV infection, show that most individuals engaging in risky sexual behaviour are well informed about their theoretical risk of infection, even if they do not perceive themselves to be at high risk personally (DiClemente et al, 1986; Fitzpatrick et al, 1990; Gold et al, 1991; Gold and Skinner, 1992; Gold et al, 1992; Hays et al, 1992; Kelly et al, 1992b; Weinstock et al, 1993; Church et al, 1993). This suggests that knowledge about risk is necessary but not sufficient to lead to safe behaviour, and that personal perception of risk is an important determinant of safer sexual behaviour (James et al, 1991).

2. Attitudes to condom use. Condoms are used by adolescent boys for their value as contraceptives rather than to for their efficacy in reducing the risk of transmission of HIV (Orr and Langefeld, 1993). The practice of condom use depends upon their popularity amongst peers and is also associated with beliefs about allowing spur-of-the-moment sex (Kegeles et al, 1988). Conversely, negative views about condoms reduce the likelihood of their use (Valdiserri et al, 1988; Magura et al, 1990; Fitzpatrick et al, 1990; Kelly et al, 1992b; Weinstock et al, 1993). Enjoyment of unprotected intercourse is a significant predictor of both persistent risky behaviour and of change from low to high risk in gay men (Stall et al, 1990; Hays et al, 1992). Impulsivity and risk-taking have been reported to be more common among heterosexuals who do not use condoms attending a genito-urinary medicine clinic (Clift et al, 1993). Negative attitudes to condom use are not uncommon among injecting drug users ((White et al, 1993). Attitudes to condom use vary between the sexes. Women tend to report more negative views about asking their male partners to use condoms, fearing it might compromise their relationship, and feeling generally less empowered to negotiate safer sex (Cohen et al, 1992). In general, condoms are perceived by women as being under the man's influence, suggesting that the development of methods under the woman's control, such as the female condom or other barrier contraceptives and viricides should be urgently pursued.

3. Emotional state and psychological distress and problems. The evidence for an association between mood states and unsafe sexual behaviour is complex and, at times, contradictory. The presence of psychological stressors, such as adverse life circumstances and poor parental support, has been reported to be associated with risky sexual behaviour in US adolescents, and surprisingly, also the presence of high levels of self-esteem (Walter et al, 1991). Unsafe behaviour in HIV seronegative gay men has been reported to be positively correlated with optimism, anger, low emotional control, poor acceptance of sexual orientation (Perkins et al, 1993b), low self-esteem (Horn and Chetwynd, 1989) and depression (Kelly et al, 1991b; Kelly et al, 1993a). Change from low to high sexual risk in gay men requesting information about their HIV status has been linked with mental distress and denial–fatalism coping strategies (Beltran et al, 1993). Low mood has been found to be associated with unsafe sexual encounters in young gay men, while the opposite was the case for older gay men (Gold and Skinner, 1992).

4. Demographic factors. Several demographic factors have been associated with unsafe sexual behaviour including lower educational levels, poverty and belonging to an ethnic minority group (St Lawrence et al, 1990; Dublin et al, 1992; Peterson et al, 1992). Black and Hispanic women in the US report lower condom use with their partners (Weinstock et al, 1992) and US Hispanic gay men are more likely to be involved in unsafe sexual acts (Doll et al, 1991). In Africa, HIV infection has been reported to be more common in women, and in those who were separated or widowed (Barongo et al, 1992). A number of studies have identified younger men as more likely to engage in unsafe sex (Ekstrand and Coates, 1990; Kelly et al, 1990; Hays et al, 1990b), while others have found no links with age (Connell and Kippax, 1990; Davies et al, 1992). Data from the UK indicated that recent HIV infections may disproportionately affect gay men aged 19 years or under (Evans et al, 1993).

5. Knowledge of HIV status. Knowledge of seropositivity has sometimes been found to be associated with the adoption of safer sexual behaviour (McCusker et al, 1989) but this finding is by no means universal (Ostrow et al, 1989a; Heyward et al, 1993; Otten et al, 1993) (see Chapter 5).

6. Alcohol and substance use. An association between drug and alcohol use and unsafe sexual behaviour has been reported in many studies involving gay men and heterosexuals (Stall et al, 1990; Doll et al, 1991; Gold et al, 1991, 1992; McKusker et al, 1990; Ostrow et al, 1990; McEwan et al, 1992; Booth et al, 1993). For example, greater sexual risk has been particularly associated with the use of amphetamines (Klee, 1992) and crack (Fullilove et al, 1990; Ellebrock et al, 1992). Other studies, however, do not confirm this link between alcohol or drug use and risky sexual behaviour (Gold et al, 1992; Gold and Skinner, 1992; Myers et al, 1992; Temple et al, 1993). Even when an association is found, it is not always possible to establish the causal direction. Drugs and alcohol may be taken to facilitate a pre-existing intention to have unsafe sex, or the use of substances may have a direct effect in reducing inhibitions and increasing sexual arousal. Alternatively, both unsafe behaviour and substance use may result from a third factor such as search for excitement or risk-taking. Another reason for this link could be a chance event, as both sexual encounters and drugs and alcohol are available in similar settings. Crack cocaine has been associated with greater risk of unsafe sexual behaviour (Booth et al, 1993).

7. Type of relationship. Having a regular, monogamous or important partner is associated with unprotected sex in gay/bisexual men (Fitzpatrick et al, 1990; McKusick et al, 1990; Adib et al, 1991; Hunt et al, 1992), injecting drug users (Rhodes et al, 1993), women, including female (Evans et al, 1991; Wermuth et al, 1992; De Graaf et al, 1992) and male sex workers (Gibson and Aggleton, 1993). One obvious problem in such cases is that while one partner may assume the relationship to be monogamous, this may in fact not be so, with the consequent risk of infection for the unsuspecting partner.

8. Perceived social norms. Social and cultural norms are important in determining safer sexual behaviour. Among gay men, the perception that insistence on safer sex is not acceptable within one's peer group and the absence of peer support for safer sex have been found to be predictors of high risk sexual behaviour (Kelly et al, 1990; Stall et al, 1990; Adib et al, 1991; Kelly et al, 1992c). Conversely, changes to lower risk behaviour are associated with the perception that social norms favour safe sex (Centers for Disease Control, 1991; Hays et al, 1992).

9. Intrapersonal factors. Gold and co-workers have studied the role of cognitive and situational variables in safe and unsafe sexual encounters in a series of surveys involving gay and heterosexual men (Gold et al, 1991, 1992; Gold and Skinner, 1992). A finding which held for younger and older gay men as well as heterosexual men was the tendency to use heuristics, 'rules of thumb', to make judgements about their probable risk in different situations. Gold et al (1991; 1992) produced a taxonomy of different heuristics related to high-risk sexual behaviour such as '. . . if he was HIV positive he wouldn't do this'. The most commonly used of these rules was the so-called *sickness heuristic* an example of which is 'he looks so well he could not possibly be infected'. The sickness heuristic is based on the idea that people who are ill or have infectious diseases tend to look ill or show some sign of disease and in many situations this rule works. Like other heuristics, however, the sickness heuristic is not universally true and applied in the wrong situations, such as in HIV disease, it can lead to serious errors. Nor are heuristics necessarily rational or adaptive. Anyone with even a passing knowledge of HIV infection would realize that the sickness heuristic is not appropriate in HIV infection but, unfortunately, people tend to use heuristic rules habitually, automatically, and uncritically. Certainly amongst the individuals interviewed by Gold et al (1991;1992) there was widespread use of inappropriate heuristics despite the fact that most were very well informed about HIV infection. As in other situations, information is not sufficient to change behaviour and other explanations involving information processing and state dependent learning must be sought. Similar findings about the concerning the beliefs and assumptions about the health status of the partner in unsafe encounters have been reported by Keller (1993).

In summary, a variety of factors have been identified that play a part in the occurrence of risky sexual behaviour. The include: (1) perception of personal HIV risk; (2) attitudes to condom use; (3) emotional state; (4) substance use; (5) intrapersonal factors; (6) perceived social norms; and (7) type of relationship. The extent to which these factors act independently or together to determine sexual behaviour is not always clear, but identification of their contribution may assist in the development of intervention to prevent the spread of HIV infection.

Determinants of unsafe injecting drug use

Efforts to promote changes in injecting drug use in the direction of lower risk activities have met with some success (Stimson, 1991; Watters et al, 1994)), but there are substantial numbers of drug users still involved in unsafe behaviours. Some of the factors associated with persistent risky behaviour are reviewed here.

1. Knowledge of HIV status. In a London study involving over 100 HIV seropositive injectors, borrowing and lending of injecting equipment was marginally less likely for those aware of their status (Rhodes et al, 1993), and results from a large European give some support to this finding (Desenclos et al, 1993). Large-scale studies, however, suggest that amongst drug users in treatment, changes in behaviour may be unrelated to HIV testing and counselling (Higgins et al, 1991)

2. Perception of risk. It has been argued that the risk of HIV infection is perceived by drug users as one possible undesirable event amongst many other risks related to their urge to obtain drugs, including the possibility of arrest, attack, withdrawal or overdose (Connors, 1992), and so concern about HIV alone may not be sufficient to lead to behaviour change.

3. Involvement in treatment for drug problem. There is good evidence to indicate that both the risk of seroconversion and of persistent unsafe behaviours are greater in injectors not in contact with treatment facilities compared with those receiving treatment (Metzger et al, 1993), although it is not clear whether treatment itself, as opposed to other factors which might have contributed to seeking help in the first place, are responsible for the differences. On the other hand, Ross et al (1993), in a report from Australia, found drug users who had never been involved in treatment to be younger and to have a lower level of risky behaviours than those currently or previously in treatment, suggesting that the two groups were at different stages of their drug careers.

4. Demographic factors. In the UK, women have been reported to be in greater risk than men, and in the US, black women at greater risk than white women (Stimson, 1991; Magura et al, 1993). Race in the US shows a marked association with the infection, as do socioeconomic levels, unemployment and area of residence (Stimson, 1991).

5. Use of other drugs. The use of crack cocaine by injectors is associated with an increase in high risk sexual and drug injecting behaviours, and thus with greater risk of acquiring and transmitting HIV (Booth et al, 1993).

6. Emotional state and psychological distress. As with unsafe sexual behaviour, needle risk behaviours have been reported to be associated with higher levels of depression and anxiety, low self-esteem, and low confidence in decision-making (Simpson et al, 1993). Hartgers et al (1992) reported differential effects of psychological morbidity on needle sharing in relation to serostatus, with only those individuals who were HIV seronegative showing an association.

7. Prison experience. There is good evidence that imprisonment can be an important factor in the transmission of HIV infection. In some parts of the world, the proportion of seropositive prisoners is substantial, European figures ranging from 11 per cent in Switzerland to over 25 per cent in male inmates in Spain (Harding, 1990). In addition, injecting drug use and equipment sharing are common (Bird et al, 1992; Turnbull and Stimson, 1994), and access to clean equipment, and education and counselling are minimal (Gore and Bird, 1993; Turnbull et al, 1993; Dixon et al, 1993), in spite of official WHO recommendations (WHO, 1987).

In summary, the determinants of unsafe drug use are similar to those found for unsafe sexual behaviour, such as perception of risk, emotional state and substance use. In addition, involvement with drug treatment programmes and prison experience can also play a part.

6.3 Psychological and behavioural prevention of HIV infection

6.3.1 Introduction

Efforts to change HIV risk behaviours to reduce the spread of the infection have tended to rely on established models of health promotion, ranging from campaigns directed at the general public to interventions aimed at particular groups, such as gay men or injecting drug users. Few interventions have been theory-driven (Kelly et al, 1990; Catania et al, 1990b; Thornton et al, 1994), and the majority of initiatives have made use of *ad hoc* techniques and local resources.

Evaluating preventive interventions is not always easy. Many factors can influence behaviour change, and it is not always possible to isolate the relative contribution of a particular procedure or approach, especially in the long term. Ideally, a randomized design should be used, comparing alternative interventions, or a new intervention against the routine approach, but scientific procedures are not always feasible in the conditions where many educators and health practitioners work. Outcome measures can include a wide range of indicators. The most important indicator, actual reduction in the rate of HIV infection and AIDS, may not be easy to establish in the short term because of the incubation period and the time delays before symptoms develop. Alternative surrogate indicators will need to be considered, such as surveys of reported behaviours, perceived self-efficacy to engage in safe behaviour, and rates of other sexually transmitted diseases.

One important aspect of the evaluation of prevention strategies concerns the question of cost. Soderlund et al (1993) reviewed the cost of six different prevention strategies, including mass strategies, person-to-person education, social marketing of condoms, use of genitourinary medicine clinics, blood transfusion, and needle exchange programmes. Costs varied substantially depending on the countries studied, approach and methods used, and length of time the programme was in operation. Person-to-person programmes were the most costly. However, costs need to be considered in parallel with their efficacy, and this is an area of research which has so far been rather neglected (Gray, 1991).

It is sometimes assumed that with the advent of vaccines to prevent the spread of HIV, the need for behaviour change will become less pressing. In fact, the development of vaccine trials research raises many complex ethical and practical problems (Lurie et al, 1994) and will require the continuation of research into the assessment of risk behaviour, promotion of trial participation, and maintenance of low-risk behaviours (Grinstead, 1994).

6.3.2 General preventive interventions

Media campaigns

The effects of media campaigns on HIV risk reduction in the general population are difficult to assess and there have been few attempts at a systematic evaluation of their efficacy. There are some notable exceptions, however, such as the case of the national campaigns developed in Switzerland (Stutz et al, 1991). Reports of the efficacy of media campaigns suggest that there is an increase in condom use in young people at first sexual intercourse (Wielandt, 1993), although there is a tendency for this to decline over time (Ku et al, 1993). In spite of such campaigns, concern about the infection remains low in the general population (DiClemente et al, 1988; Kappel et al, 1989) and there is a parallel lack of substantial behaviour change (Melnick et al, 1993). A demonstrable consequence of HIV media campaigns has been the association between publicity and the number of people seeking HIV testing, in particular in response to television-based campaigns (Beck et al, 1990; Ross and Scott, 1993), suggesting an increase in anxiety about the possibility of being infected, which is not necessarily followed by behaviour change (Sherr, 1990). The increase in HIV testing after media campaigns does not appear to lead to the identification of a substantial number of new cases, suggesting that those coming forward for testing are in general anxious individuals with a history of low-risk behaviours (Ross and Scott, 1993). The mass media remains a potentially important method of increasing awareness about HIV infection (Kalichman and Hunter, 1992) but their role in promoting behaviour change needs to be complemented by more individualized and focused interventions.

Risk reduction and young people: the role of school and college

Adolescents and young adults are the most sexually active group and thus a clear target for risk reduction education. Schools offer the advantage of access to this group at risk. While there may be political and other obstacles to the provision of sex education and education about HIV infection in schools, there is good evidence for their acceptability and effects (Kirby et al, 1991; Jemmott et al, 1992). For example, Walter and Vaughan (1993) have described the results of a six-lesson HIV prevention curriculum for students aged 12 to 20 in New York City. Over 1200 students of both sexes were included in the study, about half of them receiving the experimental intervention and the rest acting as controls. More than 70 per cent were Black or Hispanic. The risk reduction lessons included: information about HIV infection and prevention techniques; self-assessment of risk behaviour and of appropriate preventive resources; correction of misperceptions about the behaviour of their peers; role play to empower students to negotiate delay in the initiation of sexual intercourse and to encourage condom use. Results at the three-month follow-up showed significant effects favouring the experimental intervention in terms of knowledge, beliefs about risk, barriers and norms, self-efficacy and some reported risk behaviours (monogamy, condom use). As in other studies (Kirby et al, 1991; Jemmott et al, 1992) the positive change in knowledge and beliefs that resulted was not accompanied by substantial reductions in some risk behaviours, suggesting that further approaches are needed for individuals who experience particular difficulties initiating or maintaining safer behaviours.

Counselling, HIV testing and behaviour change

HIV testing is not uncommon in developed countries. US national surveys indicate that about 20 per cent of the adult population has been tested at least once, including about 60 per cent of men who have sex with men, 46 per cent of male and 73 per cent of female injecting drug users, and 35 per cent of heterosexual men and women having unprotected intercourse with multiple partners (Berrios et al, 1993). The value of HIV testing and counselling in terms of promoting low risk behaviours has not been conclusively established (Cates and Handfield, 1988; Beardsell, 1994). Whether this reflects the inherent limitations of the process, or whether it is an indication of the failure of pre- and post-test counselling as currently practised, is an open question.

Higgins et al (1991) reviewed 66 studies with data about the behavioural effects of HIV testing and counselling, and found that behavioural changes in the direction of lower risk activities were apparent in many longitudinal studies of gay/bisexual men, injecting drug users, pregnant women and others, but the changes were often unrelated to the experience of HIV testing and counselling. Recent work on the incidence of sexually transmitted diseases following post HIV test counselling is disappointing. Zenilman et al (1992) studied over 1200 HIV tested and counselled genitourinary department attenders, about half of whom were seropositive, and found that almost 10 per cent acquired at least one definite sexually transmitted disease during the follow-up period, with no differences by serostatus. More disturbing still are the findings of Otten et al (1993) who in a similar study found the rate of sexually tranmitted diseases between the pre- and post-test follow-up period to have decreased among those who were HIV seropotive but more than doubled in the seronegative group.

In summary, while for some individuals HIV testing and counselling may be associated with behaviour change, such change can occur in the absence of testing, and failure to change behaviour can persist in spite of it. The relationship between testing and behaviour change is therefore a complex one, and likely to be influenced by self-selection bias, peer group norm perceptions, and by the actual process of counselling. The effects of the latter may well be modest, and efforts should be made to identify the ingredients that promote behaviour change and to enhance their efficacy.

6.3.3 Targeted preventive interventions

Interventions for gay/bisexual men

In spite of the substantial changes in sexual behaviour reported by many surveys of gay/bisexual men, it is clear that the initiation and maintenance of safer sex behaviour continues to be problematic for a proportion of men, and that efforts are being focused on the search for interventions with longer-term efficacy (Ekstrand, 1992).

1. Community-based interventions. In a series of innovative studies, Kelly and co-workers (Kelly et al, 1991c, 1992c; Kelly, 1994) have shown the value of community interventions to modify sexual behaviour in gay/bisexual men. Key opinion formers in the gay community were identified and trained to discuss safer sex activities with friends and acquaintances, showing that the intervention led to a substantial and persistent decline in rates of unsafe sexual behaviour among subjects in the experimental compared with the control cities.

2. Small group interventions. A number of controlled investigations using cognitive behavioural principles have been evaluated. A 12-week group intervention programme including education about HIV risk, identification of triggers to unsafe behaviour, teaching and practice of cognitive and behavioural skills to manage difficult situations, assertiveness training, sexual negotiation skills, and training in problem-solving strategies (Kelly et al, 1989; Kelly and St Lawrence, 1990) was evaluated using an experimental versus waiting-list design. The results showed significant and lasting effects for the intervention in terms of decrease in the frequency of unprotected anal intercourse, risk knowledge, and behavioural skills dealing with sexually coercive situations. The importance of skills-training is highlighted by the study of Valdiserri et al (1989) comparing group-based intervention including a lecture on safer sex with a lecture and skills training, the latter resulting in much greater increase in condom use.

3. Individual interventions. Interventions based on cognitive behavioural principles have been used to develop individually tailored help for people requiring more intensive assistance or for those whose problems would not be easily tackled in group settings (Thornton et al, 1994). For example, some individuals experiencing difficulties developing and maintaining safer sex also have problems in other areas concerned with impulse control, such as eating and weight or alcohol consumption. Similarly, low self-esteem and mood disorders may contribute to inconsistency in safer sex behaviour (see above), and cognitive behavioural techniques of proven value for these kind of disorders can be used.

Interventions for heterosexual men and women

World-wide, heterosexual spread is the most common form of transmission of HIV (Mann et al, 1992; Easterbrook and Hawkins, 1993), and therefore there is urgent need for the development of effective intervention strategies targeted on heterosexuals.

1. Small group interventions. Interventions based on the cognitive behavioural model have been employed with young runaway adolescents of both sexes in a controlled investigation in residential shelters in New York City. The results showed a decline in unsafe sexual behaviours and increase in condom use (Rotheram-Borus et al, 1991) and Kelly (1994) has described a similar approach for young women.

2. Clinic-based individual interventions. Allen et al (1992) described the value of providing education using videotapes, HIV testing and counselling, and free condoms and spermicide to child-bearing women in Rwanda. More than 1400 women were included and followed up for up to two years. Condom use increased after intervention, in particular among seropositive women, and the rates of gonorrhoea decreased. Condom use was particularly increased when male partners were also counselled and HIV tested. Although the changes were statistically significant, levels of condom use remained relatively low, with about 36 per cent and 16 per cent of seropositive and seronegative women using them at follow-up. Similar results were reported by Heyward et al (1993) in a study of women in Kinshasa, Zaïre. As discussed above, men and women have different perceptions and attitudes about the use of condoms, and the relative failure of the these studies focused on women's use of condoms is not surprising. Empirical evidence for gender differences in attitudes to condom use is provided by the study by Cohen et al (1992) comparing three different programmes to promote condoms among genitourinary medicine clinic attenders: (a) 'condom skills' with emphasis on the mechanical aspects, (b) 'social influences' focused on negotiation with partners, and (c) 'distribution' providing participants with unlimited supplies of condoms. Rates of sexually transmitted diseases at follow-up were significantly reduced for men in the first two programmes, but none of the interventions had effects on the rates in women. The need for development of methods of HIV prevention which women perceive as their own is therefore urgent (Ehrhardt, 1994).

3. Couple counselling. A follow-up of 144 heterosexual couples discordant for HIV serostatus, where the majority of those with HIV infection were men, shows the value of personal counselling and support (Padian et al, 1993). No uninfected partners seroconverted over the follow-up period, and condom use and abstinence increased significantly over time. Couple counselling remains a need in the case of men with haemophilia and HIV infection and their partners. While condom use was greater in those who were HIV seropositive (Catalán et al, 1992b) there was evidence for continuing unsafe sexual behaviour in this group of individuals and their partners (Dublin et al, 1992; Chorba et al, 1993), highlighting the need for couple-based interventions.

Interventions for injecting and other drug users

Most interventions to reduce the risk of HIV spread through drug injecting have been aimed at encouraging behaviours carrying lower risk, although there has been concern about finding ways of discouraging the use of drugs in the first instance (Stimson, 1991). It is sometimes difficult to identify the specific factors which have led to behaviour change, both general and specific interventions possibly contributing. General educational strategies and peer-group norm awareness may have resulted in high levels of knowledge among injectors about transmission and prevention methods, and some of the changes in injecting behaviour documented in drug users (Peters et al, 1994), although sexual behaviour change has been far less substantial (for review see Stimson 1991). Some specific interventions are reviewed below.

1. *Drug treatment.* People in treatment programmes show evidence of risk reduction, as in the case of methadone treatment (Ball et al, 1988; Chaisson et al, 1989), although it is generally agreed that a planned intervention and counselling, and not just the supply of methadone are required (Martin et al, 1990).

2. *Syringe exchange.* There is good evidence for the value of syringe exchange programmes, facilitating access to needles and syringes in a community-based way (Battjes et al, 1991; Heimer et al, 1993; Gruer et al, 1993; Keene et al, 1993; Watters et al, 1994), but it is generally agreed that access to syringes needs to be supplemented by information and counselling (Van den Hoek et al, 1989).

3. *Syringe decontamination.* A parallel approach to syringe exchange, which has resulted from the legal restrictions imposed on access to syringes and needles, is the use of bleach to decontaminate injecting equipment (Watters et al, 1991), a method that has been suggested for developing countries (Stimson, 1991).

4. *Psychoeducational interventions.* For drug users in contact with treatment centres, psychoeducational interventions aimed at improving knowledge about HIV transmission, and to enhance social skills and self-efficacy when dealing with potentially risky situations have been shown to be effective (El-Bassel and Schilling, 1992; Malow et al, 1994; Sorensen et al, 1994), stressing the need to develop multimodal approaches.

5. *Outreach work.* Many injecting drug users are not in touch with treatment centres and may not be motivated to give up their drug use, but may be accessible to specifically designed interventions to prevent HIV spread (Stimson, 1991). Evaluation of street outreach programmes developed in the US shows that substantial proportions of drug users can be reached in this way, and that information about HIV, condoms, and bleach kits can be made available to them, providing an essential link in the chain of education for prevention (Serrano et al, 1993).

Interventions to prevent vertical transmission

Prevention of mother-to-child spread of HIV infection depends on the early identification of the infection in the mother. It can be argued that knowledge of the mother's HIV status allows the woman, her partner, and their medical advisers to consider a range of options which can affect the risk of transmission to the unborn child.

1. *Antenatal HIV testing.* There is evidence that among women with HIV, the infection is identified in a substantial proportion of cases at the antenatal clinic (Davidson et al, 1989), and in view of the increase in prevalence of infection in pregnant women in developed (Nicoll et al, 1994) and developing countries (Mann et al, 1992), there is concern about the best way to identify cases of infection. Selective offer of the HIV test to women thought to be at risk of infection has been recommended (Department of Health, 1992), but there is good evidence that many HIV infected women are unaware of their being at risk or are unwilling to disclose information about risk behaviours (Landesman et al, 1987; Wenstrom and Zuidema, 1989). Universal offer of the test with pre-test counselling at the antenatal clinic appears to be a more effective way of identifying HIV seropositive women than selective offer of the test (Barbacci et al, 1991), and the policy of offering the test to all women is becoming widespread, and is acceptable to women and to midwives (Meadows et al, 1993b, c).

2. *Use of anti-retroviral medication.* Preliminary reports about the value of anti-retrovirals to prevent infection of the unborn child have been recently released. Zidovudine given to mothers for about 11 weeks during pregnancy and labour, and for 6 weeks to the babies led to a transmission rate of 8.8 per cent, compared with 25.5 per cent in the untreated group (Centers for Disease Control, 1994a, b). If the results are confirmed in further studies, in the absence of side-effects to the infant, the potential for the prevention of vertical spread will be greatly enhanced.

3. *Termination of pregnancy.* The option of terminating the pregnancy is another possible choice facing the woman with HIV infection. Many factors will influence her choice, including her perception of the risk of the baby being born infected, access to other methods of reducing this risk, and the nature of the supports available and counselling received. In developed countries, a majority of women in this predicament choose to continue the pregnancy (Selwyn et al, 1989; Johnstone et al, 1990).

4. *Method of delivery.* There is evidence that Caesarean section may reduce the risk of transmission (European Collaborative Study, 1994), and if confirmed in further studies, this finding may have significant effects on obstetric practice, and add to the evidence in favour of identifying pregnant women with HIV infection.

5. Breast feeding. Breast feeding has been known to be a mode of transmission of HIV for some time, and in developed countries it is recommended that breast feeding is avoided by HIV seropositive mothers (Department of Health and Social Security, 1989). In contrast, in developing countries the argument has been that the risks to all babies resulting from widespread avoidance of breast feeding would be greater than the gain to a few, although this view has been questioned (Ziegler, 1993).

Interventions to trace the contacts of people with HIV infection

Contact tracing and notification have been an essential part of the control of sexually transmitted diseases, and their use in the prevention of the spread of HIV has much potential, although there has been concern about its ethical and practical aspects (Potterat et al, 1991; Bayer and Toomey, 1992).

Partner notification includes the range of public health activities through which sexual and injection-sharing partners of seropositive individuals are notified and counselled about their risk, and offered access to services. There are two main modes of contact tracing, depending on whether the HIV infected person contacts and notifies partners, or whether health workers make contact with partners in confidence, the latter being the more effective (Landis et al, 1992; Spencer et al, 1993). Potential advantages of contact tracing include the identification of infected individuals and provision of health care (Pattman and Gould, 1993), prevention of spread to others, and its cost-efficacy (Gieseke et al, 1991; Holtgrave et al, 1993). Partner notification has been found to be acceptable to those contacted (Jones et al, 1990), although the threat of domestic violence against women with HIV infection needs to be carefully considered (North and Rothenberg, 1993). Staff involved in HIV prevention are sometimes understandably apprehensive about the practical and ethical consequences of contact tracing (Keenlyside, 1991), and careful consideration needs to be given to the development, implementation and monitoring of partner notification programmes (Potterat et al, 1991).

Interventions aimed at commercial sex workers

Commercial sex workers, both female and male, can play an important part in the spread of HIV (Estebanez et al, 1993; van Haastrecht et al, 1993; Hart and Whittaker, 1994; De Graaf et al, 1994), although their role has tended to be overemphasized (McKeganey and Barnard, 1992; Ward et al, 1993), while that of their clients and partners has not always been adequately noted (Day et al, 1993; Barnard et al, 1993). Prevention of HIV infection in commercial sex workers cannot be considered in isolation from the complex social, legal and economic problems they experience (Estabanez et al, 1993). The Consensus Statement issued by the WHO (1989) stresses the need to encourage governments to recognize the presence of prostitution and to develop interventions to decrease health risks, including HIV. Interventions aimed at changing risk behaviours in commercial sex workers need to be designed in consultation with them, and must take into account the social and legal constraints they face. The practical difficulties involved in doing research in this field may explain the limited number of published investigations on the efficacy of interventions. One example of research is that by Fox et al (1993) who have provided information on one such intervention for female sex workers in Honduras. Over a 10 week period talks on sexually transmitted diseases, including AIDS, and free condoms were given to all female sex workers attending a genitourinary medicine clinic, and information was obtained about their sexual behaviour before the talks and four months later, using diaries and questionnaires. Knowledge about HIV transmission and condom use increased significantly during the study period.

Interventions for new populations at risk: the case of the mentally ill

People with severe mental illness are at increased risk of HIV infection, several investigations showing small but worrying rates of HIV infection and risky behaviours in psychiatric populations (Baker and Mossman, 1991; Cournos et al, 1991; Brown, 1991; Sacks et al, 1992; Kelly et al, 1992a; DiClemente and Ponton, 1993; Susser et al, 1993; Empfield et al, 1993; Cournos et al, 1994; Kalichman et al, 1994; Ayuso-Mateos et al, 1994). There are encouraging reports showing the value of preventive interventions aimed at the mentally ill. In a sample of psychiatric out-patients and using a randomized design involving a brief behavioural intervention compared with a waiting-list control condition, Stevenson et al (1994) showed significant advantages for the experimental intervention in terms of HIV-related knowledge and intentions to reduce risky behaviours, as well changes in unprotected sex and condom use. Non-randomized interventions like those described by Lauer-Listhaus and Watterson, (1988) and Sladyk (1989) have also demonstrated the value of psychoeducational intervention for psychiatric patients. It is not altogether surprising that the kind of approaches which have been found to work in other populations are also effective when applied to the mentally ill: dealing with the anxieties of staff about their patients being involved in sexual activities may prove a harder task.

6.4 Psychological prevention of HIV disease progression

6.4.1 Psychological factors and immune function

The impact that psychological factors can have on immunological function is now well established (for a review see Ader, 1988) although the relevance of psychoneuroimmunology to HIV infection remains unclear. There is, however, considerable circumstantial evidence to suggest that some role for a psychological influence in HIV infection might be expected (Gorman and Kertzner, 1990; Antoni et al, 1990). Not only does the brain directly affect the immune system through sympathetic nervous system innervation (to the thymus, spleen, and lymph nodes), but many of the immune system cells possess neurotransmitter and neurohormone receptors. More direct evidence comes from changes in immune responses using psychological manipulations such as classical conditioning (Ader and Cohen 1975), hypnosis (Hall, 1983) and relaxation training (Kiecolt-Glaser et al, 1985; 1986). Psychological factors have also been shown to be important outside of laboratory settings. For example, psychological stressors have been shown to increase the susceptibility to infectious diseases such as upper respiratory tract infections, particularly the common cold (Stone et al, 1987; Evans et al, 1988b; Evans and Edgerton, 1991).

There is also evidence for a link between emotional state and immune function. Several animal studies have found that T cell production is modulated by the relative activation of the frontal lobes (Renoux et al, 1983; Nevou et al, 1986) with left-sided activation up-regulating and right sided activation down-regulating production. Comparable findings for natural killer cell activity, although not for T cell subsets, have been reported in humans (Kang et al, 1991). These findings are particularly relevant because of the well established observation that emotional experience in humans is lateralized, with negative emotions, such as depression and anxiety, being controlled by the right cerebral hemisphere and positive emotions by the left (Davidson, 1984; Silberman and Weingartner, 1986). The implications of this are that negative affect (e.g. anxiety and depression) may have the effect of down-regulating immune responses with the consequence that psychological interventions aimed at improving mood could have a beneficial impact on immunological function. Although these ideas have considerable appeal, they should be treated as speculative at this stage.

6.4.2 Psychological factors, immune function and HIV

Despite much speculation, there is little direct evidence that psychological factors are important in either the susceptibility to, or rate of progression of, HIV infection. For this reason, most physicians remain sceptical of the importance of psychological factors. In stark contrast to the scepticism common amongst medical practitioners, the role of psychological factors in the delay or prevention of HIV disease progression is widely accepted by many people with HIV. In a survey of people who had been known to be HIV seropositive for more than five years and remained well, 94 per cent attributed their continued health to psychological factors (Troop et al, 1994).

To date, there have been few studies published on psychoneuroimmunology in HIV infection. Perhaps the most important reason for this is that the methodological problems in establishing a clear link between psychological factors and immunological functioning are formidable and difficult to overcome with a clinical population. For example, susceptibility to infection, an area in which psychological factors may be as important as they are in other infectious diseases, would be almost impossible to study in HIV infection. Identifying and studying individuals who are to likely to be exposed to infection and seroconvert presents considerable practical and ethical problems. The alternative strategy of deliberate infection, a method frequently used in common cold research, is clearly out of the question.

Another important methodological problem is that immunological function may be affected by a wide range of social and behavioural factors including substance use (drugs, alcohol, caffeine, and tobacco), nutrition, sexual activity, aerobic fitness, sleep patterns, medication, social class, occupation, and age (Ader, 1988; Goodkin et al, 1994). In many experimental studies, these factors would be considered to be random errors which, provided a large enough sample size is used, should not have an undue influence on the outcome of the study. In psychoneuroimmunological research the same factors are almost certainly systematically related to both the psychological factors and the measures of immunological function. For example, someone who is depressed is likely to be less active (i.e. have lower aerobic fitness), have less sex, poorer sleep, and may use more alcohol and drugs. To establish a link between depression and immunological function, all these factors would need to be taken into account.

Nor is the choice of measures of immunological function straightforward. There are a wide range of measures that could be used and it is not always clear which are the most relevant in any particular case. In many studies in HIV infection, the sole measure used has been CD4 count because this measure is regularly taken and easily available. Although CD4 count is of established importance in HIV disease, it may not be the most appropriate measure for psychoneuroimmunological research, particularly when short-term experimental manipulations are involved. Lymphocyte count measures, such as CD4, are relatively unreactive over the short term (Stein et al, 1991), but may be more informative over longer periods. In contrast, the responsivity of different lymphocyte subsets (e.g. lymphocyte proliferation to mitogen and natural killer cytotoxicity) may be much more sensitive. Responsivity measures may be more sensitive to psychological influences but they are also more difficult, more time-consuming and more expensive to measure. In addition, there are large individual variations, significant diurnal variations and the samples must be fresh when assayed. There may also be systematic variation between immunological assays taken on different days and for this reason, in group studies, blood taken from each group should be analysed at the same time.

The choice of psychological measures also present difficulties. Although state measures may show good relationships with immunological measures cross-sectionally, it would be surprising if measures of transient mood states had strong predictive associations longitudinally. Mood states are only likely to be important in long-term prediction if they are maintained over a prolonged period or in as much as they reflect durable psychological characteristics. For this reason, relatively stable psychological features such as personality, dispositional style (e.g. coping mechanisms) and social support should be included in addition to measures of mood.

The design of the study is also important. To show that psychological factors influence immune functioning, it is essential that a longitudinal design is used. Longitudinal designs are by definition more time consuming, expensive and difficult to run than simple cross-sectional studies.

6.4.3 Research evidence

Despite these methodological difficulties, several studies have been published which attempt to show the importance of psychological factors in HIV infection. Table 6.1 summarizes those studies which include measures of both psychological and immunological function in HIV infection. Studies reported at

Table 6.1 Summary of research into the psychoneuroimmunology of HIV infection

Authors/group	Design	Psychological measures	Immunological measures	Authors' conclusions
Antoni et al, 1991; 1991a University of Miami	71 well gay/bisexual men were assessed at intervals in the 5 weeks prior to HIV serostatus notification and followed up for 5 weeks.	Coping style (COPE) Anxiety (STAI) Mood states (POMS) Intrusive thoughts (IES)	Lymphocyte subset counts. Lymphocyte responsivity. Cortisol β-endorphin.	Among the HIV+ subjects, cortisol levels and lymphocyte responsivity were negatively associated with psychological distress both before and after serostatus notification.
Burack et al, 1993 University of California, San Francisco	330 HIV+ (non-AIDS) gay/bisexual men were assessed and followed up with semi-annual assessments up to 66 months.	Depression (CES-D)	Rate of decline of CD4 count.	Depression is associated with a more rapid decline in CD4 count.
Goodkin et al, 1992a University of Miami	62 HIV+ (asymptomatic) gay/bisexual men were assessed cross-sectionally	Life events (LES) Social support (SPS) Coping style (COPE) Mood states (POMS)	Natural killer cell responsivity.	Active coping was positively associated with natural killer cell activity.
Goodkin et al, 1992b University of Miami	11 HIV+ (asymptomatic) gay/bisexual men were assessed cross-sectionally.	Life events (LES) Coping style (COPE)	Lymphocyte subset counts.	High levels of life events and passive coping style were associated with lower lymphocyte counts.
Ironson et al, 1990 University of Miami	46 well gay/bisexual men were assessed at intervals in the 5 weeks prior to HIV-1 serostatus notification and the 5 weeks afterwards.	Anxiety (STAI) Intrusive thoughts (IES)	Lymphocyte subset counts. Lymphocyte responsivity. Natural killer responsivity.	There was a dissociation between psychological and immunological responses in the HIV+ but not the HIV− groups.
Kemeny et al, 1994 MACS study, Los Angeles	45 HIV+ (asymptomatic) gay/bisexual man who had recently suffered a bereavement were compared with 45 matched non-bereaved controls.	Mood states (POMS)	Lymphocyte subset counts. Lymphocyte responsivity. Neopterin.	There are differences between the bereaved and non-bereaved men on any immunological measure. In the non-bereaved group, those reporting depressed mood showed lower CD4 counts and lower proliferation response to PHA.
Kessler et al, 1991 MACS study, Chicago	1059 HIV+ (asymptomatic) and 1084 HIV− gay/bisexual men assessed semi-annually up to 5 times	General life events AIDS-specific life events	CD4 as a percentage of all lymphocytes. Onset of thrush and/or fever.	There were no significant associations between the psychological and immunological measures.

University of Columbia, New York	HIV− gay/bisexual men were assessed at four time points over a 2 year period.	anxiety rating scales	CD4 and CD8 count.	associations between the psychological and immunological measures in either the HIV+ or HIV− groups.
Lyketsos et al, 1993b MACS study, all sites combined	1809 HIV+ (non-AIDS) gay/bisexual men were assessed semi-annually for up to 8 years.	Depression (CES-D)	Rate of decline of CD4.	Depression was not significantly associated with a more rapid decline in CD4 count.
Nokes and Kendrew, 1990	31 HIV+ (AIDS) gay/bisexual men were assessed and followed up over 6 months.	Loneliness	Number of AIDS-related infections.	There was no significant association between loneliness and the number of AIDS-related illnesses.
Perry et al, 1992 Cornell University Medical College, New York	221 HIV+ (non-AIDS) patients of both sexes and mixed risk factors were assessed at baseline, at 6 months and at 1 year.	Depression (BDI) Brief Symptom Inventory Anxiety (STAI) Intrusive thoughts (IES) Social support (ISEL) Hardiness (HQ) Life events Personality Disorder Questionnaire + clinical ratings	CD4 and CD8 count.	There were no significant associations between the psychological and immunological measures.
Rabkin et al, 1990b University of Columbia, New York	124 HIV+ (non-AIDS) gay/bisexual men were assessed at baseline and at 6 months follow-up.	Hamilton Anxiety and Depression rating scales Demoralization Hopelessness Social conflict Grief Life events	CD4 and CD8 count.	There were no significant associations between the psychological and immunological measures
Solano et al, 1993 Institutio Italiano di Medicina Sociale, Rome	100 HIV+ (asymptomatic) subjects of both sexes and mixed risk factors were assessed at baseline and at 6 months and 1-year follows-ups.	CD4 count.	Denial and repression were negatively associated with CD4 count and fighting spirit positively. Hardiness and social support, in interaction with baseline CD4, were also associated with CD4 count.	

MACS = Multicenter AIDS Cohort Study. HIV+ = HIV seropositive; HIV− = HIV seronegative.
Questionnaires used in more than one study include: COPE = Coping Orientations to Problems Experienced; STAI = Spielberger Stait–Trait Anxiety Inventory; POMS = Proile of Mood States; IES = Impact of Events Scale; BDI = Beck Depression Inventory; CES-D = Center for Epidemiologic Studies Depression scale; LES = Life Experiences Studies Depression scale; LES = Life Experiences Survey; HQ = Hardiness Questionnaire.

conferences which have not subsequently been published are not included. The majority of studies included gay or bisexual men so the implications of the findings are not necessarily generalizable to other risk groups. The area of greatest consensus is that if psycho-neuroimmunological factors are important in HIV infection, the crucial time will be in the asymptomatic stages of disease, although this assumption is not supported by any direct evidence. For this reason, all but one study excluded people with a confirmed diagnosis of AIDS. In some cases, only those with CDC stage II disease were included which meant that even mild signs such as lymphadenopathy were treated as an exclusion criterion. Most of the studies also used a longitudinal design.

The studies listed in Table 6.1 can be broadly divided into two types. First, there are the larger studies which, for the most part, use pre-existing cohorts and a relatively narrow range of measures. Second, there are the smaller studies which tend to use specially recruited cohorts, a broader range of measures and employ a more sophisticated experimental design. Of the larger studies (i.e. sample size greater than 100), only Burack et al (1993) reported a significant longitudinal association between a psychological (in this case depression) and an immunological measure (rate of decline of CD4 count). None of the other large studies (Kessler et al, 1991; Kertzner et al, 1993; Lyketsos et al, 1993b; Perry et al, 1992; Rabkin et al, 1990b) found any such association. In most of these, however, although the sample sizes were large, the range of both the psychological and immunological measures were quite limited. In addition, in most, CD4 count was the sole immunological measure, although clinical measures such as the first onset of symptoms or the start of prophylactic treatment were also included, and none used measures of immune responsivity. Similarly, most of these studies were restricted to one psychological measure (either life events or depression) and only the Perry et al (1992) and Rabkin et al (1990b) studies used a broader range of measures. None of these large studies used both a broad range of psychological and immunological measures.

Of the smaller studies (sample size less than 100) all found some association between psychological factors and immunological measures with one exception (Nokes and Kendrew, 1990). This study was the only one reported which included people with AIDS, used limited psychological measures and had no direct immunological measure. The remaining small studies generally included a broader range of psychological measures, most included measures of immune responsivity and the measurement of confounding factors was carefully assessed and taken into account in the analysis. In most cases, however, these smaller studies were either cross-sectional or involved short follow-up periods. Only one study (Solano et al, 1993) reported a significant association between psychological and immunological measures over a period of up to one year. This may suggest that the relationships between psychological state and immunological function are only transient.

The are no firm conclusions to be drawn from these studies, but the balance of evidence suggests that there is little, if any, effect of mood state on CD4 count over periods of a year or more. Whether more durable psychological characteristics such as personality and dispositional style, are stronger predictors is still uncertain. There is, however, an accumulation of evidence that psychological factors are important over a period of a few weeks on some aspects of immune function such as natural killer cell function and lymphocyte proliferation. Whether these changes are durable and whether they have any direct relevance to disease progression in HIV is still not known. Many of the discrepancies between the studies in this area are almost certainly due to differences in methodology. Size is not the most important factor. It may not be possible in a large study to include the necessary breadth of assessment. Most importantly, a range of both psychological (including state, dispositional, interpersonal and personality) and immunological (including lymphocyte count and responsivity) measures should be used in a longitudinal design. In addition, information about confounding factors (e.g. drug and alcohol use, behavioural and lifestyle patterns) which are known to affect the immune system should be collected and controlled for either experimentally or statistically.

In addition to those studies examining the relationship between psychological and immunological measures, there have also been a small number of intervention studies. Intervention studies are potentially of great importance in this area. If properly conducted, using a good experimental design, many of the methodological problems associated with longitudinal, correlational studies may be resolved. The four intervention studies reported to date are summarized in Table 6.2. In each case, the interventions were short term and the follow-up periods were short. Three of the intervention packages involved cognitive or behavioural stress reduction methods. Two of these (Auerbach et al, 1992; Coates et al, 1989) found no immunological benefit from stress reduction. In one case (Auerbach et al, 1992), this negative finding is unsurprising as there were no psychological benefits either and in the other case (Coates et al, 1989) no psychological measures were reported so it is unclear whether any significant psychological changes were seen. The remaining study was well designed and reported a positive outcome from the intervention. Antoni et al (1991b) found that the short-term stress associated with notification of a positive HIV result was ameliorated by stress management in the weeks before receiving the result and that this had a beneficial impact on immunological function. LaPerriere et al (1990, 1991) using a similar study design found significant benefits for aerobic exercise.

Although two well-designed studies have reported short-term immunological benefits from psychological interventions, the efficacy of such interventions in delaying disease progression over the longer term is unknown. One consistent assumption from all these studies, however, is that if there is an effect of psychological factors on disease progression it is in one direction: poor mental health will lead to poorer health outcomes. This being the case, worrying overmuch about whether psychological factors influence health becomes something of an academic issue. Poor mental health (e.g. depression, unhappiness, anxiety, worries, etc.) is undesirable in itself and should be dealt with using the appropriate psychological or pharmacological means. Any beneficial impact on the disease progression is an added bonus.

Table 6.2 Summary of psychoneuroimmunological interventions to delay the progression of HIV infection

Authors/group	Design	Psychological measures	Immunological measures	Authors' conclusions
Antoni et al, 1991b University of Miami	47 well gay/bisexual men were randomly assigned to a cognitive-behavioural stress management programme or a waiting-list control, 5 weeks prior to notification of HIV serostatus and 5 weeks afterwards.	Coping style (COPE) Anxiety (STAI) Mood states (POMS) Intrusive thoughts (IES)	Lymphocyte subset counts. Lymphocyte responsivity. Cortisol. β-endorphin.	HIV+ subjects who underwent the stress management course showed no significant increase in depression but did show increases in CD4 and natural killer cell counts. Controls showed increased depression and no change in CD4 or natural killer cell counts.
Auerbach et al, 1992 Health Establishment Institute of California	26 HIV+ asymptomatic gay/bisexual men were randomly allocated to 8-week behavioural intervention or to a waiting-list control.	Mood states (POMS) Depression (BDI) Personal Views Survey HIV distress inventory	CD4 count.	There were no differences in CD4 count between the treatment group and controls but there were also no differences between the groups on the psychological measures.
Coates et al, 1989 University of California, San Francisco	64 HIV+ gay/bisexual men (excluding those on medication and those with specified opportunitistic infections) were randomly allocated to 8 2-hour sessions of stress management or to a waiting-list control.	None reported.	Lymphocyte subset counts. Natural killer cell responsivity. Lymphocyte responsivity.	There were no differences between the treatment group and the controls in lymphocyte number or function.
LaPerriere, et al 1990, 1991 University of Miami	50 HIV+ asymptomatic gay/bisexual men were randomly assigned to 5 weeks of aerobic training or to waiting list control prior to HIV serostatus notification.	Anxiety (STAI) Mood states (POMS)	Lymphocyte subset counts.	HIV+ controls showed increase in anxiety and depression and a reduction in natural killer cells following serostatus notification. HIV+ exercisers showed no changes and did not differe from the HIV-group.

MACS = Multicenter AIDS Cohort Study. HIV+ = HIV seropositive; HIV− = HIV seronegative.
Questionnaires used in more than one study include: COPE = Coping Orientations to Problems Experienced; STAI = Spielberger State–Trait Anxiety Inventory; POMS = Profile of Mood States; IES = Impact of Events Scale; BDI = Beck Depression Inventory; CES-D = Center for Epidemiologic Studies Depression scale; LES = Life Experiences Survey; HQ = Hardiness Questionnaire.

6.5 Summary

Behavioural change in the direction of lower HIV risk activities remains the main target of prevention strategies aimed at the containment of the epidemic of HIV infection. Risk behaviours are common and their modification is not easy. A variety of factors contribute to their persistence. In the case of unsafe sexual behaviour, risk perception, attitudes to condom use, emotional state, demographic factors, use of alcohol and other substances, intrapersonal factors, perceived social norms, and type of relationship, have been implicated in unsafe sexual behaviour. A similar pattern of determinants has been put forward in the case of unsafe injecting drug use. Psychological interventions to modify unsafe behaviours are discussed next, including the role of media campaigns, school and college education, and HIV testing, as well as targeted interventions for different groups at risk and in different settings.

Prevention of progression of HIV infection by psychological and behavioural means is discussed in the second part of the chapter, with emphasis on reviewing the empirical evidence about the role of psychological factors on immune function and health changes in people with HIV infection. The methodological and practical problems involved in this area of research are discussed.

7 The emotional cost of caring: impact on professional staff and volunteers

7.1 Introduction

That caring for a severely ill person may at times be extremely demanding and distressing cannot be seriously doubted and in this respect HIV disease is no exception. Indeed, caring for a person with serious HIV disease may present additional stresses which result from its medical complexity, perceived risk of infection, social stigma and ethical and political dilemmas. In HIV infection, almost any organ or system can be affected, leading to the involvement of many professionals from medical, nursing, social work and mental health specialties, as well as voluntary workers. The ability of these health workers to cope with persistent exposure to caring for people with debilitating and severe conditions, and to face the repeated experience of death vary between individuals and within an individual at different times. Many factors are likely to affect a person's ability to cope, including: (a) personal and motivational issues, such as previous experience of illness and death, and reasons for choosing to work with people with HIV; (b) the nature of the job and the degree and length of exposure to losses due to HIV; and (c) the work setting and the nature of the supports available.

Other factors may also add to the emotional pressures on care workers. The stigma attached to many of their patients may also be extended to them, so that their relatives and peers may become unsupportive or downright rejecting. Fears of contamination can play an important part in the development of emotional difficulties. Finally, the ethical and legal questions raised by HIV can affect health workers' willingness and ability to provide care (Maj, 1991; Silverman, 1993) (see Chapter 8).

There have been empirical investigations of the impact of caring for people with HIV infection and some of this work will be reviewed here. There is, however, a dearth of systematic research into how best to prevent and minimize the adverse emotional consequences for care workers and volunteers.

7.2 Psychological impact on professional staff

7.2.1 Emotional reactions and factors associated with stress

Wofsy (1988) noted that health care staff go through several stages in adjusting to the reality of AIDS. First, HIV is seen as someone else's problem. Next, demands for a risk-free environment follow, with a series of 'prove to me' challenges: prove to me that it cannot be transmitted by saliva, that it is safe to eat in a restaurant, that an infected health worker will not infect others, or that my child cannot get it from a classmate. Eventually, there is a general recognition that HIV is here and is not going to go away. Acceptance tends to lead to intellectual interest, and after reading, asking and listening, the focus changes to concern and compassion for the person with the infection. This astute observation remains empirically untested.

The impact of HIV infection on health workers has been assessed in numerous studies (Eakin and Taylor, 1990) in order to estimate how this will effect the quality of care given to people with HIV infection. However, after a decade of living with AIDS, research into occupational stress associated with HIV has not yet moved from descriptive and clinical observations, experiential accounts or questionnaire surveys, to controlled studies or testing of specific hypotheses. There are very few reports concerning carers from developing countries, where the problem is at its most severe and where resources are limited.

In some early reports of in-patient units caring for their first patients with HIV, fear, avoidance, denial of emotional response, and identification even to the point of believing themselves to be affected by the illness were described among the staff (Polan et al, 1985; Rosse, 1985; Cummings et al, 1986) alongside frequent instances of unprofessional behaviour (Lerton, 1983; Glazer and Dudley, 1985). These included nurses and other health care workers choosing to resign rather than care for people with AIDS, refusal to handle specimens from infected patients, domestic and maintenance staff refusing to enter or touch anything in rooms of people with HIV infection, and inappropriate infection control in routine contacts with people with HIV infection or with those thought to be infected.

Investigations of specific sources of stress pinpoint several themes. General anxiety about patients and their care, fears related to dealing with particular medical crises and procedures (e.g. cardiac arrest or dealing with incontinence), and stress due to negative attitudes of own families and friends to their HIV work was reported in a study of 500 nurses (Klonoff and Ewers, 1990). Similarly, stigma, suffering and the terminal nature of AIDS were identified as major sources of stress by a group of nurses, social workers, doctors, dentists and psychologists, while the opportunity to provide comfort, support and education to patients with HIV illness were perceived as very satisfying (Nashman et al, 1990).

The stress of working with people with a life-threatening illness and with dying people, and having to deal with their psychological and physical problems are not unique to HIV care staff. Comparisons between staff working in oncology and AIDS care have found that a similar proportion, between a third and one-half, report these stresses in both groups (Catalán et al, in press). The experience of nurses working with people with haemophilia is somewhat different. Those who had worked with persons with haemophilia for 10–15 years were particularly vulnerable to feelings of guilt for having participated in the treatment that resulted in HIV infection. The areas of greatest distress were failures of patients to take steps to prevent transmission, and experiencing repeated losses, as patients died from the consequences of the infection (Gordon et al, 1993).

Descriptions of psychological distress obtained in psychiatric and psychotherapeutic practice evoke parallels with signs and symptoms of post-traumatic stress disorder (McKusick and Horstman, 1986; Silverman, 1993). Recurrent intrusive thoughts, dreams, flashbacks, avoidance of the stimuli associated with the stressor (e.g. avoidance of people with HIV illness, avoidance of clinical duties, or career changes), exaggerated fears of becoming infected, emotional numbing and detachment, have been described and sometimes labelled as *compassion fatigue*. Some of these reactions have been likened to the *vicarious traumatization* that has been reported in psychotherapists working intensively with survivors of sexual abuse and violence (McCann and Pearlman, 1990).

The term 'burnout' (Mayou, 1987) has become popular to describe the consequences of work-related stress, not just in relation to health care, but for almost any occupation. It tends to be used in a rather imprecise way, usually making it synonymous with tension or stress. There have been attempts to operationalize the concept, and Maslach (1982) has identified three components to burnout: emotional exhaustion, depersonalization, and lack of personal accomplishment. *Emotional exhaustion* refers to a feeling of lack of capacity to offer psychological support to others. *Depersonalization* describes a sense of indifference towards patients and colleagues. *Lack of personal accomplishment* indicates feelings of dissatisfaction with professional competence. A report by McKusick and Horstman (1986) concerning staff involved in HIV care found that after working with people with AIDS, 36 per cent of physicians experienced an increase in depression, 34 per cent in anxiety, 39 per cent felt overworked, 46 per cent reported more stress, and 38 per cent more fear of death. In another report, Ross and Seeger (1988) found that burnout affected 30–40 per cent of hospital staff caring for people with AIDS, despite the reported intellectual stimulation they gained in the course of their work. Major contributors to burnout included concern about the young age of the patients, uncertainty about their emotional needs and inability to deal with them, and the neurological aspects of AIDS and dying patients.

Nurses providing AIDS care have been found to suffer burnout less frequently than nurses working in cancer care but their burnout was more severe (Bennett et al, 1991). It has been reported that staff in these care groups have levels of psychological morbidity similar to those of their patients (Catalán et al, in press). Over a third of health workers in oncology and HIV care, regardless of care groups, reported levels of psychological morbidity above caseness level on the General Health Questionnaire (Goldberg and Hillier, 1979), a proportion similar to that reported for medical patients and general practice attenders using the same instrument (Goldberg and Huxley, 1992). In Catalán et al's study, about a fifth of all care workers showed substantial levels of burnout. Compared with gay health workers, heterosexuals working with people with HIV were more likely to experience burnout. As the large majority of people with HIV in this study were gay/bisexual men, it may be that gay health workers found it easier to relate to them, and experienced greater sense of achievement and work satisfaction. The suggestion that gay health workers experience less work-related stress in HIV care, is consistent with the findings reported in studies of volunteers mentioned below.

The proportion of total working time spent in HIV care has been found to be a risk factor for burnout, and to correlate with levels of depression (McKusick and Horstman, 1986). Spending less than 60 per cent of the working week on HIV has been claimed to be the threshold for avoiding psychological distress (Miller, 1988). In one study, nurses from hospitals with high admission rates for people with AIDS, who would be expected to be better informed and have greater experience of caring for people with HIV, were found to be less willing to care for patients with AIDS than nurses from hospitals with moderate or low admission rates (Kempainnen et al, 1991). The authors suggested that the pressures caused by heavy workload in such hospitals may overburden staff and contribute to cause emotional stress.

7.2.2 Managing and preventing work-related stress

There have been no systematic reports of interventions to prevent or reduce work-related emotional stress in HIV settings, and what evidence there is, is based on description of services or surveys of health workers. Common-sense suggestions have included, for example, encouragement to ensure that care is shared between professionals both in hospital and in the community, to reduce the impact on individuals. Staff involvement in the care of people with other medical problems, as opposed to exclusive involvement in HIV, has also being recommended. Continuing professional education and updating about HIV, and participation in team decision-making is also regarded as important in reducing stress (Volberding, 1989). Mutual staff support groups contributed to a dramatic drop in turnover rates of nurses in an AIDS unit (Bartnof, 1989). Staff groups may help to reduce an individual staff member's sense of isolation, allow staff to see how colleagues cope, and lead to greater team cohesion.

It is likely that the needs of different professional groups, such as doctors and nurses, will require different interventions. For example, the emotional stresses faced by junior medical staff involved in caring for patients with chronic medical problems who are well informed about their condition and are able to challenge the doctors' clinical decisions, are likely to be different from those of their more senior colleagues who have been exposed to the death of many of their patients, or the stresses faced by nursing staff providing palliative care to distraught patients.

For most health care workers, recognition of situations that lead to distress or to working difficulties within the team, and development of strategies to deal with them could be achieved by means of staff group meetings. It is sometimes useful to include an outside facilitator, with no direct involvement with the team other than at the time of the group meetings, although groups can function well without such a person. In the group meetings, it is best to focus discussion on work-related issues, rather than on personal emotional problems, even if individual staff reactions have personal significance and relate to previous traumas or difficulties. On occasions, individual health workers may, in the course of their work, identify problems within themselves requiring psychological help. In such cases it is best to seek assistance outside the work setting, rather than through professional support groups.

7.3 Psychological impact on volunteers

Voluntary organizations have made a key contribution to care of people with HIV infection. In each area, membership of these organizations ranges from a few dozen to several hundred people. Volunteers are involved in distributing food, providing information hotlines, helplines, education about prevention, and legal and political advocacy. Provision of emotional support and befriending of people with HIV infection has been an important area of voluntary work. An example of the work of volunteers is provided by 'buddies', trained volunteers who befriend and support people with HIV infection on a personal basis, according to individual needs. This support often lasts until the death of the person and often beyond death through involvement with relatives.

Organizations involving gay/bisexual men in developed countries have played a crucial role in the development of volunteer systems. Services provided by volunteers in San Francisco reduced the cost of care per patient with symptomatic HIV infection from \$150 000 to \$40 000 per year (Omoto and Snyder, 1990). Apart from the indirect financial contributions, volunteers work in ways which are not possible for paid carers. They offer a personal and continuous relationship with a substantial degree of flexibility. A survey of one volunteer project in the US found that almost all the volunteers visited at least once a week, more than half provided transport at least once a week and spoke on the phone at least twice a week. Shopping, cleaning and preparing meals were done less often. Over 60 per cent of volunteers spent six or more hours weekly donating their services (Velentgas et al, 1990).

The reasons why people become volunteers has received only limited attention. Claxton et al (1994) found that the most common reasons for volunteering were related to a specific interest in HIV rather than a general interest in voluntary work. For instance, wishing to help overcome the prejudice experienced by people living with HIV infection, wanting to find out more about HIV, and helping others in a situation they could identify with, were the most commonly endorsed reasons. This finding is consistent with the observation made by Titmuss (1971) that volunteering is not an act of charity, and that it has much more to do with relationships. Volunteer activity offers a sense of belonging and contributing, and thus provides very powerful incentive for those who participate. Titmuss suggested that giving to strangers opens an outlet for the contribution that the individual wishes to make to society, and affirms that the kind of society we want to live in, is one which is just, fair and caring.

It is not known to what extent personal motivation and altruistic feelings may contribute to reduce emotional stress in volunteers. Available information from the few studies published to date, suggests that, despite the demands of HIV-related care, the mental health of volunteers, as a group, is not significantly affected, and that only a proportion experiences difficulties. Burnout and psychiatric morbidity have been found in approximately one-fifth of volunteers (Maslanka, 1992), although some studies have reported rates as high as 40 per cent (Guinan et al, 1991). Burnout is a common reason for dropping out of volunteering (Calvert, 1991), although Claxton et al (1994) found that self-reported burnout was lower among 'buddies' (25 per cent) than among health care staff working with people with HIV/AIDS (over a third) (Catalán et al, in press). 'Buddies' also reported lower levels of anxiety or depression than health care workers. Factors which were associated with high levels of psychological distress in volunteers were: age (older 'buddies' being less distressed); 'wanting to feel needed'; poorer health status of the person being helped; and dissatisfaction with the training received. Volunteers who are themselves living with HIV infection report, as expected, poorer physical health but are at no greater psychological risk (or advantage) than their seronegative colleagues (Hamel et al, 1991a, b). On the other hand, volunteers providing emotional, as opposed to practical support, reported gaining a sense of personal effectiveness, emotional and social support, and knowledge about themselves (Guinan et al, 1991).

Compared with health care workers, several factors are likely to contribute to the reported lower levels of burnout in volunteers. Self-selection is one such factor: by the nature of their roles, volunteers would be less likely to fear 'occupational' HIV infection, feel less discomfort about sexual issues surrounding the infection, or the social stigma sometimes evoked by caring for people with AIDS. In addition, volunteers spend less time providing support than professional carers, for whom the amount of time spent in direct patient care can be a risk factor for emotional stress. A national Canadian survey found that distress in non-professional carers increased with years of HIV experience (1–2 years) and percentage of time devoted to HIV-related work (>50 per cent) (Lamping et al, 1991).

7.4 Attitudes to patient care and knowledge about HIV

7.4.1 Surveys of attitudes and knowledge amongst health care staff

Knowledge and attitudes to HIV have been measured by questionnaire surveys of health workers, by examining hospital policies and by the experiences of people with HIV infection. Attitude surveys have typically enquired about the following: views about risks involved in casual contact with those with HIV infection; willingness to be involved in various aspects of the care of patients with HIV, from counselling about HIV antibody test to terminal care; the integration of patients with HIV infection with other patients in hospital; the degree of confidence and competence when asking about HIV infection risk activities; willingness to care for people in different HIV transmission groups; views about homosexuality and substance misuse; and concern with social stigmatization through caring for patients with HIV infection. Knowledge about HIV transmission, occupational risk and personal fear of becoming infected, and infection control measures, have been assessed in numerous studies involving primary care staff (Boyton and Scambler, 1988; King, 1989c; Boyd et al, 1990; Lewis et al, 1987), across medical specialties (Searle, 1987; Paine and Briggs, 1988), among hospital staff (Gordin et al, 1987; Pomerance and Shields, 1988; Klimes et al, 1989) and dentists (Gerbert, 1987).

These studies are mostly of local significance and do not yield surprising results. Usually it is found that a variable number of staff are not well informed about HIV transmission risk and occupational infection control measures. The themes that have repeatedly emerged centre around the fear of becoming infected by HIV at work, social stigmatization due to being involved in the care of those with HIV infection, unease about the sexual issues surrounding the infection, and a sense of professional inadequacy, as well as of reward and challenge (Eakin and Taylor, 1990).

The diagnosis of AIDS has the potential to elicit a negative judgement about patients and unease among people on whom they may depend for their physical care and emotional and social support. A patient with AIDS, compared with an identically described patient said to have leukaemia, evoked much more negative attitudes (Kelly et al, 1987; St. Lawrence et al, 1988). The person with AIDS was considered to be more responsible for his illness and more deserving of what had happened to him; to be experiencing more pain, but to be less deserving of sympathy and understanding; to be more dangerous to others; and more likely to require quarantine measures. The respondents (doctors and psychologists) were also less willing to interact socially with AIDS patients. Support for measures overriding civil liberties in order to control the AIDS epidemic has been expressed by a proportion of health workers (e.g. making sexual relations between men illegal; treating patients with HIV infection according to society's rather than to the patients' needs and interests) (Boyton and Scambler, 1988).

Attitudes to the care of people with HIV infection appear to be part of a complex interaction of a number of factors. These include: knowledge about HIV infection; having had previous contact with people with HIV infection; presence of homophobia; negative views about drug users; concern about occupational risk of infection; occupation; length of experience and years since training was completed; medical specialty; and age. Studies of hospital workers have demonstrated the link between levels of knowledge and attitudes, with better informed staff expressing more positive attitudes towards AIDS patients and their care (Gordin et al, 1987; Pomerance and Shields, 1988; Klimes et al, 1989; Henry et al, 1990). In a British study, having had previous contact with patients with HIV infection and having graduated in the UK in the past 10 years was associated with the greatest knowledge and the most positive attitudes towards AIDS among general practitioners in London (King, 1989c, d). Interestingly, most general practitioners were more confident in handling psychosocial problems than physical ones and they were accepting of all HIV positive patients with the exception of drug users. Similarly, in a nationally representative sample of Danish doctors, nurses and nursing aides, a strong association was found between attitudes to those with HIV infection and HIV transmission knowledge, as well as the number of personal contacts with gay men and with those living with HIV infection. Positive change in attitudes was more apparent in those who had known six or more people living with HIV infection (Krasnik et al, 1990).

7.4.2 Effect of staff attitudes on patient care

Negative attitudes to patients with HIV infection, no matter their cause or origin, are likely to be associated with reduced quality of care, and sometimes with the actual denial of care. For example, a state-wide survey of primary care physicians in California found that 32 per cent felt uneasy about treating gay men in their practice. The degree of homophobia was closely linked with the doctors' levels of knowledge with regard to HIV infection (e.g. 'Do you know a screening test for AIDS?'), application of knowledge (e.g. clinical assessment of a suspected case), and skills (e.g. sexual history-taking and counselling) (Lewis et al, 1987). Doctors in primary care with less positive attitudes or less understanding of the psychological and social consequences of HIV infection, desired less clinical involvement with such patients (King, 1989c). For instance, they were less prepared to counsel patients over the long term, found it difficult to obtain help for patients with HIV infection from other health workers, welcomed their patients receiving all their care in hospital, believed that counselling patients' partners was not their responsibility, and would prefer not to have known patients with HIV infection.

Surveys of US dentists indicated that 63 per cent would rather refer those with AIDS to other dental professionals (Gerbert, 1989). However, the experience of patients with HIV infection in California showed that the denial of care was less common (1.3 per cent HIV positive men and 10.8 per cent men with AIDS) than the attitudes of dentists had suggested (Gerbert et al, 1989). This discrepancy reflects the well-established observation that there is a low correlation between attitudes and behaviour. There are also economic factors (dentists assuming that the AIDS patients will not be able to pay), and selectiveness on the part of the patients (approaching only the dentists already known to treat those with HIV infection). People with HIV infection are understandably sensitive about the sympathy and confidentiality the health staff can provide and when they perceive that these qualities are lacking, they will not approach them (Mansfield and Singh, 1989; Mandal et al, 1991).

Reports from the US suggest that high proportions of doctors remain unwilling to treat patients with AIDS. One survey found that 23 per cent of junior hospital doctors and trainees in general practice said they would not look after such patients if they had the choice. Similar attitudes remain amongst more senior staff and 19 per cent of patients with AIDS were refused care by a medical specialist and 39 per cent of patients by a surgeon (Shapiro et al, 1992). In contrast only 4 per cent doctors in France and 14 per cent in Canada indicated a preference not to treat AIDS patients. These differences were not explained by lesser experience, self-perceived competence or more deficient training of doctors in the US (Shapiro et al, 1992).

Inadequate knowledge can be easily changed by professional education and training. McKinnon et al (1990), for example, achieved good levels of knowledge simply by issuing all staff with an information booklet. Attitudes, however, are more difficult to change, more time consuming, and the change is less likely to be maintained (Santana et al, 1991). Staff education and training about HIV has been widespread but there has been little or no evaluation. Educational interventions have included various forms of didactic teaching and participative learning (Gerbert et al, 1988a; Santana et al, 1991), dissemination of printed material and questionnaires (Wachter et al, 1988), telephone or computer feedback (Gerbert et al, 1988a), discussions with people with AIDS, and visits to the families of dying patients (Goldman, 1987; Stanford, 1988).

Results of evaluations of educational interventions show short-term changes in attitudes, knowledge, perception of risk and reported care behaviour. However, the evaluation of interventions designed to change attitudes is limited without randomization and control groups to exclude the effects of selection bias, and in the absence of follow-up to identify attitude change among health workers occurring with time and more contact with patients with HIV infection. One example of a randomized trial of educational interventions for groups of hospital staff was reported by Gallop et al (1992). The study showed that in order to change attitudes, and not just knowledge, group discussions about the information given were necessary. Change in homophobic attitudes and fear of infection needed the presence (on video or in person) of a person with HIV infection discussing his illness and experience of hospitalization.

7.5 Occupational HIV infection

7.5.1 Fear of occupational infection

The perception of occupational risk of HIV infection is increased by the serious, fatal nature of the infection and by the stigma surrounding the disease. Fear and concern about acquiring HIV infection is widespread among health workers. For example, 57 per cent of medical emergency personnel (Smyser et al, 1990), 44 per cent of Danish doctors and nurses (Krasnik et al, 1990), 36 per cent of an acute hospital workers (Henry et al, 1990) and 40 per cent of mental health and drug workers (Dow and Knox, 1991) have been reported to be anxious about acquiring HIV infection in the course of their work. Uncertainties about the risks of transmission were also reported among general practitioners (Anderson and Mayon-White, 1988). Knowledge about occupational transmission and inactivation of the virus is also limited (Sibbald and Freeling, 1988).

Fear of occupational infection is often associated to overestimating the risk of casual transmission of HIV, and to ignorance about infection control measures. Some of the fears should be, therefore, amenable to change through education. However, use of infection control procedures can lower the risk of HIV transmission but can not eliminate it completely, particularly because of accidental needle-stick injuries. It has been argued that perhaps only about a third of HIV exposures can be prevented, while the remaining two-thirds are unavoidable (Marcus et al, 1988). As long as there is a genuine risk that HIV can be transmitted at work, the health workers' anxiety will persist. Therefore, realistic aims of education and training are to reduce the risk of infection to the lowest possible level, and to ensure that unrealistic fear of infection does not compromise the quality of patient care. Discussion in small groups or work teams, with opportunities to ask questions and deal with feelings about the factual information being given, is better suited to achieving these aims than lectures (Gerbert et al, 1988a, b).

7.5.2 Surveillance and risk of infection to health care workers

The occupational risk of HIV infection became a major concern for health workers, their doctors and their employers in 1984, when the first case of seroconversion after percutaneous exposure to HIV-infected blood at work was documented (Lancet, 1984). Countries with well-developed health services have developed and established procedures for reporting occupational exposure to HIV within the established systems for monitoring injuries at work. Local centres may report details and outcome of each significant exposure to a central registry or may report exposures which result in infection to national HIV and AIDS surveillance centres. For instance, in UK a national system of surveillance was set up jointly by the Association of Medical Microbiologists and the Public Health Laboratory Service Communicable Disease Surveillance Centre (CDSC) in 1984 (CDSC, 1984). Prospective surveillance involves recording the details of incident and exposure in standard manner, providing information about immediate management and the result of the health care worker's baseline HIV antibody test, and assessing the significance of the exposure to HIV. Staff with exposures assessed as significant should then be managed according to good practice guidelines (see below). The outcome of significant exposure incidents, including HIV antibody tests at six weeks, three months, and at a minimum of six months after the exposure, is also reported to the surveillance body.

Occupational transmission of HIV has been reported and confirmed in cases of percutaneous inoculation or contact with an open wound, broken skin, or mucous membranes with blood or blood contaminated body fluids, or with concentrated virus in certain laboratory settings. Estimates of seroconversion rates following percutaneous exposure to HIV infected blood (the most common type of exposure) range from 0.10 per cent (Ippolito et al, 1993) to 2 per cent (95 per cent confidence rates from 0.006 to 7.15 per cent) (Heptonstall et al, 1993) in European countries and the US. The overall risk of becoming HIV positive after one percutaneous injury has been estimated as 3 in 1000 (Working Group of the Royal College of Pathologists, 1992). The risk has been estimated to be higher for certain types of percutaneous exposures. A seroconversion rate of 3 in 58 (5.8 per cent) (Tait et al, 1992) observed in a small study in South Africa has not been adequately explained, one possible explanation being that only high risk exposures were reported by the health workers.

The estimation of transmission rates may be affected by biological factors, observational bias, and sampling variation (Heptonstall et al, 1993). Biological factors include the volume of the inoculum and the concentration and perhaps the strain of the virus present. Antigenaemia increases as disease progresses, but may be changed by anti-retroviral therapy, which may also affect the efficacy of post-exposure prophylaxis. Observational bias may result from differences in thresholds for reporting exposure incidents, definitions of significant exposures, and in surveillance methods for case ascertainment.

Percutaneous injury is responsible for the largest proportion of HIV infection acquired at work by health carers in US, 80 per cent of whom are nurses (Gerberding, 1991). It has been estimated that 37 per cent of exposures to HIV could have been avoided by the use of appropriate disposal of sharp objects and needles (Marcus et al, 1988). However, in some settings (operating theatres and casualty) the finite risk of transmitting HIV is multiplied by repeated exposures, by delayed awareness of skin punctures (Matta et al, 1988) and by the higher prevalence of blood-borne infections in the patient population (Gerberding, 1991). Among all admissions to US hospitals from July 1989 to June 1990, 0.9 per cent patients were estimated to be HIV seropositive (one in every 115 patients) and about a third of these patients with HIV infection was re-admitted with a diagnosis not suggestive of HIV (Stafford et al, 1991). In a casualty department, 6 per cent of patients were found to be infected with HIV (Kelen et al, 1991). Accidental exposures to HIV are also more likely when the staff are more tired, working too fast, or if they are nervous, inexperienced, and if sharp instruments and needles are handled by more than one person at a time instead of being passed in a tray.

The number of documented cases of HIV transmissions following occupational exposure since 1983, is less than 70 world-wide, and another 120 are cases of possible occupationally acquired HIV infection in health care staff (Heptonstall et al, 1993) This figure may be an underestimate due to the criteria used by the Centers for Disease Control for the acceptance of cases as occupationally acquired infection (Williams, 1991).

7.5.3 Management of occupational exposure to HIV

People exposed to a significant risk of HIV infection need to be counselled about HIV and followed up at least over the next six months (Heptonstall et al, 1993). A significant exposure is defined as one in which a person sustains: (a) a percutaneous exposure (skin is cut or penetrated by a needle or scalpel, trochar, tooth, or bone spicule) to blood known or found to be HIV infected, body fluid or laboratory fluid known to contain live virus; or (b) a mucocutaneous exposure (the eyes, inside of the nose or mouth, or broken skin) to blood known or found to be HIV-infected or laboratory fluid known to contain live virus.

Guidelines for good practice for the management of significant exposures suggest that, as soon as possible after the incident, the person is counselled regarding transmission risk from the incident and about the use of zidovudine prophylaxis. Follow-up at six weeks, three months, and at a minimum of six months after exposure, needs to be discussed as well as the need to report interim illness. The staff member must have an assurance of confidentiality and that follow-up will not restrict employment. They will be given advice about future insurance and advised to avoid further possible transmission (protected sexual intercourse, avoidance of pregnancy, blood, organ, and semen donation). Informed consent for HIV testing is sought and a blood sample for a baseline HIV test is taken. Blood sample from source of the exposure is also taken if identifiable and available for testing. Hepatitis B and C and other risks are managed appropriately. Follow-up appointment is arranged and a report should be sent to Public Health Laboratory Service Communicable Disease Surveillance Centre. Thereafter, the worker should have continuing access to advice and support. The effects of prophylaxis, if zidovudine has been taken, should be monitored. HIV tests should be repeated at six weeks, three months, and at a minimum of six months' post exposure. The management and outcome should then be reported to the Public Health Laboratory Service Communicable Disease Surveillance Centre.

If the exposure has not been assessed as significant, the person should be given appropriate reassurance. Other infection risks need to be considered such as hepatitis B and tetanus, and future hepatitis B exposure risk needs to be considered and managed appropriately in their case. Completely effective post exposure prophylaxis is not yet available. Zidovudine is generally recommended but it does not always prevent seroconversion. The Communicable Disease Surveillance Centre in the UK (Department of Health, 1992) and the Centers for Disease Control in Atlanta (CDC, 1990) state that at present zidovudine cannot be considered a necessary part of post exposure prophylaxis (Tokars et al, 1993). The absence of other likely preventive interventions means that in practice most health workers involved in significant occupational exposure incidents choose to take zidovudine prophylactically.

7.5.4 Staff with HIV infection and risk to patients

The risk of transmission of HIV from health worker to patient is unknown but generally considered to be low. 'Look back' investigations and testing of more than 19 000 patients who have been treated by HIV seropositive staff HIV failed to identify cases where patients had been infected (Robert et al, 1993). In spite of the limitations of this kind of study, where testing patients for HIV is voluntary, and only those who opted to be tested were followed-up, 'look-back' studies established that the overall the risk to patients from HIV-infected surgeons and dentists is very low. Unfortunately, look-back studies are also unlikely to detect the infrequent but highly infectious individual who might pose a substantially higher risk to patients (Mishu and Schaffner 1993). With the exception of a dentist from Florida with AIDS who infected five patients in his practice (Cieselski et al, 1992; Centers for Disease Control, 1991b) there are no other documented instances to date. In the case of the Florida dentist, the specific mechanism of transmission was never discovered as there had been no breakdown of recommended infection control.

In the UK, health care workers have a professional obligation to seek medical advice and HIV testing, if they believe they may have been exposed to HIV infection, in whatever circumstances (Department of Health Expert Advisory

Group on AIDS, 1994). If they test positive, the health workers must seek appropriate expert medical and occupational health advice. They must not perform, and cease to perform, 'exposure-prone procedures'. These are procedures in which injury to the health worker could result in worker's blood contaminating the patient's open tissues.

If it is established that the worker has performed exposure-prone procedures, the local director of public health should be informed, in confidence, by the health worker or by a physician at the worker's request. The director of public health then should consult Department of Health and decide whether a patient notification exercise is called for. This means writing to all patients who may have been exposed to infection and offering them reassurance, counselling and HIV testing if they so wish. A doctor or occupational health physician who knows that an infected health worker has not sought or followed advice to change practice, and/or is continuing to perform exposure-prone procedures, should inform the health worker's professional regulatory body and the local director of public health.

The low risk of transmission of HIV from a health worker to a patient is yet unquantified and we need further data to underpin future policy. Bird and Gore (1993) suggested that to get relevant data, the compliance of health workers with early official guidelines to seek appropriate diagnostic testing and counselling should be assessed. For example, the interval between the report of HIV seropositivity and the diagnosis of AIDS should be longer in health care staff than in other occupations if the guidelines were followed. Secondly, the follow-up of patients who have been exposed to HIV through invasive procedures should include HIV testing. Such patients should actively consider that the only adequate reassurance is a negative antibody test, but this may uncover too some patients who had acquired the infection by other means. Thirdly, information is needed about the risks of various invasive procedures. A study using trained observers to attend operating theatres at unpredictable and random times should provide comparisons between self-reported and observer-reported injuries and blood contamination. While of interest, these proposals raise complex practical and ethical questions requiring further public and professional discussion.

7.5.5 Infection control: universal precautions versus routine screening

HIV infection has re-opened the debate about the dangers and dilemmas of occupational cross infection (during the giving or receiving of care) which developed at the turn of the century in relation to syphilis (Meyer, 1993). After recognition of the problem, it took time to control syphilis effectively through technical innovation (rubber gloves were developed), personal prophylaxis, education and regulation. These efforts led to the development of a strategy remarkably similar to the 'universal precautions' approach applied to HIV today. The directions from which this common end point was approached, however, were diametrally different for the two infections. With syphilis, doctors initially took no precautions and such measures slowly evolved over time. With HIV the early years were marked by wearing of protective suits, masks, and goggles for such tasks as patient transport, with subsequent relaxation of much of this 'isolating armour'.

The need to protect themselves (and other patients not infected by HIV) interacts with the health workers' attitudes to management of patients. There are two main approaches to occupational HIV infection control. The first one is to treat all patients as if they were HIV seropositive and therefore, all staff are advised to take the appropriate protective infection control measures ('universal precautions') (Centers for Disease Control, 1988; Department of Health Expert Advisory Group on AIDS, 1990). The second favours routine screening of hospital patients despite the medical, legal and ethical problems associated with it. Neither approach guarantees complete protection against the transmission of HIV: universal precautions do not prevent accidental needle-stick injuries and a negative HIV test result does not guarantee that the person is infection-free as the person may not yet have seroconverted.

Among doctors, attitudes to infection control tend to vary according to their medical specialty (Paine and Briggs, 1988). There is a disparity between expert opinion, which is largely accepted by advisory professionals, and the views of clinicians (Boyton and Scambler, 1988). For instance, the majority of clinicians feel that patients in high risk groups should be screened before hospital admission. The expert opinion is that there are very few circumstances in which patients should be routinely screened. There is debate about possible exceptions, as in the case of candidates for transplantation and pregnant women. In both groups testing with consent has been argued to help the management of the patient rather than to protect staff (Searle, 1987).

The philosophy of 'universal precautions' has been found to be difficult to implement and has sometimes been universally ignored. Junior doctors in casualty were observed to comply with it on only 16 per cent of occasions and to err most in the handling and disposal of needles (Hammond et al, 1990). Emergency department personnel were seen to discard needles as recommended only half of the time, and a third of the time needle re-sheathing occurred (Henry et al, 1991). Self-reports from junior doctors (Woolley et al, 1991) and general practitioners (Boyd et al, 1990) indicate that more that 50 per cent ignore advice to not re-sheath needles. There is debate suggesting that appropriate re-sheathing techniques are safer than no re-sheathing for the ultimate disposal of needles (Anderson et al, 1991). The need for technological innovation in infection control has resurfaced and efforts are underway to produce safer needles and syringes, and puncture-resistant gloves to supplement the rubber glove revolution of a century ago.

Currently, marked variations exist in the policies and practices regarding HIV antibody testing amongst, for example, infectious diseases teaching hospitals and acute hospitals in the US (Henry et al, 1988). Thirty-three per cent of all the US infectious diseases hospitals and 57 per cent of acute hospitals in Minnesota estimated that the consent of the patient was rarely obtained when an HIV antibody test was ordered. Fifty per cent of infectious diseases hospitals and 37 per cent of acute hospitals reported having a policy recommending, but not requiring, that the physician obtain consent from the patient and provide information on risk reduction. Post-test counselling was not provided to more than half of the patients tested in hospitals with that policy. The value of testing was lost to the patients and the opportunity to counsel on risk reduction in the interests of public health was missed.

The debate about routine screening of patients versus universal precautions continues. In the US, the case of the Florida dentist with AIDS who infected five of his patients and the CDC reports that nearly 5800 health workers are infected with HIV (Breo, 1990) have led to calls for mandatory HIV testing of both doctors and patients. The US Senate passed legislation effectively requiring those health workers and dentists performing surgical and other invasive procedures to be screened for HIV infection and if found to be seropositive to be barred from performing such procedures (Morris, 1991).

In the UK, the Department of Health has resisted the pleas for introduction of routine HIV testing of health care workers on basis of cost and unproven benefit. The average cost of testing a health care worker for HIV has been estimated at £120 (Rogers et al, 1993). This includes the use of an enzyme-linked immunoassay for HIV four times a year, counselling before and after testing, and hospital out-patient overheads. Annual costs for all hospital doctors and clinical staff would be about £8 million in 1995. All hospital doctors, midwives, nurses and all dentists could be screened at annual cost to the National Health Service of £65.7 million. If screening were to be confined to staff working within specialties in which invasive surgery is practised the cost would be £1.83 million (Tolley and Kennelly, 1993).

7.6 Summary

The severe health problems seen in people with advanced HIV infection, their young age, and the stigma associated with the condition, together with fear of infection, are important sources of stress for professional carers. However, their levels of work-related stress may not be different from those found in staff dealing with comparable illnesses, such as cancer. Good team work and formal support structures, such as team meetings, may help to prevent work-related stress. The amount of time spent in direct patient care may also be a factor in staff stress. Voluntary workers are subject to comparable pressures, but they appear to suffer lower levels of stress. Motivational factors are likely to be one reason for the difference.

The studies of health workers' knowledge and attitudes towards HIV point to a need for continuing staff training and education, both for their own and the patients' benefit. Exposure to professional acquaintance with HIV positive people promotes better attitudes towards their care and a more realistic assessment of the risk of HIV transmission at work. Fear of infection in health care settings remains an emotive issue among some staff, and education and training are essential to deal with staff anxiety and to minimize the risk of occupational infection. Systematic surveillance of accidental exposure incidents shows that the risk of occupational infection is low, and there guidelines for good practice to ensure that such incidents are rare, and that they are managed appropriately.

8 Ethical and legal issues

. . . he knew that the tale he had to tell could not be one of final victory. It could only be the record of what had had to be done, and what assuredly would have to be done again in the never-ending fight against terror and its relentless onslaughts, despite their personal afflictions, by all who, while unable to be saints but refusing to bow down to pestilences, strive their utmost to be healers'

Albert Camus, *The Plague*

8.1 Introduction

Each new disease raises new ethical and legal dilemmas, or at least presents old issues in new guises and in this regard, AIDS is no exception. In this chapter, some of the ethical and legal issues that have been raised by AIDS will be addressed.

8.2 Historical perspective

The response of societies to contagious disease throughout history has not always been very creditable. The victims of disease have frequently been abandoned, isolated from the rest of society and blamed for their own condition. In other cases, whole sections of society, usually socially marginalized groups, have been blamed for wilfully spreading disease and scapegoated by the rest of society. Sadly, the case of AIDS has shown that, despite improved medical understanding, the traditional historic patterns of response to infectious disease remain alive and well.

8.2.1 Isolation and abandonment

Perhaps the most common response to the fear of infectious disease is to isolate or to abandon those who are ill. In extreme cases, such as the Black Death of 1347–50 when perhaps one third of the population of Europe died (Ziegler, 1969), abandonment of the ill was widespread. Families would forsake their dying relatives, priests abandoned their parishes and physicians avoided the sick. In attempts to try and control the spread of disease, whole communities would either flee to unaffected areas, often taking the plague with them, or attempt to exclude the outside world. It would be hard to condemn people for behaving this way in an attempt to avoid a probable and unpleasant death. In the Middle Ages, isolation and abandonment of the sick were the only known ways of controlling the spread of disease, and even then they were extremely ineffective. Indeed, throughout much of history, the only way to avoid many infectious diseases has been to exclude those infected from society: the case of leprosy as recorded in the Bible provides another example.

For many diseases, however, including AIDS, isolation of the infected and exclusion from society serves no useful purpose as there is no significant risk of infection from normal social intercourse. Despite this, isolation has been, and is being, practised around the world with people with HIV infection. Perhaps the most extreme case is Cuba where mandatory testing results in the enforced imprisonment of people found to be HIV seropositive (Bayer and Healton, 1989). Such methods employed by national governments are thankfully rare. More common is a lower level of avoidance and isolation in which people with HIV infection are discriminated against in the workplace, in health care settings and in society at large. Even medical practitioners, who should be well-informed about the risks, sometimes fail in their professional responsibilities in this regard. Defoe, retelling the story of London's Bubonic Plague of 1666 said 'It is true, when the infection was at its height . . . there were very few physicians which cared to stir abroad to sick houses. . .'. There are also many examples of the medical profession responding to health crises with great courage and self-sacrifice. In the plague that struck Athens in the fifth century BC, Thucydides, himself a victim, reported how physicians, ignorant of the causes and with no effective treatment, 'died most thickly, as they visited the sick most often . . .' Nearly 2500 years later in the London of 1987, despite widespread national publicity, the Terrence Higgins Trust, reported that many family doctors were refusing to treat people living with AIDS (Hencke and Veitch, 1987). They included one family doctor who refused to approach the corpse to certify the cause of death of man who had had HIV, and another who refused to examine a patient with AIDS, would not touch the bottle of pills the patient had been using, and issued a new prescription without any diagnosis (Hencke and Veitch, 1987). Although discrimination on grounds of HIV infection is illegal in some countries, notably the US, protection elsewhere against such action is unusual. In the UK, for example, it would be lawful to refuse to employ someone simply because they were HIV seropositive. On a wider scale, discriminations against people with HIV is common. As Dr Jonathan Mann, then director of the World Health Organizations's AIDS programme said 'As anxiety and fear cause some to blame others, AIDS has unveiled thinly disguised prejudices about race, religion, social class, sex and nationality' (Veitch, 1988).

8.2.2 Blaming the victim

Blaming the victim too has a long and dishonourable tradition. Practised particularly against diseases which afflict marginalised or otherwise oppressed minority groups, blame is most strong when the disease is also associated with behaviours or lifestyles which are widely disparaged. AIDS, at least in the developed world, is predominantly found amongst gay/bisexual men and injecting drug users. The widespread prejudices against homosexuality and drug use have lead to HIV and AIDS being seen as just recompense for leading a 'deviant' lifestyle or even a punishment from God. Perhaps the most prominent British exponent of this view is Mr James Anderton who, speaking whilst Chief Constable of Greater Manchester, referred to AIDS as a 'self-inflicted scourge' and went on to claim that gay men and injecting drug users were 'swirling round in a human cesspit of their own making' (Perera, 1987). Blaming the victim may be thought of as a manifestation of the 'Just World' hypothesis (Learner, 1980). Learner argues that there is a widespread irrational belief that the world is a just place and that good and evil are always appropriately rewarded. The corollary of this belief is that, if bad things happen, they must be the fault of the victim. Such is the strength of this belief, that people may believe it about themselves. That is, someone who becomes ill with AIDS, may feel that it is their own fault.

A common, though less extreme version of blaming the victim is reflected by the often-heard term of 'innocent victim', used most frequently with regard to a child or person infected through blood products. In the UK, the concept of the 'innocent victim' reached its zenith in 1988 when the Princess Royal, in a speech to the London World Summit on AIDS, said 'The real tragedy is the innocent victims, people who have been infected unknowingly by a blood transfusion . . . but possibly worst of all, those babies who are infected in the womb . . .' (Veitch, 1988). The corollary of having innocent victims is that others must be guilty and are, therefore, responsible for their own illness.

8.2.3 Scapegoating

A further response by society to infectious disease is to scapegoat particular groups of people. During the Black Death, minority groups were blamed for spreading the plague through the poisoning of wells or the sale of contaminated food. In Spain, the Arab population was persecuted and throughout Europe, pilgrims were held in deep suspicion and often excluded from the towns and cities. The prime scapegoats, as ever, were the Jews. Widely regarded as maliciously spreading the disease, many thousands were killed in retribution on a scale not seen again until the 20th century (Ziegler, 1969). Such responses to disease are extreme but even today, blaming groups of people for spreading HIV is commonplace. As Sontag (1988) points out, infectious diseases are invariably seen to come from elsewhere, usually abroad and are spread by foreigners. Sontag quotes the Director General of India's Medical Research Council who said 'This is a totally foreign disease and the only way to stop its spread is to stop sexual contacts between Indians and foreigners'. Inevitably, travellers from abroad, the modern equivalent of the medieval pilgrim, are blamed for the spread of disease across the world. Even the US, which has a generally good record on human rights, prohibits entry to people with HIV infection.

8.2.4 Repressive public health measures

In response to the fears and prejudices of their populations, governments are often tempted to introduce repressive measures against the ill on the grounds of public health. Victorian England of the 1860s saw an attempt to control the spread of syphilis in the army and navy through the introduction of a series of measures instituted under the Contagious Diseases Acts (Sieghart, 1989). Under these Acts of parliament, women in garrison towns and naval ports, who were believed to be prostitutes, could be detained against their will, subject to medical examination and compelled to accept a treatment which was frequently ineffective and often dangerous. It is of note that the men who used these women's services received no equivalent treatment.

Not only were the measures contained in the Contagious Diseases Acts deemed to be unjust and arbitrary, they made almost no impact on the spread of the disease. During the First World War, in response to the huge morbidity amongst servicemen resulting from sexually transmitted diseases, a Royal Commission was set up to investigate the problem. The Commission recommended the setting up of clinics providing free treatment where people could go on a voluntary basis with their confidentiality guaranteed. The new voluntary scheme proved far more effective than the previous measures and remains in place, with some modifications, to this day.

In the case of AIDS, although many governments have considered the use of repressive public health measures (compulsory HIV testing and mandatory registration, isolation or treatment), the lessons of the past have been widely accepted. The WHO has been particularly important in promoting the importance and efficacy of voluntary public health measures and their statements to this end have been widely influential (WHO, 1988).

8.3 Human rights

The belief that people have rights is an ancient one but the nature and form of these rights has long been disputed in a debate that continues to this day. Are human rights universal or do they vary from culture to culture and from one time period to another? Are human rights inherent and inalienable?

8.3.1 International law

Despite the continuing controversy, since the end of the second world war there have been a series of binding internationally agreed statements of human rights. The international law on human rights has been set down in the United Nations Charter (1945), the Universal Declaration of Human Rights (1948) and the 1976 Helsinki agreements on 'Civil and Political Rights' and 'Economic Social and Cultural Rights'. In addition, there have been a series of global treaties addressing specific issues and several regional agreements on human rights.

Among the many human rights internationally accepted are the right to life, health and privacy (Table 8.1) and these rights are held to apply to everyone regardless of sex, race, religion or other status.

Although these rights are widely accepted and legally binding, in practice few countries adhere fully to the agreements and violations of the code are common.

Table 8.1 A summary of some of the internationally agreed human rights. (Adapted from Sieghart, 1989.)

- a right to life
- a right to health
- a right to liberty and security of person
- freedom from inhuman or degrading treatment or punishment
- freedom of movement
- a right to privacy
- a right to marry and found a family
- a right to work
- a right to education
- a right to social security, assistance and welfare

Whilst the violation of these human rights is both morally wrong and in breach of binding international law, in reality there are few effective means of enforcement for any nation which chooses not to abide by the code.

Some rights, such as 'freedom from inhuman or degrading punishment' are absolute' and may not be limited under any circumstances. Others, such as the 'right to life' are limited. The death penalty is, for example, acceptable under the code, provided the court that passes sentences is properly constituted. Other limitations to human rights may be justified if they are in the public interest and this includes public health interests.

Despite the very real limitations in the applications of the internationally agreed code of human rights, it serves two useful purposes. First, in spite of the wide variations in culture, race and religion across the world, it has proved possible for the vast majority of nations to agree on a common standard of human rights. Second, the code represents a standard against which it is possible to judge the response of all nations to new challenges issues such as the emergence of the AIDS pandemic.

8.3.2 Human rights and HIV

Within the guidelines of the international code of human rights, some public health responses to the HIV pandemic are clear violations. Sieghart (1989) argues that the list of prohibited responses would include mandatory HIV testing, compulsory registration of people with HIV, quarantine or other isolation, exclusion or expulsion of citizens by a state on the grounds of HIV and discrimination on the grounds of HIV serostatus. Only in the most extreme circumstances (for example, if the survival of the nation were at stake), could these rights be suspended and it is difficult to see how this defence could be justified in the case of AIDS.

Further health responses would be acceptable under international law, such as anonymous HIV testing to study the prevalence of the disease, and the monitoring of the spread of disease through the mandatory reporting of cases, providing the right to privacy is maintained. In some cases, states which fail to apply certain measures might be considered negligent. These would include a failure to ensure clean blood supplies and clean medical equipment or a failure to provide public health information about HIV.

Other public health responses might be justifiable on the grounds of a conflict of interest between parties. The right to privacy, as followed within professional rules of medical confidentiality, or the right to liberty, could be suspended on the grounds of protecting others. Similarly, the right to work could be suspended for an individual if their health condition made their work practices unsafe to others or if they fail to follow, or are negligent in applying medical advice on hygiene precautions. It is in these cases, where there is a conflict between the human rights of different parties, that most important ethical dilemmas arise.

There are, of course variations in the ways in which different nations interpret human rights with resultant variations in the implementation of public health measures. The case of gay bath houses is a good example of this. In San Francisco, the role of bath houses in spreading the infection has been well documented (Shilts, 1987) and they were closed in the mid 1980s on public health grounds. Later, the bath houses were re-opened but subject to regulation. In other countries, such as Sweden, bath houses were closed permanently. Elsewhere, (e.g. the Netherlands) bath houses remain open and unregulated on the grounds that to do otherwise would be an invasion of privacy (Bayer and Healton, 1989). In these cases, different nations have weighed the balance between the right of privacy and the protection of others and come to a variety of conclusions. Despite this, in most cases, an attempt has been made, within the accepted framework of human rights, to produce a just outcome. A major exception to this is the UK where homosexual acts in public between consenting men are illegal, and as bath houses are considered to be public places, they are, and always have been, illegal.

8.4 Medical ethics

Medical practitioners have always been faced with ethical dilemmas in their clinical practice and some of the earliest records of the profession concern ethical and professional codes of conduct. The most famous of these is the Hippocratic Oath, which, amongst other commitments, obliges the physician to treat those in need and to maintain confidentiality.

Traditionally, medical conduct has been guided as much by professional ethics under peer supervision as by external legal considerations and, in recent years, other health professionals have adopted professional and ethical systems that are broadly similar to the traditional medical approach. In many cases, professional ethical guidelines are more restrictive than the law and in some cases there may be conflict between the two. Whilst there has always been a debate about what constitutes ethical behaviour for medical professionals, new diseases have always set new challenges and raised new issues with regard to the limits of ethical practice. In this regard, AIDS has been no exception and following the recognition of the disease in 1981, professional bodies of many health care professions around the world have issued new statements or policy documents specifying the ethical and professional expectations with specific regard to AIDS. In the 1988, both the American Medical Association (AMA) and the General Medical Council (GMC) (revised in 1993), the body that governs the ethical and professional standards of all practising physicians in the UK, issued general guidelines for ethical issues with regard to HIV infection and AIDS. Adapted summaries of both sets of recommendations are presented in Table 8.2 and both bodies came to broadly similar conclusions. Professionals who seek ethical guidance from either of these organizations are strongly advised to consult the original documents which include the full guidelines. The main difference between them is that the AMA guidelines do not address the issue of consent to treatment in the specific context of AIDS. In both cases there were some issues for which general guidelines would not be appropriate or could not be agreed but there were four main areas of concern: the doctor's duty towards patients, the duty of doctors infected with the virus, issues of patient consent and confidentiality. Each of these shall be considered in turn.

8.4.1 The duty of health care workers towards patients

The GMC guidelines state that doctors are obliged to treat people with HIV and AIDS with the same standard of medical care which they would apply to other patients. Whilst doctors may refuse to treat someone on the ground of lack of expertise or inadequate facilities, it is categorically stated to be unethical to refuse to treat someone on the grounds of personal risk. That is, a doctor may not refuse a patient solely because of fear of infection. Similarly, the GMC considers it unethical to refuse treatment on the grounds of moral judgement about the patient's activities or lifestyle. It would, therefore, be considered unethical to refuse to treat people on the grounds that they were gay or that they injected drugs. It would also be unethical to refuse to treat any one else perceived as being at high risk of having HIV infection, regardless of whether the doctor was aware of their HIV serostatus. Similar statements have been produced in other countries (e.g. the American Medical Association Council on Ethical and Judicial Affairs, 1988).

That there is an obligation to treat is by no means universally accepted. Not only does an obligation to treat interfere with the health care workers freedom of choice, it also forces them to take risks with their health (Annas, 1988) and, therefore, could be said to violate their human rights. Certainly it is expecting much of anyone to put themselves at serious risk of illness and death with the terrible consequences that may have for themselves, their friends and family. Health care workers who employ invasive procedures with their clients do expose themselves to a small but not insignificant risk (Marcus et al, 1988) and some reluctance to treat may be understandable if not ultimately justifiable. In practice, psychiatrists and other mental health professionals are at low risk of infection by HIV from their patients and only in relatively unusual circumstances (e.g. needle-stick injuries and physical assault involving exposure to infected blood) is there any significant risk. For this reason, it would only be ethically acceptable for a mental health professional to refuse to treat someone with HIV in exceptional circumstances.

8.4.2 The duties of health care workers infected with HIV

Although there have been few reliably reported cases of patients infected with HIV by health care workers, the risks of some medical procedures are very real. The most famous case involved a Florida dentist who allegedly infected a series of his patients with HIV (Centers for Disease Control, 1991b). In this case, it has been alleged that the dentist flagrantly violated routine infection control procedures and may even have deliberately infected his patients, although there is no direct evidence to substantiate these claims. This is the most clearly documented case and it is now known, from the close match between the viral strains of dentist and patients, that he was the source of the infection (Ou et al, 1993). The Florida case appears to be something of an exception, however, and investigations into other dentists who have practised while being HIV seropositive have found no cases of transmission (Dickinson et al, 1993). Indeed, there are few, if any, other reliable cases of health care workers infecting their patients even when the most invasive procedures have been used. Investigations in the US into the patients of two surgeons who were HIV seropositive found not one single case of HIV transmission out of over 1500 patients who were followed-up (von Reyn et al, 1993; Rogers et al, 1993).

The GMC guidelines of 1988 state that it is unethical for doctors in the UK who are infected with HIV or believe themselves to be infected to continue to practise solely on the basis of their own assessment of the risk to patients. In such cases, doctors are required to have regular medical supervision and seek specialist advice about the extent to which they should limit their professional practice. If advised to restrict or, in extreme cases, terminate their clinical practice, they are obliged to follow that advice. Similar guidelines have been produced by the American Medical Association with the additional recommendation that practitioners should disclose their HIV seropositive status to their patients if there was any 'identifiable risk'. In July 1991, the US Senate made it a criminal offence for health care workers with AIDS who perform invasive procedures to fail to disclose their serostatus to their patients.

After the GMC guidelines had been published, a series of incidents were widely reported in the British media in which practising surgeons who had died of AIDS or who had stopped practising because of HIV were identified in the press. One health authority, Mid-Glamorgan, initially tried to suppress the cause of death of their employee, a surgeon, for fear of causing alarm, although ultimately without success (Johnson, 1993). In each case, all patients who had undergone surgery were invited to receive counselling with a view to assessing their personal risk and, where appropriate, have an HIV test. Although no figures have yet been published on this case, past experience suggests that the risk of infection is extremely low in cases like this.

In response to these incidents, new guidelines were published by the Department of Health (1991) which instructed all health care workers who were HIV

Table 8.2 Summary of the ethical guidelines provided by the General Medical Council and the American Medical Association

	General Medical Council (UK)[1]	American Medical Association Council on ethical and judicial affairs[2]
The doctor's duty towards patients	Doctors should extend the same high standard of treatment to patients infected with HIV that they would offer to any other patient. They may not refuse to treat on grounds of: – personal risk – moral judgement about the patient's activities or lifestyle *Exemptions*: – lack of skill or knowledge to undertake a particular treatment – conscientious objection to particular treatments	Doctors may not ethically refuse to treat a patient whose condition is within the doctor's current realm of competence Doctors are dedicated to providing competent medical service with compassion and respect for human dignity Doctors unable to provide the services required by AIDS patients should make referral to those physicians or facilities equipped to provide such services
Duties of doctors infected with the virus	Doctors who think they may have been infected must seek testing and counselling Doctors who are found to be HIV seropositive must – seek specialist advice about limiting their professional activities – must follow the advice given – must not rely on their own assessment of risk to patients Doctors called upon to advice colleagues about modifying their professional practice have a duty to report colleagues who do not follow that advice	A doctor who knows that he or she is seropositive should not engage in any activity that creates a risk of transmission or the disease to others A doctor who has AIDS or who is seropositive should consult colleagues as to which activities the physician can pursue without creating a risk to patients

Consent to investigation or treatment	Treatment may only be carried out with the patient's consent HIV testing should not be undertaken without consent *Exemptions* – when HIV testing is imperative to secure the safety of others In the case of children, the consent should be sought from the parents. If the parents refuse, consent may be sought from the child provided the child is considered competent to make the decision. If the child is not competent, some circumstances may make it ethical to test without consent	No specific recommendation
Confidentiality	Confidentiality should be maintained in the same way as usual Communication with other health professionals should only be with consent *Exemptions*: – it is acknowledged that circumstances may justify breaking confidentiality but these are not specified	Doctors are ethically obligated to respect the rights and privacy and of confidentiality of AIDS patients and seropositive individuals *Exemptions*: – where there is no statute that mandates or prohibits the reporting of seropositive individuals to public health authorities and a doctor knows that a seropositive person is endangering the third party, the doctor should: (i) attempt to persuade the patient to cease endangering the third party (ii) if persuasion fails, notify the authorities (iii) if the authorities take no action, notify the endangered third party

[1]Adapted with permission from the General Medical Council (1988, 1993).
[2]Adapted with permission from the American Medical Association (1988).

seropositive to cease all invasive procedures immediately. In addition, when a health care worker who is HIV seropositive has been involved in invasive procedures, health authorities will be obliged to contact all patients who may have been put at risk over the last 10 years to offer counselling.

Confidentiality for the health care worker seems to be a very low priority in such cases. In the UK, it has been frequently been the case that the names of HIV infected health care workers are given to the media. The media in turn have usually publicized both the names of the health care workers concerned and publicized whatever details of the person's private life they could discover. A similar lack of restraint has been seen elsewhere. In the Florida dentist case, perhaps the most widely publicized case of an HIV-infected health care worker, details of his private life were widely reported as well as allegations that he had acted unprofessionally or even maliciously despite the paucity of direct evidence to substantiate these claims.

In addition to the risks of infection that patients may face from health care workers during invasive procedures, there is also the theoretical risk that cognitive impairment caused by HIV may result in incompetent and even dangerous treatment. This might include not only an increased risk of HIV transmission, but an unacceptably poor level of health care. To date, no cases have been reported where health care workers have been so cognitively impaired that they present a danger to their patients. In practice, HIV-1 associated dementia is very much an end stage disease (Chapter 4) and health care workers who have demented, are unlikely to be well enough to work. There is, however, the risk that cognitive deterioration, not amounting to a clinical dementia, could result in impaired clinical performance and for this reason it has been argued that HIV infected professionals should be monitored in their performance (Gostin, 1991).

The GMC places a further duty upon doctors. If a doctor has been approached by a colleague with HIV infection for advice and counselling about their ability to practice, the doctor is obliged to ensure that the advice is followed. If the doctor finds the advice is not being followed and that patients are may be being put at risk, the doctor must inform the GMC. That is, doctors, and by analogy other health care workers, have a duty to monitor the performance of colleagues who they know to be HIV seropositive with a view to ensuring that their practice is safe.

8.4.3 Consent to investigation or treatment

Whilst it is widely accepted that a doctor should only treat a patient with their informed consent, in the sphere of mental health, the ability to consent may often be compromised giving rise to a host of ethical difficulties. The definition of informed consent varies from society to society. In the US, informed consent requires that enough information is given to satisfy a 'prudent patient'. In the UK, the requirement for informed consent differs and the amount of information given is determined by what a 'reasonable' member of the relevant health profession would consider appropriate (Boyd 1989). Clearly, there may be differences between the information that a 'prudent patient' and a 'reasonable health care worker' might find sufficient.

Perhaps the area where consent has proved to be the most problematic is in the area of consent to be tested for HIV infection. Under international law, testing for HIV without consent would be a violation of the right to privacy. Although this right is not absolute, the grounds for waiving it, such as a danger to others or public health needs, are probably not met in the case of AIDS. The public health defence, if tested in the courts, would probably fail on two grounds (Sieghart, 1989). First, an HIV test is not an effective way of assessing whether the person carries the virus as they may not have seroconverted at the time of testing or they may be infected at any time after the test. Second, there is no effective cure for HIV so there is no obvious benefit to the patient from having the test. Further, provided good hygiene practices are followed, there is no significant risk of infection to others. In contrast, the disadvantages that result from compulsory testing are significant and might include ostracization from friends, family and employers with consequent financial losses. In addition, many health authorities, including the WHO, argue that mandatory HIV testing would be counterproductive and might deter people from seeking medical advice. The prohibition on testing for HIV without informed consent also applies if blood is taken for other medical reasons. That is, blood sampled for other medical need may not be subsequently tested for HIV unless the explicit consent of the patient is obtained.

Anonymous blood testing for epidemiological research, with informed consent, does not violate privacy and is, therefore, acceptable under the code of human rights (Sieghart, 1989). For statistical sampling reasons, seeking consent in such cases might bias the data collected and a totally random sample would give more reliable information about sero-prevalence. Although somewhat controversial, anonymous HIV testing without explicit informed consent, may be acceptable provided that blood is already being sampled for other medical needs and that the information is in the public interest. In such cases, although no consent has been sought, it is not clear how an individual's human rights would be infringed by this practice.

Problems arise when a patient is unable to give consent. For example, if a patient is unconscious, an HIV test, or other medical treatment could be performed without consent, provided it was medically necessary to do so. In such cases, the consent of a relative is not sufficient in its self. In practice, it is difficult to think of a situation in which an HIV test would be medically necessary but such cases might exist and would certainly occur if there were some effective treatment or cure for HIV.

In the case of children, the right to consent is often held by the parents or guardians and the child's explicit consent is not always needed although there are differences in how the law applies in such cases. The GMC recommends that the doctor should judge whether the child is able to give informed consent if so, the child's consent will suffice. Difficulties may arise when there is conflict between the parents wishes and the doctor's judgement of what is medically necessary. In such cases, for example, when the parents refuse a blood transfusion for their child on religious grounds, the British courts have typically overridden the parents' wishes.

The case of someone who is unwilling or unable to consent to medical treatment because of mental handicap or mental illness is more difficult. In the UK, the Mental Health Act does not allow for the compulsory treatment of physical illnesses although people may be detained and treated without their consent for their mental illness. That is, people with a mental illness or who are mentally handicapped, have the same protection under UK law as anyone else with regard to HIV testing or other physical procedures. Only in the case of urgent medical need or danger to others, can these rights be waived and then it may be necessary for the doctor justify the decision in court. If there arises a conflict between the interests of a patient and others, Krajeski (1990) suggests that several factors should be taken into account. These include, 'Who will benefit? The patient, other patients or staff?', 'Is there a sound medical rationale for testing?', 'Is there a reasonable and appropriate intervention that could be implemented on the basis of the result?' and 'What are the foreseeable consequences or testing or not testing'.

8.4.4 Confidentiality

The tradition of maintaining confidentiality between doctor and patient is an ancient one that goes back at least as far as Hippocrates. The Hippocratic Oath contains the clause: 'All that may come to my knowledge in the exercise of my profession or outside of my profession or in daily commerce with men, which ought not to be spread abroad, I will keep secret and never reveal'. Not only is confidentiality supported on ethical grounds, there are extremely good practical reasons for it to be maintained. The protection of confidentiality not only encourages people to seek medical help where they might otherwise be reluctant to do so, it also allows patients to be frank and forthcoming about the details of their health. Particularly in the case of illnesses that attract social approbation, such as sexually transmitted diseases, the rule of confidentiality has proved an effective way of encouraging people to seek treatment. Such is the importance of confidentiality, that nowadays, explicit guidelines for the maintenance of confidentiality exist, not only for members of the medical profession, but also for all other health professionals. In addition, medical confidentiality is clearly supported under the international code of human rights under the right to privacy.

Despite this, the right to confidentiality is not absolute. The GMC recognizes one circumstance in which it is justifiable to violate confidentiality: when others are put at risk. Even under these circumstances, confidentiality may only be breached when there is a 'serious identifiable risk to a specific individual'. Further, the doctor is expected to have discussed the situation with the patient with a view to ensure that either the person at risk is informed or that the risk is eliminated. In many circumstances, the clinicians can use their relationship of trust with the patient in a constructive way that will allow the dilemma to be solved, albeit at some personal cost to the parties concerned (Boyd, 1992).

Cases where there is a conflict between confidentiality and the safety of others have been addressed in the courts in cases unrelated to HIV. The now famous case of *Tarasoff* v. *Regents of the University of California* involved a psychologist whose patient murdered a woman having told the psychologist that he intended to do so. The court found that, on the basis of his training and knowledge of the patient, the psychologist was capable of anticipating the murder and had failed in his 'duty to warn' the victim. Whilst similar cases have not reached the courts in many other countries, the decision in the Tarasoff case is consistent with both international law and medical ethics and similar decisions should be expected in comparable cases in other countries. There is some question as to how far the 'duty to warn' extends. In the Mirin case (Beckett, 1991), a psychiatrist repeatedly warned his patient's ex-girlfriend that the patient had violent intentions towards her and on several occasions admitted him for treatment. The patient ultimately killed his ex-girlfriend and despite the psychiatrist's efforts, at the subsequent legal proceedings, the psychiatrist was deemed negligent in his 'duty to warn' in that he had failed to protect her. Similar cases have not yet occurred in the case of HIV infection and rulings in other countries might be quite different. What is clear, however, is that balancing the rule of confidentiality against the protection of others is an area of enormous potential difficulty for health professionals not only in terms of ethics but in terms of legal responsibilities.

That there is a duty of care for health professionals is widely accepted but difficulties arise particularly when the nature of risk is uncertain or when the person at risk is not clearly identifiable. In the Tarasoff and Mirin cases, both the risk and the victim were clearly identifiable. That is, the health care worker knew who the victim was likely to be and what their patient was likely to do. In many cases, such situations may be fraught with difficulties and the information upon which the clinician is expected to act may be uncertain in that the nature of the risk is unclear or the identity of the person at risk is unsure. In addition, the consequences of breeching confidentiality may be to destroy the therapeutic relationship with the patient altogether and may end up in putting more people at risk. For example, revealing the HIV status of a patient to his or her partner may result in the break-up of that relationship. As a consequence, not only may the clinician–patient relationship be damaged and the patient may be more reluctant than ever to reveal his HIV status to future partners, thereby putting more people at risk.

It should be noted that the GMC does not accept that it is justifiable to inform other doctors or other health professionals without the patient's consent even when they are directly responsible for the patient's care. Whilst every effort should be made to explain the difficulties involved in ensuring adequate health care when the doctor is not fully informed, if the patient still refuses to consent, then the patient's wishes should be respected.

8.4.5 Suicide, assisted suicide, and euthanasia

Clinical experience suggests that many people with HIV infection contemplate suicide as an option for when their health or their quality of life become so poor that they feel they would rather be dead. In practice, most of the people who say they might kill themselves, do not formulate clear plans of intent and probably will not do so. Others may seek the help of friends, family or medical professionals to give them the means to kill themselves, or even ask them to administer the means, to end their lives. Because of the legal and ethical difficulties, there is little reliable information available on how many people actually do kill themselves or are 'helped to die' but anecdotal evidence suggests that suicide or assisted suicide occurs in a small but significant minority of cases.

The issue of suicide in people with HIV infection is dealt with in detail in Chapter 3. Perhaps the most common ethical dilemma for mental health professionals confronted with a suicidal patient is whether to intervene or not. If a patient wishes to commit suicide as a result of mental illness, there is a clear duty to treat that patient. In the UK, the 1983 Mental Health Act would allow such a patient to be detained for assessment and treatment and such circumstances are covered by similar legal and ethical guidelines in many other countries. The dilemma arises when it is unclear whether the patient is really mentally ill or has made a rational and uncoerced decision to end their life. In this case, it may be both unlawful and unethical to attempt restraint. Situations such as this usually occur when the patient is very ill and is often motivated by fear of further suffering and the wish to avoid an undignified death. Such fears are sometimes misguided and may be relieved by frank discussions of future care options. In particular, much of the suffering and loss of dignity that is so often feared may be alleviated by good palliative care. Despite this, some patients may still make a rational decision to kill themselves.

In terms of law, aiding or abetting suicide is widely prohibited and in some societies, suicide itself is illegal. Therefore, a health professional who assists directly or indirectly in a patient's suicide is likely to be acting unlawfully and might expect to be prosecuted. Not only is assisting suicide illegal, in almost all cases it will be a breach of professional ethics. In recent years a series of books have been published which are, in effect, do-it-yourself manuals for euthanasia. Perhaps the most famous of these is *Final Exit: the practicalities of self-deliverance and assisted suicide for the dying* by Derek Humphrey, the director of the Hemlock Society, a voluntary euthanasia society based in the US. The book reached number one in the bestseller charts in the first week of its publication in the US. A similar publication in the UK, *Guide to self-deliverance* published by the Voluntary Euthanasia Society in England resulted in the prosecution of its authors on the grounds of a conspiracy to assist suicide. More recently, *How to die with dignity*, published by the Scottish Voluntary Euthanasia Society was withdrawn following conflicting legal advice (Dyer, 1991).

In some cases, assisting suicide goes beyond self-help manuals. In the US, there was a widespread public and professional outcry against Dr Jack Kevorkian who assisted Mrs Janet Adkins, a patient with early Alzheimer's disease, to end her life using his 'suicide machine'. Within a few days of knowing her, Dr Kevorkian connected Mrs Adkins to the machine which she used to kill herself using a lethal injection of pentothal and potassium chloride (Dyer, 1991). The outcry in this case was not so much about the use of euthanasia, but that

Dr Kevorkian assisted Mrs Adkin's suicide after knowing her for such a short time. Further, it is alleged that Dr Kevorkian failed to check the accuracy of her diagnosis or assess her fitness to make the decision (Cassel and Meier, 1990). The case of Dr Quill, contrasts significantly with this (Quill, 1991). Dr Quill had had a long-standing professional relationship with 'Debbie' that started before she developed leukaemia. Dr Quill, prescribed barbiturates to Debbie, fully knowing her intention to kill herself. In neither case were the physicians prosecuted, though in other countries, including the UK, they would almost certainly have been charged with murder. Dr Kevorkian, who freely admits to having helped 20 seriously ill patients end their lives, has subsequently been prosecuted in Michigan for other cases. In the widely publicized trial that followed, Dr Kevorkian was acquitted. Within days of the jury's decision, two further events brought the illegality of assisted suicide in the US into question. The Michigan Commission on Death and Dying produced a report that broadly supported Dr Kevorkian's arguments and US District Judge Barbara Rothstein overturned a law that forbade assisting suicide (Roberts, 1994). Judge Rothstein based her decision on a ruling on abortion by the Supreme Court in 1992. Quoting from the ruling she said 'Like the abortion decision, the decision of a terminally ill person to end his or her life *involves the most intimate and personal choices a person can make in a lifetime* and constitutes a *choice central to personal dignity and autonomy*'. These developments suggest there may be a trend towards liberalising legal restraints on physician assisted suicide in the US.

Voluntary active euthanasia (from the Greek *eu* 'good' and *thanatos* 'death'), sometimes referred to as 'mercy killing', in which medication is administered by a physician with the intention of killing the patient, is also universally outlawed and contrary to most established codes of medical ethics. Despite this, public support for euthanasia is high. Helme (1992) reported that 69–75 per cent of Britons believed that euthanasia should be permitted under certain circumstances and similar figures have been reported from other countries. Whether many physicians would be prepared to perform euthanasia is another matter. A survey in the UK found that 60 per cent of physicians had been asked by their patients to hasten their deaths and 12 per cent had taken active steps to do so (Ward and Tate, 1994). Nearly half of the physicians in the same survey said that they would be prepared to perform euthanasia if it were legal. A survey of physicians in San Francisco working with people with AIDS found that nearly a quarter would be likely to grant a patient's initial request for assistance with suicide (Slome et al, 1992). What little evidence there is suggests that many people with HIV infection are keen to have euthanasia and assisted suicide as an option. Tindall et al (1993) found that 90 per cent of their sample of Australian gay men with advanced HIV disease wanted the option of euthanasia available for themselves. Certainly, the issue of euthanasia has grown in political prominence in recent years. In the US, the states of California, New York, Oregon and Washington have all recently held referenda on the subject and in the UK, a 10-minute rule Bill was put before the House of Commons in the last parliament. In each case, the attempts to legalize euthanasia were defeated.

In The Netherlands, although euthanasia is against the law, if guidelines set out by the Royal Dutch Medical Association are followed, no legal action will be taken. These guidelines include that the patient must be suffering unbearable physical or mental distress, and repeatedly, without coercion, express a wish to die. The patient must fully understand and explicitly reject other treatment options. In addition, the wish to die must be in writing and a second, independent physician should be consulted. Throughout this procedure, the family should be informed and the method of death must be such that the family is not caused avoidable distress. If these guidelines are followed, the physician may then proceed to kill the patient through the administration of drugs, most commonly through intravenous administration of benzodiazepines in combination with curare derivatives (Laane, 1993). Once the process is complete, the physician must report the circumstances of the death to the police who, provided there are no grounds for believing the guidelines were violated or that the death was in any way suspicious, will log the report but take no further action. The Dutch experience shows that the majority of people who request euthanasia are elderly, suffering from disseminated cancer and in their own homes (Commissie Onderzoek Medische Praktijk inzake Euthanasie, 1991). The most important reasons for requesting euthanasia were 'futile suffering', 'avoidance of humiliation' and 'unbearable suffering'. Pain was a factor in 40 per cent of cases but the main factor in only 1 in 20 (Van der Wal et al, 1992). It is still unclear how commonly euthanasia is practised in the Netherlands. Van der Maas et al (1991) found that around 2 per cent of all deaths in 1990 were due to euthanasia or assisted suicide and this proportion has increased since. A further 25 per cent of cases are not registered (Van der Wal, 1994). Failure to register euthanasia may occur for a variety of reasons but may be most common in those cases where euthanasia is more questionable.

The toleration of euthanasia in the Netherlands arose from a series of court cases and until 1993 there was no legislation to support the practice. In 1993, however, the Dutch Senate narrowly passed a law enforcing the voluntary guidelines that had been in use since 1984. Ironically, the act of formalizing the law on euthanasia has had the effect of increasing the number of prosecutions. Until 1993, no more than four physicians in any year had been prosecuted but in the first 6 months of the new law, 14 physicians were under investigation.

Euthanasia has also been used in the Netherlands with people with AIDS and the empirical reports that have been presented to date, based on the reports of physicians and relatives, have been favourable (Van den Boom et al, 1991). In is unclear how many people with AIDS in The Netherlands have considered euthanasia but from the general population it seems that for everyone who choses euthanasia, at least three times as many seriously consider it as an option (Van der Maas et al, 1991). This estimate is consistent with Van den Boom et al's (1991) findings from interviews with relatives of people who had died with AIDS. They found that more than a fifth had elected for euthanasia and three times as many had discussed the option with their family.

In other countries, although voluntary active euthanasia is illegal, physicians or family members who are found guilty are often treated leniently provided they are seen to have acted on compassionate grounds. The recent case of

Dr Nigel Cox illustrates this. Dr Cox, a consultant Rheumatologist at the Royal Hampshire County Hospital, Winchester in the UK, admitted administering a lethal injection of potassium chloride to a Mrs Boyes, who was terminally ill. Mrs Boyes, a long-time sufferer from rheumatoid arthritis, had developed ulcers on her arms and legs, a rectal abscess which penetrated to the bone, fractured vertebrae swollen joints and gangrene. Despite pain killers (diamorphine at 50 mg per hour, finally increased to 100 mg per hour), she remained in extreme pain and as one of her nurses reported: 'She howled and screamed like a dog whenever anyone touched her'. A few days before her death, she pleaded for tablets or an injection to end her life. With the patient still in extreme pain, Dr Cox administered the injection and recorded his actions in the medical notes (Dyer, 1992). A nurse involved in the case reported the entry to the hospital management who informed the police. Dr Cox was charged with attempted murder and, were it not for the fact that the true cause of Mrs Boye's death could not be established (her body had been cremated), Dr Cox would have faced a murder charge and a mandatory life sentence. At the trial, the jury, several of whose members were in tears, returned a majority verdict of guilty. The judge, Mr Justice Ognall, acknowledging the difficulties of what he referred to as a 'wholly exceptional' case, passed a suspended sentence of 12 months which allowed Dr Cox to leave the court a free man.

Whilst Dr Cox received much support from the general public, the response from other physicians, was more mixed. Despite a sympathetic editorial in the *British Medical Journal* (Smith, 1992) there was a critical response from many other doctors, especially from those involved in palliative care in the hospice movement. In particular, it was argued that the levels of analgesia used were inadequate and that they should have been increased until the pain stopped, even if that meant the patient would be unconscious (Rosen, 1992; Tapsfield and Amis, 1992; Willis, 1992). Other physicians were more supportive of Dr Cox's actions and emphasised the importance of individual choice (Allebone, 1992) and the exceptional nature of the case, particularly the fact that increasing analgesia had the paradoxical effect of increasing Mrs Boyes's pain (Dixon and Morely, 1992). What emerges from this debate, is that in the UK at least, there is no consensus amongst medical practitioners about what someone in Dr Cox's position should have done.

Despite the controversy in the medical profession, there has been a broad consensus in the political response in the UK. A report from the House of Lords select committee on medical ethics, rejected the case for legalizing euthanasia and the government published a white paper endorsing the committee's position (Government response to the report of the select committee on medical ethics 1994). This means that there will be no change in law on euthanasia or assisted suicide in the UK in the foreseeable future.

In addition to voluntary active euthanasia, Beckett (1991) describes other forms of euthanasia on which there is more variation in different legal systems. These include: 'double effect euthanasia', 'voluntary passive euthanasia' and 'involuntary passive euthanasia'. Double effect euthanasia, involves administering pain-killing or other medication in sufficient dosage that it might be expected to hasten death. In the absence of firm information, it is uncertain how common double effect euthanasia really is but anecdotal reports suggest it is far from uncommon and may even be the most frequently used form of euthanasia. One reason this may be so is that it is widely believed that aiding a patient's death with what is seen to be a standard treatment provides the physician with a degree of legal protection. The case of Dr Stephen Lodwig illustrates this. In 1990, Dr Lodwig was sent to trial on the charge of murder following his administration of an injection of lignocaine and potassium chloride to a terminally ill patient. The charges were dropped when it was revealed that medical trials using this combination were under way in the London teaching hospital where he had been trained. The other reason why double effect euthanasia may be the most common way of assisting patient death is that it allows the physician to avoid directly confronting the issue of killing someone together with the moral and emotional consequences of doing so.

Involuntary passive euthanasia involves the withdrawal of treatment which keeps a person alive when that person is unable to give informed consent. This might occur when the patient is unconscious with no prospect of recovery. Unlike active euthanasia, passive euthanasia is often lawful if there is no realistic possibility of recovery. In the US, the case of Ms Nancy Cruzan who lay in a coma for eight years sustained by tube feeding is perhaps the best known case of this. In 1988, Ms Cruzan's parents sought to exercise her right to refuse treatment so that she might be allowed to die. In 1990, the US supreme court ruled that there was insufficient evidence to prove that Ms Cruzan would herself have chosen to die; a decision which prevented the termination of treatment. Subsequent testimony from Ms Cruzan's friends and colleagues persuaded a lower court that, under her present circumstances, she would indeed have wished to die and treatment was withdrawn shortly afterwards leading to her death two weeks later (Jennett and Dyer, 1991).

In the Cruzan case, much emphasis was placed on attempting to determine the wishes of the patient, whereas similar decisions in the UK have concentrated much more on pursuing the 'best interests of the patient'. Although these concepts are clearly related, the difficulty of establishing someone's wishes when they are incompetent to express them may sometimes make the withdrawal of treatment more difficult in the US than in the UK. The case of Mr Tony Bland provides a recent example of this. Mr Bland was 18 in 1989 when he suffered hypoxic brain damage, secondary to thoracic crush injuries during the Hillsborough Football Ground disaster, leaving him in a 'persistent vegetative state'. He was kept alive by artificial means and, with no prospect of recovery, his family and physicians sought permission from the courts to cease treatment so that he might be allowed to die 'with the greatest dignity and least of pain, suffering and distress' (Tomkins, 1993). In 1993, the House of Lords, the highest court in the UK, decided that it was lawful to withdraw treatment in this case even though Mr Bland was unable to give consent to doing so himself. In his judgment, Lord Goff said that in deciding such cases, the four safeguards proposed by the medical ethics committee of the British Medical Association should be considered. These guidelines are that every effort should be made at rehabilitation for at least six months after the injury, that the diagnosis of persistent vegetative state should not be considered or confirmed until at least 12 months and the diagnosis should be made by at least two other independent doctors. In addition, the wishes of the patient's immediate family should be given great weight. The importance of delaying the diagnosis in these cases was emphasized recently by a report on 43 consecutive patients who had been admitted to a specialist unit in a vegetative state (Andrews, 1993). Of these 43, 11 regained awareness, in one case three years after the initial brain injury.

Whilst these rules provide useful guidelines for withdrawing treatment, they do not deal with the another form of passive involuntary euthanasia in which treatment is withheld because it is not deemed to be in the interest of the patient. In the case of AIDS, it is unusual for patients to be in a persistent vegetative state. It may often be the case, however, that a patient could be kept alive a little longer if all available medical options were applied and pursued aggressively although the end result would not be in doubt. In practice, such decisions are made frequently and guided by the medical lore that

> *thou shalt not kill; but need'st not strive*
> *Officiously to keep alive* (Clough, 1850)

Voluntary passive euthanasia also involves the withdrawal of treatment but with the informed consent of the patient. In most cases, there is little difficulty, either ethically or legally, in following a patient's wishes not to receive treatment, even if the treatment may be lifesaving. Indeed, treating a patient against their wishes would, in most circumstances, be a violation of their human rights and therefore ethically unacceptable. In practice, of course, it may be extremely difficult for most health workers to watch someone die who they feel could benefit from their help. The only major exception to respecting the patient's wishes occurs when the patient is not deemed competent to make the decision. This would be the case when people are mentally impaired or are suffering from a mental illness. In these circumstances, psychiatrists or other mental health professionals may be called upon to determine whether the patient is indeed competent to make decisions about their treatment. In the case of someone who is mentally ill, depressed or suicidal, it may well be justified on ethical grounds to override a patient's wishes although the legal standing of such decisions vary from country to country.

8.4.6 Advance directives or living wills

'Advance directives', also known as 'living wills' are a way in which patients may express their wishes about their future medical care under circumstances in which they would not be able to be involved in the decision-making process. In this way, patients are able to specify treatments they would and would not be willing to accept and under what conditions. The objective of advance directives is not to replace active participation of patients in medical decisions but to provide a clear statement of their views for when they are unable to express them themselves. The use of advance directives began in the US where the right of self-determination is a paramount consideration in medical care and where problems may arise when a patient's views are not known and cannot be determined. At present, advance directives have legal standing in 40 states in the US but no legal authority in many countries, including the UK. Despite this, the principles of advance directives are popular and more than 90 per cent of out-patients in a recent survey from the US favoured their use (Emanuel et al, 1991). Increasingly, advance directives are popular elsewhere, particularly amongst people who foresee a premature death, including people with HIV infection. In the UK, the Terrence Higgins Trust provides a self completion form for people with HIV to write their own living will. The Trust's living will includes sections for the terminal stages of physical illness, permanent mental impairment and permanent unconsciousness. In each case, the form provides two options: to be kept alive for as long as possible using whatever forms of treatment that are available or to limit treatment to palliative care. In addition, the form allows the person to specify a 'health care proxy' who is empowered to make decisions on behalf of the patient when the patient is no longer able to do so.

Despite their popularity, even in the US where they have some legal standing, advance directives are frequently ignored. Experience from the US suggests that in up to a quarter of cases, the wishes expressed in advance directives are not followed. In a recent report, Danis et al (1992), found that overruling advance directives is largely due to the physician's belief that following the directive would have excluded the possibility of treatment that was beneficial or because of decisions by the patient's family. The lessons from this study are that full and frank discussion between he patient, doctor and next of kin are necessary if living wills are to be complied with.

8.5 Clinical research

The AIDS pandemic has resulted in an unprecedented response from the scientific community and patient groups and a greater concentration of research effort has been focused on a single medical issue than ever before. Inevitably, the raised profile of this scientific enterprise has raised questions over the ethical acceptability of certain aspects of research.

8.5.1 The ethics of clinical trials

The current system of clinical trials with legal controls has been developed over the last 50 years to ensure that new treatments are both effective and safe. The safeguards and controls that are in place throughout the Western world have been developed as a result of much experience over the years, often motivated by disastrous examples, such as the thalidomide case, where the evaluation of the drug's safety failed badly. Currently, controls are so strict that developing a new drug to the stage where it is safe to market takes many years and is extremely expensive. Although the current systems for regulating drugs reduce the likelihood of unsafe treatment becoming widely available, the cost is at the price of delaying potentially effective treatments. In the case of AIDS, much concern has been voiced from activist groups that the time taken to license new treatments is so long that even if an effective cure were found now, it would not be readily available before many thousands of people had died. For people facing their own death in a short period of time, existing licensing systems must seem excessively cautious and frustratingly inappropriate. Certainly, in the case of people who are near death, there seems some justification for relaxing some of the safety controls for new treatments, but although many researchers are sympathetic to this dilemma, it seems unlikely that any changes will be made in the immediate future for legal reasons. The case of zidovudine is of relevance here. In the mid 1980s the Food and Drug Administration in the US was under considerable pressure from HIV activist groups to license zidovudine, and finally did so at the earliest opportunity. Latterly, some activist groups (in some cases the same ones), have condemned the FDA for prematurely licensing a toxic drug. Some extreme groups have even argued that zidovudine, not HIV, is the cause of AIDS and that use of the drug is part of a conspiracy to kill gay men. With pressure to speed up the licensing of new drugs and continuing pressure to ensure their safety, the temptation for the regulatory authorities will be to maintain the tried and trusted status quo.

The ethical justification for regulatory systems for licensing new treatments is straightforward. It is that it would simply be unethical to condone the use of treatments which were either unsafe or ineffective. The gold standard for determining the efficacy of a new treatment is the randomized double blind placebo controlled clinical trial. As part of this procedure, some people will be given an inert treatment (the placebo) even when the researchers have reason to believe (from uncontrolled studies, animal and laboratory work), that the new treatment is effective. For this reason, it has been argued, clinical trials are unethical. The main problem with this argument, is that it presumes that the question the trial is attempting to answer (i.e. 'Is this treatment effective?') is already known (Wald, 1993). If this were the case, then the trial would most certainly be unethical. There are, however, many examples of treatments which appear promising on the basis of animal studies, laboratory work and uncontrolled trials which simply do not work when tested in a controlled trial. For this reason, provided that the trial is properly conducted and is asking a question about the efficacy of a treatment where reasonable evidence does not already exist, the trial can surely be justified on ethical grounds.

Efficacy is not the only criterion by which a treatment should be judged. The potential harm that a treatment may cause should also be considered. In some cases, it may be that a treatment is known to be safe but not known to be effective. For example, giving pregnant women supplements of folic acid, a normal constituent of diet, may or may not be effective in preventing the development of neural tube defects in their unborn children as has been claimed, but it is certainly safe (Wald, 1993). In this example, the case for encouraging pregnant women to take the supplement is strong in that it will do no harm and may have extremely beneficial effects. Similarly, many complementary therapies (although by no means all) are quite harmless and may even do some good, at least in terms of psychological well-being. Problems do arise through the use of complementary therapies on those occasions when patients are encouraged to abandon the use of established treatments or are misled by false claims offering treatment or cure. In many countries, there is simply no effective regulation of complementary therapies.

Given that there are established methods of evaluating new treatments, a further question arises: 'What treatments shall we try out?' This is not a trivial question in that the number of potential pharmaceutical agents that could be examined is infinite. Further, a double blind placebo controlled trials is extremely expensive and may take several years to complete. In practice, most therapeutic agents will be excluded on the basis of preliminary studies in animals or in the laboratory although many will still remain. The remaining agents and the decisions about which ones to pursue further will be made in the light of prevailing scientific opinion through an established system of peer review. Even after these initial stages, there are so many pharmaceutical agents that it may be worthwhile proceeding to a full-scale clinical trial. In fact, so many drug trials are under way in HIV infection that it has become increasingly difficult to obtain patients for a new trial who are not already taking other active agents. In addition, many patients wish to try as many experimental treatments as possible in order to keep well and there is considerable resentment that conventional clinical trials preclude this possibility. One suggested solution to this is to run parallel track designs in which patients would be permitted to a take a range of new pharmaceuticals. In this way, the introduction of new therapeutics could be speeded-up considerably and patients would be given a greater choice in deciding which treatments they would like to try. Against this, some of the clarity of interpretation of the traditional placebo controlled trial would be lost and regulating authorities in most countries have proved reluctant to change existing rules.

In most cases, the interest of commercial companies will coincide with the views of the scientific establishment in that they will not wish to spend money on a drug which, in the opinion of the experts, will not work. Sometimes, however, this system can go seriously wrong. In 1985 MicroGeneSys developed a vaccine for use against HIV using the viral envelope protein, gp120. With preliminary evidence of its efficacy, albeit widely disputed, MicroGeneSys approached the National Institutes of Health (NMH) in the US for support for further development. At the same time, MicroGeneSys employed a company of Washington lobbyists to pursue their interests. The result was that in 1992, $20 million was added to a defence bill forcing the army to spend this sum on the gp120 vaccine, effectively bypassing the established system of scientific peer review. The result of this behind-the-scenes lobbying caused an outcry amongst the scientific community and in the media, with the *New York Times* referring to the debacle as 'Madness on Capitol Hill'. As Dr Bernadine Healy of the NMH put it, 'I don't know how you can go to a patient and say "We're giving you this drug because a lobbyist chose it"'. Amid much embarrassment, Congress backed down and gave the army the choice of continuing with the gp120 trial or using the money for other AIDS-related research (Roberts, 1992). The ethical question that this raises is what is the most effective way of selecting which areas of research to pursue and which to put off? Whilst the system of peer review itself is flawed, a system which at least attempts to evaluate the scientific evidence is surely better than one in which decisions are based on who employs the most effective lobbyist.

8.5.2 Quality of life

It is becoming increasingly recognized that the traditional measures of evaluation used in medicine such as survival and symptom reduction, are not sufficient to evaluate the efficacy of medical treatments. In the realm of infectious diseases, the success of medicine in the past has been such that a total cure has been the expectation. In the case of AIDS, the prospect of a cure in the near future is not good and other ways of measuring improvement are needed. Although treatment may not show improvements in conventional survival measures, there may be significant benefits in terms of symptom relief, functional performance, psychological and social well-being. This broader range of outcome measures is usually known collectively as 'quality of life'. It is noteworthy that much of the research into the evaluation of quality of life has been conducted in the field of oncology where the treatments are often of only marginal effectiveness and where the side-effects of treatment may be so adverse that the decision to treat or not to treat becomes enormously difficult. In the case of AIDS, the approach to the evaluation of treatment more usual to that of oncology, rather than of infectious disease, presents the more appropriate paradigm.

Details of how quality of life may be measured are dealt with in Chapter 4. This section will address the issues of why it is important to measure quality of life. Historically, there have been two main justifications for measuring quality of life. First, there is the position that argues that prolonging survival is not sufficient on its own to justify the use of a treatment and that broader indices of the impact of treatment should be made on ethical grounds. Second, there is the position which seeks to evaluate treatments on an economic basis to allow decisions about cost-effectiveness of competing treatments to be made. Although these approaches are not mutually exclusive, the historical trend has been for the economic and ethical approaches to quality of life measurement to run on parallel courses with relatively little overlap.

The ethical case for measuring quality of life is well illustrated by the cases of Mr Tony Bland and Ms Nancy Cruzan. In each case, life could have been prolonged indefinitely but both were in persistent vegetative states with no hope of recovery. In each case, the courts' decisions that the treatment could be withdrawn was strongly influenced by each person's presumed quality of life. In less extreme cases, the balance between the beneficial impact of a treatment and its adverse side effects may be finely poised and it is here that quality of life measurement is most useful. For example, in the case of zidovudine, it has been reported that for people with asymptomatic HIV infection, there is a small but transient drop in quality of life in the first few months of treatment amongst those on the active medication compared with those on placebo but no difference after a year (Wu et al, 1991). If zidovudine were effective in people with asymptomatic infection, then this small drop in quality of life might well be justified but as the Concorde double blind placebo controlled trial of zidovudine study shows (Concorde Co-ordinating Committee, 1994) there is no clear benefit in terms of survival or disease progression in doing so. For this reason, there is little justification for accepting the small, albeit transient drop in quality of life that is seen in this case. In contrast, zidovudine appears to be effective in people with advanced HIV disease, not only in terms of prolonging life, but also in maintaining quality of life (Wu et al, 1990). This finding is encouraging as it was conceivable that zidovudine might have prolonged survival but at the cost of a low quality of life.

It is not the case that quantitative information from quality of life assessments in clinical trials will always answer questions about whether it will be beneficial to receive a treatment or not. Quality of life measures are still relatively blunt instruments and it would be unwise to place undue emphasis on them whilst making individual clinical decisions. Rather, the aim of quality of life studies is to provide information to both patients and doctors to allow an informed discussion over future treatment options, thereby increasing patient autonomy and doctor–patient discussion.

8.6 Summary

The response of societies around the world to AIDS shows many of the failings in dealing with illness that previous generations have shown. These include discrimination against the sick, blaming them for their ill health, scapegoating sections of society and the introduction of repressive public health measures. Despite this, important lessons from the past have been learned particularly with regard to the efficacy of voluntary public health provision. In addition, the established system of international law has provided both a common statement of human rights and a standard with which it is possible to evaluate our treatment of people with HIV infection.

In the realm of medical ethics, the dilemmas faced by health workers are those they have always faced but presented from a new perspective by the fresh challenges of AIDS. Foremost of these are the duties of health care workers to their patients, issues of consent and confidentiality. In addition, issues of death, palliative care and euthanasia have been raised in a context where many people want to maintain as much control as possible over their dying.

In many areas of health care, ethical and legal issues remain unresolved and will remain so indefinitely. Current professional codes of conduct and legal precedent do, however, leave today's health care workers with a surer framework of guidance than ever before.

9 HIV infection: clinical manifestations and treatment

Brian Gazzard

9.1 Introduction

The acquired immune deficiency syndrome (AIDS) is the most talked about and written about condition in contemporary medicine. As a new disease with novel manifestations which are still appearing more than 14 years after the epidemic, it is a fascinating medical phenomenon. As an epidemic which was followed from its inception, it provides a unique opportunity for epidemiologists to learn about the spread of infectious diseases. As a condition which stigmatizes the sufferer and frightens the general public, it provides endless concern to sociologists and ethicists. As a condition which causes neurological damage and leads to psychiatric disorder, it interests psychiatrists and psychologists. Most importantly, as a pandemic which is at present unchecked and for which there appears to be no immediate prospect for early treatment or prevention, it provides a timely reminder of the frailty of human knowledge and our inability to institute effective global concerted action to improve health.

9.2 Epidemiological overview

Ten years have passed since the first reports of AIDS (Centers for Disease Control, 1981) and the numbers of cases was estimated to be 1.3 million by the WHO in December 1990, who also believe that a further 8–10 million people are infected with the causative virus, human immunodeficiency virus (HIV) (Chin, 1990). Three geographical patterns of epidemic have emerged. In pattern one countries (Western Europe, Australasia, and North America) the epidemic started in gay men and has spread to injecting drug users and more slowly into the heterosexual population. In pattern two countries (much of Africa and Latin America) the epidemic is occurring in heterosexuals. Vertical spread and spread by blood transfusion is also common. In the third pattern (large parts of Asia) there were fewer cases at the beginning of the epidemic but the numbers are now rapidly increasing because of transmission by injecting drug users and spread in women employed in the sex industry in some countries, as in India.

9.2.1 Efficiency of transmission by different routes

Gay/bisexual intercourse

The most important features determining transmission rates amongst gay/bisexual men are multiple partners and unprotected receptive anal intercourse.

Table 9.1 Risk of seroconversion with different sexual activities for a group of homosexual males (from Kingsley et al, 1987.)

	Population (6 month exposure)	Seroconversion	Incidence ratio
Anal both	5060	190	31.6
Receptive anal	765	14	15.3
Insertive anal	1866	10	4.4
No anal	1670	2	1.0

The seroconversion rate in people practising exclusively insertive anal or oral sex is low (Kingsley et al, 1987) (Table 9.1).

Blood transfusions and blood products

Between 66 and 100 per cent of blood transfusion recipients became infected if donors were tested positive for antibodies to HIV, later became antibody positive, or developed AIDS (Ward et al, 1987). The incidence was highest in babies and those given blood from symptomatic individuals.

The prevalence of HIV infection in people with haemophilia ranges from 15 per cent to more than 90 per cent. Cryoprecipitate derived from small donor plasma pools in the UK was associated with a lower transmission rate than that seen with imported material derived from large plasma pools.

Injecting drug use

Intravenous injecting drug users now account for 40 per cent of all newly diagnosed AIDS cases in the US and 60 per cent of cases in southern Europe. High rates of transmission are associated with needle sharing, particularly in communal 'shooting galleries' where people gather together and frequently use the same syringe. HIV seropositivity and intravenous injecting drug use are strongly associated with poverty, urban decay and unemployment in the US (Friedland and Klein, 1987).

Heterosexual intercourse

The HIV virus is transmitted by vaginal intercourse with an efficiency of approximately 1 per cent although transmission is enhanced from female to male by genital ulcer disease and the male being uncircumcised (Cameron et al, 1989). Male to female transmission is increased in those with a previous history of sexually transmitted disease and those having anal intercourse in addition to vaginal sex (European Study Group, 1989). Transmission rates are probably greatest at the time of seroconversion or in late disease as AIDS develops (Goedert et al, 1987).

Vertical transmission

Between 10 and 40 per cent of babies born to HIV seropositive mothers are themselves infected with HIV, the lowest rates being found in the European cooperative survey (Mok et al, 1990). The higher rates found in parts of the US and sub-Saharan Africa may be related to the increased rate of complicated deliveries. Although transmission can occur *in utero*, most of the infection probably occurs at around the time of delivery. Whether this transmission can be reduced by Caesarean section remains controversial. Breast feeding increases the risk of HIV transmission to the newborn.

Occupational risk

Occupational risk is essentially confined to needle-stick trauma although three cases of seroconversion have apparently occurred through intact skin or mucous membranes. This appears to be very rare in prospective studies. About 0.3 per cent of health care workers seroconverted following a needle-stick injury with HIV infected blood in nine prospective studies. It is likely that this rate will vary depending upon the clinical status of the infected patient and the volume of blood transmitted. Transmission may be more likely if the recipient's T cells are activated by a concomitant infection at the time of injury. It is theoretically possible that HIV infection may occur following needle-stick injury but produce no immunological response because initial viral integration is not followed by replicative cycles. Thus, it is important that prospective studies are continued long term. The Centers for Disease Control (CDC) has recently studied a group of workers two years after such injury and have not found evidence of infection even with DNA enhancement techniques such as polymerase chain reaction.

9.2.2 Expected future patterns of the epidemic

The future pattern of the epidemic is difficult to assess because the efficacy of HIV transmission by heterosexual intercourse, the infectiousness of individuals at different stages of disease and the pattern of sexual behaviour in the population all remain unknown. However, certain future patterns can be predicted.

Gay/bisexual spread

Out of more than 662 000 cases of AIDS in the US reported in May 1988, 63 per cent were in gay men. Evidence from eight cohort studies of gay men suggest a declining incidence of seropositivity coupled with a falling frequency of other sexually transmitted diseases between 1985 and 1987 compared with the earlier part of the decade (CDC, 1987c), perhaps due to intense educational efforts in these groups of individuals. However, the seroconversion rate of 1–2 per cent per year in this community remains unacceptably high and it is possible that the rate of infection amongst younger gay men is even higher.

Heterosexual spread

The future pattern of the HIV epidemic in Africa remains difficult to assess and is crucially dependent upon educational measures and efforts to control other sexually transmitted disease. At present, the epidemic is much greater in certain urban areas but is rapidly spreading along major trading routes into the rural community. The fastest growing group of AIDS cases in the US have acquired the virus heterosexually (De Gruttrola and Mayer, 1988). Most of these individuals, however, had a partner who was in a high-risk group and there has only been a slow increase in the chance of infection when neither partner can be classified into a known risk category.

9.3 Clinical aspects

9.3.1 The virus

Epidemiology, particularly transmission by blood and blood products, suggested that the cause of AIDS would be an infection, probably a virus capable of infecting CD4 lymphocytes, which animal retroviruses were known to do. The evidence that HIV is the cause of AIDS is sufficient to satisfy most scientists, although some believe that additional co-factors may be important in predicting the rapidity of the development of AIDS.

HIV is a novel retrovirus. In addition to the standard structural genes coding the reverse transcriptase (pol) envelope (ENV) and core proteins (GAG), it has a complex regulatory gene structure which can enhance or inhibit replication (Weber and Weiss, 1988), as is found in the complex retrolentivirus group (Spuma, Visna and HTLV viruses). The HIV virus attaches to cell surfaces bearing a CD4 receptor, and then a DNA copy of the RNA viral genome is made by the reverse transcriptase enzyme. The DNA is translocated to the nucleus and formed into a circle, and then integrated into the host genome. The subsequent events which trigger replicative cycles of the virus are unclear, but replication can occur as a result of cellular signals related to activation of T cells or as a result of co-infection with another virus.

A second virus, HIV-2, closely related to HIV-1 has been isolated from patients in West Africa and Latin America. Individuals infected with this virus also developed the AIDS syndrome, but more slowly than those infected with HIV-1.

A strong immunological response most importantly of cytotoxic CD8 cells following seroconversion rapidly reduces the amount of HIV present in the bloodstream. Initially it was thought the virus then entered a 'latent phase' but more recent work has indicated that virus replication continues, particularly in lymph nodes (Weissman, 1993). Nevertheless, the patient remains asymptomatic for a variable period of years, presumably as a result of their strong immune response which checks the growth in numbers of virus.

The terminal immune deficiency associated with AIDS may be caused by mutations of the virus leading to a more virulent form which overcomes the immune response, or may be a primary failure of the immune response which allows a secondary increase in viral diversity and more rapid viral replication. Support for the former hypothesis comes from a more rapid loss of CD4 cells and the quicker development of AIDS in individuals with syncitial inducing strains of virus (SI, high fast variants), compared with those patients who only have non-syncitial inducing strains (NSI low slow variants). Similarly, recent reports indicate a blood donor and six recipients of his blood, all of whom had a surprisingly low frequency of AIDS some years later, and which is attributed to a less virulent virus having been transmitted. The alternative hypothesis is supported by the fact that immediately following seroconversion, most individuals are apparently able to suppress SI variants.

9.3.2 Classification of HIV infection and the definition of AIDS

In 1981 the Centers for Disease Control (CDC), Atlanta, Georgia, was quick to recognize an epidemic of a new disease following the initial reports of *Pneumocystis carinii* pneumonia (PCP) and Kaposi's sarcoma (KS) occurring in a group of homosexual males. The definition of acquired immune deficiency syndrome (AIDS) developed to monitor the epidemic was robust, but was formulated prior to the first description of the aetiological virus, human immunodeficiency virus (HIV) (Barre-Sinoussi et al, 1983). At any one time, between 30 and 100 times as many people have positive antibodies to this virus as have the full AIDS syndrome.

The CDC continues to modify its definition of AIDS, recognizing the importance of a positive HIV antibody test, and it has widened the number of illnesses and opportunistic infections fulfilling the criteria of immunodeficiency (CDC, 1987a) (see Tables 9.2 and 9.3). For example, dementia and marked weight loss without obvious cause, and most recently invasive carcinoma of the cervix and recurrent bacterial chest infection have been included. Perhaps more controversially, the CDC has also recently introduced a definition of AIDS depending

Table 9.2 CDC classification of HIV Infection (1987)

Group I	Acute infection
Group II	Asymptomatic infection
Group III	Persistent generalized lymphadenopathy
Group IV	Other disease
	(A) Constitutional disease: – fever > 1 month – weight loss > 10% baseline – diarrhoea > 1 month
	(B) Neurological
	(C1) Opportunistic infections diagnostic of AIDS
	(C2) Other specified secondary infections
	(D) Secondary cancers: – Kaposi's sarcoma – non-Hodgkins lymphoma – cerebral lymphoma
	(E) Other conditions

Table 9.3 Revised case definition of AIDS (CDC, 1987a)

(A) Without definitive diagnosis of HIV infection but definitive diagnosis of indicator disease

1. Candidiasis of oesphagus
2. Extrapulmonary cryptococcosis
3. Crytposporidiosis >1 month diarrhorea
4. Cytomegalovirus infection (other than liver, spleen or lymph node) in patient >1 month old
5. Herpes simplex causing pneumonitis, oesophagitis, mucocutaneous ulceration for > 1 month
6. Kaposi's sarcoma in patients <60 years
7. Primary cerebral lymphoma in patients <60 years
8. Lymphoid interstitial pneumonia affecting child <13 years
9. *Mycobacterium avium* intracellulare or *M. kansasii* (disseminated)
10. *Pneumocystis carinii* pneumonia
11. Progressive multifocal leukoencophalopathy
12. Toxoplasmosis of brain (patient older than one month)

(B) With definitive diagnosis of HIV infection (indicator disease diagnosis definitely, plus diseases above)

1. Bacterial infection (recurrent) in children
2. Disseminated coccidioidomycosis
3. HIV encephalopathy
4. Disseminated histoplasmosis
5. Isospora diarrhoea <1 month
6. Kaposi's sarcoma any age
7. Primary cerebral lymphoma age age
8. Non-Hodgkin's lymphoma
9. Any disseminated mycobacterial disease (non-*M. tuberculosis*)
10. Extra-pulmonary *M. tuberculosis*
11. Recurrent *Salmonella* septicaemia (non-*S. typhi*)
12. HIV wasting syndrome

(C) With laboratory evidence of HIV infection but presumptive diagnosis of indicator disease

1. Oesophageal candidiasis
2. Cytomegalovirus retinitis with visual loss
3. Kaposi's sarcoma
4. Lymphoid interstitial pneumonia in child <13 years
5. Disseminated mycobacterial disease (os species not defined)
6. *Pneumocystis carinii* pneumonia
7. Toxoplasmosis of brain

upon a low CD4 count (less than 200 cells per ml) as a marker of immunodeficiency, even in asymptomatic individuals (CDC, 1993).

Some workers have found the CDC definition of AIDS unwieldy and have sought to use a combination of clinical and immune parameters. One such classification, the Walter Reid, is widely used but does not improve the prognostic accuracy of the categorization compared with the CDC definition, and leaves up to 30 per cent of individuals with HIV unclassifiable. As HIV testing is not widely available in the developing world, the WHO has also introduced a simple clinical classification which is useful epidemiologically but is not sufficiently accurate as a basis for trials of treatment.

9.3.3 Clinical manifestations prior to the development of AIDS

Seroconversion illness

In individuals at risk of HIV infection followed prospectively, a seroconversion illness is common between 19 days and 3 months. This consists of a febrile illness accompanied by a non-specific rash, and sometimes meningitis, encephalitis or a myelopathy.

Extended lymphadenopathy syndrome and healthy HIV carriers

Most HIV positive patients are either perfectly well or have enlargement of the lymph nodes in several extra-inguinal sites. There is no evidence that the progression to AIDS is different in those who have lymph nodes and those who do not. Lymph node biopsy in such individuals is not usually indicated (Farthing et al, 1986).

Constitutional symptoms

Non-specific symptoms often herald the development of major manifestations of immune deficiency. The most troublesome of these is lassitude.

Weight loss

Weight loss is an important feature of HIV infection, not least because of the deterioration in the quality of life as a result of poor body image, cognitive and locomotor function. Wasting (greater than 10 per cent loss of body weight) is sufficient to make an AIDS diagnosis, and death seems to follow rapidly if weight falls below a critical level (Kotler, 1989). Weight loss may be caused by a hypocaloric diet associated with anorexia, malabsorption or an increased metabolic rate, perhaps associated with cytokine release caused by HIV infection of immune cells or opportunistic infection. The majority of patients who lose significant amounts of weight do so at the time they develop an opportunistic infection.

The most important aspect of the treatment of weight loss is rapid detection and treatment of the underlying infection. The role of dietary advice, enteral and parenteral feeding remains to be determined.

Oral disease

Buccal candidiasis produces characteristic white patches on the inner surfaces of the mouth which, on removal, leaves a raw bleeding surface. Extension of this infection to the oesophagus is common and is one of the opportunistic infections leading to an AIDS diagnosis. Buccal candidiasis is best treated by a systemic anti-fungal. Ketoconazole has the advantage of cheapness but occasionally causes severe hepatotoxicity, which appears to be less with itraconazole which is equally effective. Fluconazole is an alternative agent which may treat buccal candidiasis when given as a single dose. Relapse of infection occurs in 80 per cent of patients within three months of any treatment.

Hairy leucoplakia, which is most commonly seen on the side of the tongue, probably represents an opportunistic infection with Epstein–Barr virus. As it is asymptomatic no treatment is required.

Aphthous ulcers in the mouth, although no commoner than in the general community, tend to be persistent and very painful. They may respond to intralesional injections of corticosteroids, systemic corticosteroids, or thalidomide treatment (Youle et al, 1989).

Skin manifestations

Virus infections, including multiple dermatome herpes zoster, herpes simplex, molluscum contagiosum, and warts are common manifestations of HIV disease. Herpes viruses respond to acyclovir and molluscum contagiosum may be treated by pricking the lesion with a sharp piece of wood. **Seborrhoeic dermatitis**, which may be due to a fungal infection, is particularly common, and **acquired ichthyosis**, which is probably related to protein deficiency, occurs particularly in wasting patients.

9.3.4 Opportunistic infections and other conditions and their treatment

The opportunistic infections used by the CDC to confirm a diagnosis of AIDS are those which would be predicted to occur from a study of congenital T cell deficiencies. The majority of these are protozoa, fungi and viruses, bacteria being relatively uncommon, except *Mycobacterium avium intracellulare* (MAI). These opportunists are either ubiquitous in the environment (e.g. MAI, cryptococcus and cryptosporidium), or are reactivations of latent infections as a result of immunosuppression (e.g. cytomegalovirus: CMV, and *Toxoplasma gondii*). Whether *Pneumocystis carinii* pneumonia occurs as a result of reactivation of latent infection or recent exposure is controversial.

Respiratory infections

Pneumocystis carinii pneumonia (PCP) occurs in over 60 per cent of AIDS patients at some time during the course of the illness (Wofsy, 1987). It presents with non-specific 'flu-like' symptoms but, importantly, shortness of breath is a common feature. The chest X-ray is normal in up to 50 per cent of patients with PCP but the remainder show parenchymal lung change with a peri-hilar haze or extensive shadowing. Arterial hypoxia at rest is found in over half the patients. The diagnosis is confirmed by finding the organism in respiratory secretions or lung tissue obtained at bronchoscopy, or by sputum induction. The majority of patients respond within the first five days of treatment which is continued for between 14 and 21 days.

First-line therapy is cotrimoxazole, intravenous pentamidine, or trimethoprim/dapsone or primaquine/clindamycin combinations. Severely ill patients with an arterial oxygen of less than 8.5 Kp benefit from high dose corticosteroids. Repeated attacks of PCP pneumonia are common in patients with AIDS and, therefore, prophylaxis with cotrimoxazole, dapsone or inhaled pentamidine should be given (secondary prophylaxis). It is also standard practice to give individuals at high risk of developing PCP for the first time; for example, those with a CD4 lymphocyte subset count of less than 200 cells/mm^3 (primary) prophylaxis.

Many other opportunists and non-opportunists may produce respiratory symptoms, including cytomegalovirus (CMV), *Mycobacterium avium intracellulare* (MAI), *Legionella, pneumococcus* and *haemophilus influenzae*.

Central nervous system infections and other disorders

The central nervous system in AIDS patients may be involved by secondary complications, such as opportunistic infections, or by degenerative processes directly related to HIV infection (see Chapter 3 for review of primary central nervous system disorders). Patients may present with meningitis, a focal neurological defect presenting like a stroke or epileptic fits, or with degenerative changes of the brain, spinal cord or peripheral nerves.

(i) Meningitis

Viral meningitis is common at the time of seroconversion. There is an increased incidence of aseptic meningitis and bacterial meningitis in HIV positive patients but the commonest cause of meningitis is cryptococcus neoformans (Zuger et al, 1986). **Cryptococcal meningitis** may present insidiously with severe headache and temperature, but without much photophobia, neck stiffness or drowsiness. The diagnosis can be confirmed by finding the fungus in the cerebrospinal fluid by direct staining with Indian ink. The cryptococcal antigen test is always positive both in the cerebrospinal fluid and blood (Nelson et al, 1990). Treatment is with intravenous amphotericin or oral fluconazole, and secondary prophylaxis should be given with fluconazole (Bozette et al, 1991).

(ii) Presentation with a focal neurological defect

Acute presentation with a focal neurological defect is most commonly due to a ***Toxoplasma* abscess** usually arising as a recrudescence of latent infection. The geographical frequency of toxoplasma varies markedly related to the prevalence in the general population (Luft et al, 1983). Patients may present with epilepsy, transient ischaemic attacks or a progressive stroke. The possibility of toxoplasma encephalitis should be considered in any dementing process in an HIV positive patient. Computerized tomography (CT) usually shows multiple lesions with ring enhancement (Elkin et al, 1985). The diagnosis can only be confirmed by brain biopsy but this may be hazardous and non-diagnostic because of extensive tissue damage. Treatment is usually presumptive in those with the clinical syndrome and CT scan changes, reserving brain biopsy for those patients who had failed to respond to treatment over a period of 2–4 weeks. Combinations of pyrimethamine and sulphonamides are usually used but treatment toxicity, particularly skin rashes, is frequent. As the relapse rate of toxoplasmosis is high, secondary prophylaxis is given to all patients. In those who have positive Toxoplasma serology, primary prophylaxis should be considered when the CD4 count falls below 200 cells/ml^3. Retrospective studies have indicated that cotrimoxazole is an effective prophylactic agent.

Primary brain lymphoma usually presents in a similar way to a *Toxoplasma* abscess and CT usually shows multiple non-ring enhancing lesions. Although the prognosis of primary brain lymphoma is poor, total cranial irradiation may provide worthwhile remission in a few patients.

Progressive multifocal leucoencephalopathy (PML) caused by the JC strain of the papovavirus, is more common in HIV positive patients than in the general population (Blum et al, 1985), and the incidence is increasing as patients survive longer and the diagnosis of cerebral syndromes in HIV disease becomes more accurate. Although the CT scan appearances of PML are not distinct from those of cerebral lymphoma, on nuclear magnetic resonance imaging (MRI), the focal defects are confined to the white matter. The clinical course is very variable with rapid progression in a few patients and in others slow evolution after apparent periods of stability. This makes assessment of treatment difficult. There is no treatment of confirmed value although there are anecdotal reports of the benefit of radiotherapy or cytosine arabinoside.

Other infections which may produce focal neurological defects include **tuberculomas** and **cryptococcomas**. Most patients with these conditions are systemically ill and the organism can usually be cultured from the blood.

(iii) Degenerative nervous system conditions related to HIV infection

In addition to the primary HIV-related syndromes of dementia and other cognitive disorders which are discussed in Chapter 3, there are other neurological disorders of uncertain aetiology.

Cord degeneration. Vacuolation of the spinal cord, which may produce severe paresis and incontinence, is thought to be a direct effect of HIV infection (Petito et al, 1985).

Peripheral neuropathy. Damage to peripheral nerves during the course of HIV disease which may be due to direct HIV infection of nerve supporting structures, other opportunistic infections or complications of drug therapy. A mononeuritis or a mononeuritis multiplex, which may be a manifestation of early HIV infection, may resolve spontaneously. A painful peripheral neuropathy is a major cause of symptoms in advanced HIV disease. There is no known effective treatment, although carbamazepine and amytriptyline are often tried. The pain usually improves over several months. An ascending polyneuropathy of the Guillain–Barré type also occurs occasionally but whether the incidence is increased compared with that of the general population is unclear. Slow recovery is the rule.

(iv) Cytomegalovirus (CMV) infection of the central nervous system

Cytomegalovirus infection is the commonest cause of retinitis in HIV positive patients (Palestine et al, 1984), producing a characteristic ischaemic retina with a fluffy spreading edge. The patient remains asymptomatic until blurring of vision develops. Historical controls indicate that blindness usually occurs in untreated patients due either to macular involvement or retinal detachment.

Cytomegalovirus (CMV) inclusions are frequently found in the brain of patients presenting with a toxic encephalopathy and improvement sometimes occurs with anti-CMV treatment although the pathogenic significance of CMV inclusions is unknown. Recent evidence indicates that the painful remitting form of peripheral neuropathy may be due to CMV infection (Fuller et al, 1990). A polyradiculopathy producing flaccid paralysis of the lower limbs and bladder disturbance is also thought to be due to CMV infection.

Intravenous ganciclovir and foscarnet are both licensed for treatment of CMV retinitis. As relapse occurs rapidly on cessation of therapy, maintenance regimes are administered in the home by the patient using an indwelling central venous catheter. The major disadvantage of ganciclovir is bone marrow suppression, particularly when given with zidovudine. Foscarnet causes renal toxicity, hypocalcaemia and a possibly increased risk of seizures.

Gastrointestinal disorders

(i) Oesophageal symptoms

About 10–15 per cent of AIDS patients first present with pain or difficulty with swallowing caused by an opportunistic infection, most commonly candidiasis. In the 25 per cent of patients with discrete ulceration of the gullet, the cause may be herpes simplex virus, cytomegalovirus, or unknown (Connolly et al, 1989).

A diagnosis of **oesophageal candida** is often presumed in patients with buccal candidiasis and oesophadynia and this is sufficient for a diagnosis of AIDS. Further investigation by endoscopy is reserved for those patients who do not respond rapidly to treatment. Treatment of fungus infections and CMV has already been discussed. Large ulcers of uncertain aetiology respond to corticosteroids administered orally or by intralesional injection.

(ii) Diarrhoea

Diarrhoea is most commonly caused by opportunistic infection, although in one of the major risk groups for HIV infection, homosexual males, a variety of organisms causing diarrhoea are transmitted venereally (e.g. *Giardia*, *Salmonella*, species of *Entamoeba* and *Campylobacter* (Laughon et al, 1989).

(a) Non-opportunistic causes Bacterial causes of diarrhoea (including *Shigella*, *Salmonella* and *Campylobacter*) are more likely to be associated with a systemic upset and septicaemic illness with more frequent relapse than seen

in non-immunosuppressed individuals. Ciprofloxacin is the agent of choice for these three infections.

(b) Opportunistic causes Cryptosporidiosis is the commonest opportunistic infection causing diarrhoea in AIDS patients, although it is now appreciated that it is also capable of producing self-limiting diarrhoea in immunocompetent patients. In the immunosuppressed, a range of illness occurs, from asymptomatic infection through transient diarrhoea to massive diarrhoea of several litres a day with weight loss and death (Connolly et al, 1988). Transmission may be via animal contact, from one human to another, or via water supplies (D'Antonio et al, 1985). Immunosuppressed patients should therefore be advised to boil drinking water although whether this has any effect on the incidence of cryptosporidiosis is unknown. In addition to watery diarrhoea, cryptosporidiosis is also associated with right upper quadrant pain and infection of the bile ducts which produces appearances, on cholangiography similar to sclerosing cholangitis (Thuluvath et al, 1991).

The diagnosis of cryptosporidial diarrhoea is made by finding the organism in stool samples after concentration and staining with a modified Ziehl–Neelson stain. Treatment is mainly supportive. Oral salt and water replacement is beneficial and anti-diarrhoeal agents will reduce stool volumes. Paromomycin is associated with significant improvement in half the patients.

Microsporidiosis: Microsporidia are a large group of protozoa which produces infections in a wide variety of animals. Human infection was an obscure curiosity until Orenstein and his colleagues (1990) demonstrated that up to a third of HIV antibody positive patients, with apparently pathogen negative diarrhoea, had microsporidial infestation (*Enterocytozoon bienusi*) of the jejunum diagnosed initially by electron microscopy, but now diagnosed equally accurately by light microscopic examination of jejunal biopsies (Peacock et al, 1991) and by fluorescent tests to detect spores in stool samples. The pathogenicity of this organism is not proven as there is no effective treatment. However, it is most commonly found at a late stage of HIV disease in those with diarrhoea, massive weight loss and short survival. More recently other species of microsporidia (*Encephalitozoon cuniculi* and *Septata intestinalis*) have been shown to disseminate in the body via macrophage infection producing conjunctivitis, sinusitis and renal damage. The pathological importance of these organisms is clearer as eradication associated with symptomatic improvement occurs with albendazole therapy.

CMV colitis: Cytomegalovirus (CMV) may infect the colon producing bloody diarrhoea with abdominal pain and rebound tenderness. Sigmoidoscopy may show an acute colitis, which may extend around the whole colon. Diagnosis can be confirmed by rectal biopsy showing multiple inclusion bodies. Perforation occurs occasionally. Both licensed anti-CMV agents are effective in CMV colitis but the response is slow and relapse is frequent.

(c) Pathogen negative diarrhoea Between 10 and 30 per cent of HIV seropositive individuals with diarrhoea have no cause found despite extensive investigation. There are a number of possible causes for diarrhoea in these individuals,

including the irritable bowel syndrome, novel pathogens including pathogenic viruses, and the possibility that direct HIV infection of the gut may lead to diarrhoea (Nelson et al, 1988). Changes in villus architecture and malabsorption are associated with HIV infection in individuals with or without diarrhoea. There is continuing controversy as to whether this is due to direct infection of mucosal cells or to infection of immunologically competent cells within the lamina propria.

Kaposi's sarcoma

Kaposi's sarcoma (KS) which was first described in the late 19th century as an indolent tumour affecting the elderly, was later recognized to be endemic in Africa. It occasionally occurs after iatrogenic immunosuppression but improves if immune function recovers (Gague and Wilson-Jones, 1978). It is not thought to be a metastasizing tumour but to represent a field change in the vascular endothelium. Recent evidence indicates that the tumour is stimulated by growth factors released from HIV infected cells. This tumour is commoner in gay men than in other populations infected by HIV, and is declining in frequency. An increase in the frequency of the tumour in non-HIV positive gay men and in women infected with HIV by bisexuals, has led to the theory that an additional infective agent acting as a co-factor is important in the genesis of the condition. There is some evidence implicating CMV infection but this is by no means conclusive (Giraldo et al, 1980).

Kaposi's sarcoma lesions are purple, raised, non-tender and tend to follow the flexural creases with a predilection for the extremities, including the nose and legs. Lesions may be single, few or multiple and progress slowly or rapidly. Sometimes lesions on the legs and face become enlarged and painful, associated with cellulitis and oedema. It frequently occurs on the palate and is said to predict the presence of KS elsewhere in the gut where it is common. KS is also seen in the lungs producing progressive shortness of breath, sometimes associated with a pleural effusion. KS has been described in the heart and virtually every organ other than the brain.

9.3.5 Paediatric HIV infection

Approximately 1 million children world-wide are infected by HIV, half of whom have AIDS. Infant mortality is likely to increase by up to one-third and AIDS is likely to become the major childhood cause of death in sub-Saharal Africa by the year 2000.

Definition of paediatric AIDS

The initial CDC definition of paediatric AIDS included only children with documented opportunistic infection or biopsy proven lymphocytic interstitial pneumonitis. Less than 25 per cent of HIV infected sick children fulfilled this case definition and now a broader definition of paediatric AIDS recognizes the importance of serious bacterial infections and a presumptive diagnosis of lymphocytic interstitial pneumonitis.

Of those infants who acquire HIV vertically, one in four will develop AIDS in the first year of life. The prognosis of those who survive for at least two years is better but many are likely to develop opportunistic infections typical of adult infections in later years. In the former Soviet Union, Romania and Africa major outbreaks of HIV in children have occurred associated with inadequate sterilization of contaminated needles or failure to test blood used for transfusion.

Differences between adult and paediatric AIDS

There are a number of important differences between presentation of HIV infection in children and in adults.

1. As the fetus is infected early in development, immune tolerance may develop and there may be a long 'negative window' when the virus is present in children with no antibody response (Bernstein and Rubinstein, 1986).
2. It is recognized in adults that B cells are activated in HIV infection but have a diminished ability to respond to new antigenic stimuli. As adults have previously encountered most common bacterial infections, these are not a frequent problem. Children with HIV infection, however, are susceptible to a wide variety of bacterial infections and about 30 per cent of all cases will present with recurrent diarrhoea, otitis media, or respiratory tract infections (Bernstein et al, 1985).
3. As many of the opportunists in adults are latent infections which have not been acquired by children, the frequency of these pathogens is different. *Pneumocystis carinii* (PC) is less common but candida and primary CMV infections being more so. Primary PC infection is a major cause of death in those children developing AIDS in the first few months of life, and the possibility of providing prophylaxis from birth to all children born to HIV seropositive mothers is being considered.
4. Lymphoid interstitial pneumonitis (LIP) is a sub-acute respiratory disease occurring mainly in children (Rubinstein et al, 1986). Respiratory failure and cor pulmonale develop over a number of weeks and the chest X-ray shows nodular shadowing. Alternate day steroids improve both symptoms and prognosis. Parotid swellings, which are also a common feature of paediatric AIDS, tend to occur in association with LIP.
5. The frequency of symptomatic disease is much higher in children than in adults but this may be a problem of detection of asymptomatic HIV positive children. In one study only 2 of 200 children infected with HIV had no symptoms (Novick and Rubinstein, 1987). As more children born to HIV positive mothers are being prospectively evaluated, it is clear that some remain infected but well for a number of years after birth.
6. Perhaps because immature cells of the central nervous system are easier to infect with HIV, neurological manifestations are particularly common with very frequent developmental delay. Calcification of the basal ganglia occurs in over 50 per cent of affected children.

9.3.6 Prognostic markers for the development of AIDS

It is not known whether all patients who are HIV seropositive will ultimately develop AIDS. The risk of progression to AIDS in gay men which is slight during the first two years following seroconversion, rises to 40 per cent by eight years with a similar proportion developing lesser symptoms of infection (Moss et al, 1988). It is believed that the rate of progression to AIDS is similar for all risk groups and that most individuals will develop AIDS within 15 years of infection with HIV.

A number of laboratory markers are used to predict the development of AIDS. While the readily available measure of viral replication (HIV p24 antigen) is only of limited value, tests of immune activation (e.g. serum or urinary neopterin and beta-2 microglobulin) are more useful. Perhaps the most valuable and certainly the most widely used laboratory parameter is the CD4 count. Although CD4 cell estimates are liable to error, may be an inaccurate reflection of the number of cells in the tissue, and do not reveal abnormalities in important sub-groups of cells (e.g. memory cells), they do provide the best guide to prognosis of the currently available tests (Bowen et al, 1986) (Table 9.4). Clinical markers are also important. Thus, over 50 per cent of patients with buccal candidiasis will have developed the full syndrome within a three-month period (Klein et al, 1984). Hairy leucoplakia which is unique to HIV infection and multiple dermatome herpes zoster, may also predict the development of AIDS (Greenspan et al, 1984: Melbye et al, 1987), but are less reliable.

Table 9.4 CD4 count as percentage of total lymphocyte count and the development of AIDS

CD4 count	0–10%	10–20%	20–30%	30–40%	>40%
Proportion with AIDS after 1 year (%)	81	16	5	0	0
Proportion with AIDS after 2 years (%)	100	33	14	4	2
Proportion with AIDS after 3 years (%)	100	50	26	10	5

9.4 Management of HIV infection and the value of anti-retrovirals

9.4.1 Prevention of occupational infection

As there is no evidence for nosocomial transmission of HIV, patients need not be nursed in isolation. Blood from all patients should be treated as potentially infectious. As patients not known to be HIV positive are likely to represent an equally important risk to staff as those known to be infected, there is little point in a two-tier system of precautions. As there are a few cases of possible transmission by massive amounts of blood in contact with skin abrasions or mucous membrane, it is important that all health care personnel should develop a habit of closing all skin cuts with waterproof bandages on arrival at work (see chapter 7).

9.4.2 General advice to people with HIV infection

Many patients want advice about 'healthy living'. Although moderation of smoking and alcohol intake would seem sensible, little is known about their effects on the CD4 count or disease progression. Nutritional status can have profound effects on the immune system, and advice about intake of sufficient calories and micronutrients should be given early in disease. There is also a good deal of interest in the role of psychological and lifestyle factors and their possible contribution to disease progression, although the evidence is limited (see chapter 6 for review).

9.4.3 Anti-retroviral therapy

There are a number of points in the life cycle of HIV at which drugs might inhibit replication. At present, most treatments of HIV being developed act as inhibitors of the reverse transcriptase enzyme, but alternatives include viral entry, viral budding, inhibition of translation of viral RNA and prevention of viral assembly with proteinase inhibitors.

Zidovudine

The only licensed drug in the UK for the treatment of HIV is zidovudine (ZDV) which is a nucleoside analogue. This is phosphorylated in the cell and prevents elongation of the DNA chain being prepared from the RNA viral template by the reverse transcriptase enzyme. Dideoxycytosin (ddC) and dideoxyinosine (ddI) are also reverse transcriptase inhibitors still at an experimental stage of development.

The initial placebo controlled trial which was performed in patients who had recently had *Pneumocystis carinii* pneumonia and others with symptomatic HIV disease and a reduced CD4 count, demonstrated a reduction in mortality associated with a diminished frequency of opportunistic infection (Fischl et al, 1987). This trial has been used as evidence that patients presenting with any opportunist infection or Kaposi's sarcoma, will also benefit from zidovudine treatment. As HIV replication continues throughout the 'latent' period of infection with a slowly rising viral burden, it was logical to try anti-viral drugs at an earlier asymptomatic stage of infection, although initial placebo controlled studies had not demonstrated a delay in the development of opportunistic infection in such zidovudine treated patients (Volberding et al, 1990; Fischl et al, 1990a). Many patients who did not require treatment were also given zidovudine (Lancet, 1990), and the much larger definitive Concorde study showed that long-term treatment (on average three years) with zidovudine during the asymptomatic phase, was not translated into improvements in survival or significant delay in the onset of opportunistic infections (Concorde Co-ordinating Committee, 1994). Recent publicity has made many patients wary of starting zidovudine at all but, it is clear that treatment during the symptomatic phase prolongs life and may be associated with a reduction in the frequency of HIV-associated dementia (see Chapter 5). The prolonged use of zidovudine, particularly in those with advanced infection, is associated with development of virus with reduced sensitivity to the drug (Larder et al, 1989). Such viruses may be the reason for the transient clinical effectiveness of zidovudine.

No placebo controlled studies have been performed in children. Although many paediatricians would now give zidovudine to children with AIDS, the dose remains the subject of debate as the original studies used high dose drug often given intravenously. Zidovudine treatment in the earlier stage of disease in children remains a subject of controversy.

Initially, doses of zidovudine of between 1.5 and 1.2 gm per day were used. However, in the two recent studies of asymptomatic or patients with minor symptoms, lower doses (600 mg/day) were shown to be effective and a recent study has shown that 1 gm/day dropping to 600 mg/day produces identical survival to a group of patients maintained long term on 1 gm of zidovudine per day (Fischl et al, 1990b). The toxicity of zidovudine is markedly less at these lower doses, and therefore between 500–600 mg/day is now usually given. Even lower doses are suggested by some authors, but zidovudine levels in the cerebrospinal fluid are lower than those in plasma and worries have been expressed that these doses may not prevent HIV-associated dementia.

The major toxicity of large doses of zidovudine is bone marrow suppression. At lower doses (600 mg/day) in less ill patients, bone marrow toxicity is rare. The most frequent problem is anaemia although severe granulocytopenia is an occasional reason for stopping therapy. Thrombocytopenia is a direct effect of HIV infection and the platelet count often rises after zidovudine therapy, at least initially. A myopathy also affects a small proportion of patients taking long term zidovudine (greater than one year). In most patients, a rise in creatinine phosphokinase is a prelude to development of severe myopathy which is usually aborted if the drug is promptly stopped.

Dideoxycytosine (ddC)

In the high doses used in the initial clinical studies an unacceptable incidence of peripheral neuropathy was observed. Using lower dosages which still have an anti-retroviral effect, the frequency of this side-effect has been reduced. Dideoxycystosine however appears to be less active than zidovudine as sole therapy for HIV symptomatic patients and is likely to be mainly used in combination therapy.

Dideoxyinosine (ddI)

This agent is the active metabolite of dideoxyadenosine and has a different side-effect profile to zidovudine. The most important side-effect is pancreatitis which may be fatal. This appears to be common in those with previous attacks and is more frequent in those with advanced disease, whereas the therapeutic toxic ratio may be too narrow for its sensible use. In early disease ddI is likely to be used in individuals intolerant to zidovudine. In early disease evidence indicates that ddI and zidovudine are roughly similar in potency.

D14 (stavudine)

This is another nucleoside analogue with *in vitro* HIV activity and a favourable safety profile *in vivo*. It influences CD4 count and P24 antigen in similar ways to zidovudine, but there is no evidence to suggest that it would be markedly more clinically effective.

3TC

This nucleoside derivative of cytosine is noticeably free of side-effects. However, present studies also indicate that it has little effect in reducing the load of HIV virus in treated patients, perhaps because of the rapid development of viruses with reduced sensitivity to this compound. It might still be useful in combinations (see below).

Non-nucleoside analogues

A group of inhibitors of reverse transcriptase activity acting by a different mechanism was described by Paul Janssen. These drugs are non-toxic and active against HIV-1 but not HIV-2. Although highly active *in vitro*, results *in vivo* have so far been disappointing, as the development of resistance by HIV is extremely rapid. As they are non-toxic, it may be possible to obtain such high blood levels that even virus with reduced sensitivity may be effectively killed.

Other experimental anti-retroviral preparations

A variety of other parts of the viral life cycle provide potential mechanisms for inhibition of HIV. Although the concept that **soluble CD4** will bind in the circulation with virus and prevent attachment to cells is attractive, in practice early studies using this form of treatment have been disappointing. It is known that **alpha interferon** has a variety of antiviral effects and prevents virus budding from cells and it does have modest anti-retroviral activity in large doses.

Proteinases inhibitors have received attention lately. HIV contains a unique protease which becomes active at the time of viral budding and splits a large viral polypeptide derived from the gag gene into its constituent proteins. This protease has been successfully crystallized and its tertiary structure elucidated by crystallography. Proteinase inhibitors which have marked anti-HIV effects have been developed by molecular modelling. Non-competitive inhibitors have not proved effective and most agents are competitive and mimic the transitional states of the proteinase. These drugs do not have any activity against mammalian proteinases. Although oral bio-availability is low, sufficient drug is absorbed to produce plasma levels above the *in vitro* effective concentrations. Absorption into infected cells may be more difficult but proteinases have improved surrogate markers of HIV infection to a similar degree to that seen with zidovudine in Phase I and II studies. Unfortunately, one Tat inhibitor with promising *in vitro* activity has recently been withdrawn because of disappointing pharmacokinetics. It is likely that other potential remedies to interfere with genetic mechanisms such as **anti-sense oligonucleosides**, will suffer from similar difficulties of poor oral bio-availability and difficulties of transport into HIV infected cells.

Drug combinations

Combination therapy is attractive for two reasons. Lower doses of drug would minimize toxicity, and using additive or synergistic combinations of drugs might be expected to delay the development of viral resistance. Unfortunately, maximum doses of each drug in a combination have so far been required to produce a therapeutic effect, and combinations have not been shown to delay the development of resistance to zidovudine. Theoretically, the most attractive combinations might be a drug that interferes at an early stage of the viral cycle which would therefore prevent infection of new cells with a drug acting after integration (late phase), which would prevent successful replication of the virus in cells with an established infection. Such combinations would be a reverse transcriptase inhibitor and a protease inhibitor or alpha interferon.

Alternatively a concerted attack using several drugs targeted against the reverse transcriptase activity might produce so many changes in this enzyme that the virus is no longer viable. Although *in vitro* work suggesting this might be true has now been disproved, studies of combination treatment of several nucleosides (2, 3, or 5) are now in progress. Initial results do not indicate that such therapy is likely to represent a dramatic breakthrough.

9.4.4 The future

Drug therapy

It is clear from the plethora of trials which have appeared over the last few years that the present anti-retroviral drugs have, at best, a very modest effect in improving survival. This is likely to be due to the limited capacity of many of these compounds to inhibit viral replication effectively, and to the rapid development of viral resistance. Interesting data has suggested that in patients with virus resistant to zidovudine, the addition of a second drug might restore sensitivity to the first one, even though on genetic analysis of the virus, the resistant mutation is still present. This reversal of resistance of zidovudine has so far been seen with ddI and a number of non-nucleoside analogues. It is likely that over the next few years, a number of combinations will be used in an endeavour to utilize this fascinating finding.

Vaccination

The world is eagerly awaiting the development of a successful vaccine but the difficulties to be overcome are formidable. The virus itself is capable of considerable antigenic mutation and it is relatively unlikely that the prevalent African variant of HIV would be neutralized by antibodies produced by an envelope vaccine derived from the predominant American strain. The most important immunological events at the commonest portal of entry, the genital tract, remain unclear and so the most important properties of a successful vaccine are difficult to elucidate. Similarly, the immunological factors, which are responsible for a prompt reduction in viral load after seroconversion, remain unclear although it is likely that cytotoxic lymphocyte responses are particularly important and need to be induced by putative vaccines.

Development of previous viral vaccines has been assisted by animal models. Unfortunately these are not available for HIV as the virus only produces disease in humans. Although chimpanzees are infectable with the virus, no disease results from this infection. Sub-unit vaccines have been developed which will protect the chimpanzee from HIV-1 challenge, and some of these are now in Phase I and Phase II clinical trial. The most hopeful sign that a vaccination might be feasible have come from studying similar animal viruses such as simian immunodeficiency virus (SIV). Although inactivated whole SIV vaccines will protect primates against subsequent challenge (Murphie-Corb et al, 1989), this is mainly because of antigenic stimulation from human cellular proteins present in the culture medium.

A live, attenuated SIV (Nef deleted mutants)) has provided long-term protection against subsequent high-dose SIV wild-type challenge (Desrosiers et al, 1989). Although there are likely to be continuing reservations about the use of attenuated vaccines in a fatal disease associated with incorporation of virus into host DNA, it will be considered further in the absence of other effective measures.

The difficulties, both logistic and ethical, of trials to evaluate putative vaccines are also great as the seroconversion rate is only sufficiently high in certain under privileged areas of the world to make such a study possible. It is partly for this reason the possibility of using a vaccine to boost the immune system of patients already infected with HIV is being investigated. Although there was an initial flurry of excitement that such an approach with an envelope vaccine might be successful, more recent data does not show any clear evidence of benefit, although it is possible to show an increase in the immune responsiveness to HIV and such vaccination programmes appear to be safe.

References

Ader, R. (1988). *Psychoneuroimmunology* (2nd edn). Academic Press Inc., San Diego.

Ader, R. and Cohen, N. (1975). Behaviourally conditioned immunosuppression. *Psychosomatic Medicine*, **37**, 333–40.

Ades, A., Davison, C., Holland, F., Gibb, D., Hudson, C., Nicholl, A. et al (1993). Vertically transmitted HIV infection in the British Isles. *British Medical Journal*, **306**, 1296–99.

Adib, M., Joseph, J., Ostrow, D. and Sherman, J. (1991). Predictors of relapse in sexual practices among homosexual men. *AIDS Education and Prevention*, **3**, 293–304.

Agle, D., Gluck, H. and Pierce, G. (1987). The risk of AIDS: Psychologic impact on the hemophiliac population. *General Hospital Psychiatry*, **9**, 11–17.

Ajmani, A., Habte-Gabr, E., Zarr, M., Jayabalan, V. and Dandala, S. (1991). Cerebral blood flow SPECT with Tc–99m exametazine correlates in AIDS dementia complex stages: a preliminary report. *Clinical Nuclear Medicine*, **16**, 656–59.

Alcorn, K. (ed.) (1994). *Directory of complementary and alternative treatments in HIV/AIDS*. NAM Publications Ltd., London.

Alexius, B. (1991). Thirteen psychotic HIV–1 infected patients. *International Conference on the Neuroscience of HIV Infection*, Padua, 1991.

Allebeck, P. and Bolund, C. (1991). Suicides and suicide attempts in cancer patients. *Psychological Medicine*, **21**, 979–84.

Allebone, P. (1992). Euthanasia. *British Medical Journal*, **305**, 1224.

Allen, S., Serufilira, A., Bogaerts, J., Van de Perre, P., Nsengumuremyi, F., Lindan et al (1992). Confidential HIV testing and condom promotion in Africa. *Journal of the American Medical Association*, **268**, 3338–43.

Altamura, C., Mauri, M., Coppola, M. and Cazzullo, C. (1988). Delusional AIDS and depression. *British Journal of Psychiatry*, **153**, 267–9.

American Academy of Neurology AIDS Task Force (1991). Nomenclature and research case definitions for neurologic manifestations of human immunodeficiency virus-type 1 (HIV–1). infection. *Neurology*, **41**, 778–85.

American Medical Association Council on Ethical and Judicial Affairs (1988). Ethical issues involved in the growing AIDS crisis. *Journal of the American Medical Association*, **259**, 1360–61.

American Psychiatric Association (1988a). AIDS Policy: Confidentiality and disclosure. *American Journal of Psychiatry*, **145**, 541.

American Psychiatric Association (1988b). AIDS Policy: Guidelines for inpatient psychiatric units. *American Journal of Psychiatry*, **145**, 542.

American Psychiatric Association (1992a). AIDS Policy: Guidelines for outpatient psychiatric services. *American Journal of Psychiatry*, **149**, 721.

American Psychiatric Association (1992b). AIDS Policy: Guidelines for inpatient units. *American Journal of Psychiatry*, **149**, 722.

Anastasopoulos, D. and Tsiantis, J. (1990). *A description of mental and psychological disorders displayed by HIV positive haemophiliac and thalassaemic children and their relatives*. WHO Regional Office for Europe, Copenhagen.

Andersen, H. and MacElveen-Hoehn, P. (1988). Gay clients with AIDS: new challenges for hospice programs. *Hospice Journal*, **4**, 37–54.

Anderson, P. and Mayon-White, R. (1988). General practitioners and management of infection with HIV. *British Medical Journal*, **296**, 535–7.

Anderson, D.C., Blower, A.L., Packer, J.M.W. and Ganguli, L.A. (1991). Preventing needlestick injuries. *British Medical Journal*, **302**, 769–70.

Andrews, K. (1993). Recovery of patients after four months or more in the persistent vegetative state. *British Medical Journal*, **306**, 1597–99.

Ankrah, E.M. (1993). The impact of HIV/AIDS on the family and other significant relationships: the African clan revisited. *AIDS Care*, **5**, 5–22.

Annas, G.J. (1988). Not saints but healers: the legal duties of health care professionals in the AIDS epidemic. *American Journal of Public Health*, **78**, 844–9.

Anson, J.A., Glick, R.P. and Reyes, M. (1992). Diagnostic accuracy of AIDS-related CNS lesions. *Surgical Neurology*, **37**, 432–40.

Antoni, M.H. (1991). Psychosocial stressors and behaviourial interventions in gay men with HIV infection. *International Review of Psychiatry*, **3**, 383–99.

Antoni, M.H., Schneiderman, N., Fletcher, M.A., Goldstein, D.A. Ironson, G., LaPerrier, A. et al (1990). Psychoneuroimunology and HIV–1. *Journal of Consulting and Clinical Psychology*, **58**, 38–49.

Antoni, M.H., August, S., LaPerrier, A., Bagget, H.L. and Klimas, N. (1991a). Psychological and neuroendocrine measures related to functional immune changes in anticipation of HIV–1 serostatus notification. *Psychosomatic Medicine*, **52**, 496–510.

Antoni, M.H., Baggett, L., Ironson, G., LaPerriere, A., August S. et al (1991b). Cognitive-behavioural stress management intervention buffers distress responses and immunologic changes following notification of HIV–1 seropositivity. *Journal of Consulting and Clinical Psychology*, **59**, 906–15.

Appleby, L. (1987). Hypochondriasis: an acceptable diagnosis? *British Medical Journal*, **294**, 857.

Arendt, G., Hefter, H., Hoemberg, V., Nelles, H.W., Elsing, C. and Freund, H.J. (1990). Early abnormalities of cognitive event related potentials in patients without clinically evident CNS deficits. *Electroencephalography and Clinical Neurophysiology (Suppl.),* **41**, 370–80.

Arno, P.S. (1986). The non-profit sector's response to the AIDS epidemic: community-based services in San Francisco. *American Journal of Public Health*, **76**, 1325–30.

Ashby, M. and Stoffell, B. (1991). Therapeutic ratio defined phases: proposal of ethical framework for palliative care. *British Medical Journal*, **302**, 1322–24.

Atherton, D. (1994). Towards the safer use of traditional remedies. *British Medical Journal*, **308**, 673–4.

Atkins, R. and Amenta, M. (1991). Family adaptation to AIDS: a comparative study. *Hospice Journal*, **7**, 71–83.

Atkinson, J., Grant, I., Kennedy, C., Richman, D., Spector, S., McCutchan, J. et al (1988). Prevalence of psychiatric disorder among men infected with HIV—a controlled study. *Archives of General Psychiatry*, **45**, 859–64.

Auerbach, J., Oleson, T. and Solomon, G. (1992). A behaviourial medicine intervention as an adjuvant treatment for HIV-related illness. *Psychology and Health*, **6**, 325–34.

Avins, A.L., Woods, W.J., Lindan, C., Hudes, E., Clark, W. and Hulley, S. (1994). HIV infection and risk behaviour among heterosexuals in alcohol treatment programs. *Journal of the American Medical Association*, **271**, 515–18.

Ayers, M.R., Abrams, D.I., Newell, T.G. and Friedrich, F. (1987). Performance of individuals with AIDS on the Luria-Nebraska Neuropsychological Battery. *International Journal of Clinical Neuropsychology*, **9**, 101–5.

Aylward, E.H., Butz, A.M., Hutton, N., Joyner, M.L. and Vogelhut, J.W. (1992). Cognitive and motor development in infants at risk for human immuno-deficiency syndrome. *American Journal of Disorders of Childhood*, **146**, 218–22.

Aylward, E.H., Henderer, J.D., McArthur, J.C., Brettschneider, P.D., Harris, G.J., Barta, P.E. et al (1993). Reduced basal ganglia volume in HIV–1 associated dementia. *Neurology*, **43**, 2099–104.

Ayuso-Mateos, J.L. (1994). Use of psychotropic drugs in patients with HIV infection. *Drugs*, **47**, 599–610.

Ayuso-Mateos, J., Bayon Perez, C., Sto Domingo Carrasco, J., Sal as Jimenez, J., Olivares, D. (1989). Psychiatric aspects of patients with HIV infection in the general hospital. *Psychotherapy and Psychosomatics*, **52**, 110–13.

Ayuso-Mateos, J.L., Montanes, F., Lastra, I., Plaza, S. and Picazo de la Garza, J. (1994). HIV seroprevalence in an acute psychiatric unit. *IInd International Conference on the Biopsychosocial Aspects of HIV infection*, Brighton, 1994.

Baer, J. (1987). Case report: Munchausen's/AIDS. *General Hospital Psychiatry*, **9**, 75–6.

Baer, J. (1989). Study of 60 patients with AIDS or ARC requiring psychiatric hospitalization. *American Journal of Psychiatry*, **146**, 1285–8.

Bailey, M. (1992). Children and AIDS. In *A global report: AIDS in the world* (ed. J. Mann, D. Tarantola and T. Netter). Harvard University Press, Cambridge, Mass.

Baker, D. and Mossman, D. (1991). Potential HIV exposure in psychiatrically hospitalized adolescent girls. *American Journal of Psychiatry*, **148**, 528–30.

Baker, N.T. and Saeger, R. (1991). A comparison of the psychosocial needs of hospice patients with AIDS and those with other diseases. *Hospice Journal*, **7**, 61–9.

Baldeweg, T. and Lovett, E. (1991). Psychophysiology and neurophysiology of HIV infection. *International Review of Psychiatry*, **3**, 331–42.

Baldeweg, T., Gruzelier, J., Catalán, J., Pugh, K., Lovett, E., Riccio, M. et al (1993a). Auditory and visual event-related potentials in a controlled investigation of gay men with HIV infection. *Electroencephalography and Clinical Neurophysiology*, **88**, 356–68.

Baldeweg, T., Gruzelier, J.H., Stygall, J., Lovett, E., Pugh, K., Liddiard, D. et al (1993b). Detection of subclinical motor dysfunctions in early symptomatic HIV infection with topographical EEG. *International Journal of Psychophysiology*, **15**, 227–38.

Baldeweg, T., Catalàn, J., Lovett, E., Gruzelier, J., Riccio, M. and Hawkins, D.A. (In press a). Retrospective analysis of the effect of ZDV on neuropsychological and neurophysiological functioning. *AIDS*.

Baldeweg, T., Gruzelier, J.H., Riccio, M., Hawkins, D.A., Burgess, A.P., Stygall J. et al (In press b). Neurophysiological evaluation of zidovudine in asymptomatic HIV infection: a longitudinal placebo-controlled study. *Journal of Neurological Sciences*.

Ball, J., Lange, W., Myers, C. and Friedman, S. (1988). Reducing the risk of AIDS through methadone maintenance treatment. *Journal of Health and Social Behaviour*, **29**, 214–26.

Bancroft, J. (1989). Human sexuality and its problems (2nd edn). Churchill Livingstone, Edinburgh.

Barbacci, M., Repke, J., Chaisson, R. (1991). Routine prenatal screening for HIV infection. *Lancet*, **337**, 709–11.

Barnard, M., McKeganey, N., Leyland, A. (1993). Risk behaviours among male clients of female prostitutes. *British Medical Journal*, **307**, 361–7.

Barongo, L., Martien, B., Mosha, F., Nicoll, A., Grosskurth., Senkoro, K. et al (1992).

The epidemiology of HIV–1 infection in urban areas, roadside settlements and rural villages in Mwanza Region, Tanzania. *AIDS*, **6**, 1521–8.

Barraclough, B. and Hughes, J. (1987). *Suicide: clinical and epidemiological studies*. Croom Helm, London.

Barre-Sinoussi, F., Chermann, C., Rey, F., Charmovet, S., Gruest, J., Daugert, C. et al (1983). Isolation of a T lymphocyte retrovirus from a patient at risk for acquired immunodeficiency syndrome (AIDS). *Science*, **220**, 868–71.

Bartnof, S. (1989). Health care professional education and AIDS. In *AIDS: principles, practices and politics*, (ed. I.B. Coreless and M. Pittman-Lindenman M). Hemisphere Publishing, New York.

Barton, T.L., Rousch, M.K. and Dever, L.L. (1992). Seizures associated with gancyclovir therapy. *Pharmacotherapy*, **12**, 413–15.

Barton, S., Davies, S., Schroeder, K., Arthur, G. and Gazzard, B.G. (1994). Complementary therapies used by people with HIV infection. *AIDS*, **8**, 561.

Battjes, R., Pickens, R. and Amsel, Z. (1991). HIV infection and AIDS risk behaviours smong intravenous drug users entering methadone treatment in selected US cities. *Journal of Acquired Immune Deficiency Syndromes*, **4**, 1148–54.

Bayer, R., Levine, C. and Wolf, S. (1986). HIV antibody screening: an ethical framework for evaluating proposed programmes. *Journal of the American Medical Association*, **256**, 1768–74.

Bayer, R. and Healton, C. (1989). Controlling AIDS in Cuba: the logic of quarantine. *New England Journal of Medicine*, **320**, 1022–24.

Bayer, R. and Toomey, K. (1992). HIV prevention and the two faces of partner notification. *American Journal of Public Health*, **82**, 1158–63.

Beach, R.S., Morgan, R., Wilkie, F., Mantero-Atienza, E., Blaney, N., Shor-Posner, G. et al (1992). Plasma vitamin B_{12} level as a potential cofactor in studies of human immunodeficiency virus type 1-related cognitive changes. *Archives of Neurology*, **49**, 501–6.

Beardsell, S. (1994). Should wider HIV testing be encouraged on the grounds of HIV prevention? AIDS Care, **6**, 5–19.

Bebbington, P., Wilkins, S., Jones, P., Foerster, A., Murray, R., Toone, B. et al (1993). Life events and psychosis: initial results from the Camberwell Collaborative Psychosis Study. *British Journal of Psychiatry*, **162**, 72–9.

Beck, A.T., Ward, C., Mendelson, J., Mock, J. and Erbaugh, J. (1961). An inventory for measuring depression. *Archives of General Psychiatry*, **4**, 561–71.

Beck, A.T., Weissman, A., Lester, D. and Trexler, L. (1974a). The measuring of pessimism: the Hopelessness Scale. *Journal of Consulting and Clinical Psychology*, **42**, 861–5.

Beck, A.T., Schuyler, D. and Herman, J. (1974b). Development of suicidal intent scales. In *The prediction of suicide*, (ed. A.T. Beck, H.L. Presnik and D.J. Lettieri). Charles Press, Maryland.

Beck, A.T., Kovacs, M. and Weissman, A. (1975). Hopelessness and suicidal behaviour: an overview. *Journal of the American Medical Association*, **234**, 1146–49.

Beck, A.T., Steer, R., Kovacs, M. and Garrison, B. (1985). Hopelessness and eventual suicide. *American Journal of Psychiatry*, **145**, 559–63.

Beck, E., Donegan, C., Cohen, C., Moss, V. and Tery, P. (1990). An update on HIV testing at a London STD clinic: long-term impact of the AIDS media campaign. *Genitourinary Medicine*, **66**, 142–7.

Beckett, A. (1991). Ethical issues in the psychiatry of HIV disease. *International Review of Psychiatry*, **3**, 417–27.

Beckett, A., Summergrad, P., Manschreck, T., Vitagliano, H., Henderson, M., Buttolph,

M. et al (1987). Symptomatic HIV infection of the CNS in a patient without clinical evidence of immune deficiency. *American Journal of Psychiatry*, **144**, 1342–4.

Beedham, H.M. and Wilson-Barnett, J. (1993). Evaluation of services for people with HIV/AIDS in an inner-city health authority: perspectives of key service providers. *Journal of Advanced Nursing*, **18**, 69–79.

Beevor, A. and Catalán, J. (1993). Women's experience of HIV testing. *AIDS Care*, **5**, 177–86.

Beevor, A., Catalán, J., Barton, S. and Gazzard, B.G. (1991). Psychosocial aspects of HIV infection in women. *Ist International Conference on the Biopsychosocial Aspects of HIV infection*, Amsterdam, 1991.

Belec L., Martin P., Vohito, M. and Gresenguet, G. (1989). Low prevalence of neuropsychiatric clinical manifestations in Central African patients with AIDS. *Transactions of the Royal Society of Tropical Medicine and Hygiene*, **83**, 844–6.

Belman, A.L., Ultmann, M., Horoupian, D., Novick, B.E., Spiro, A.J., Rubinstein, A. et al (1985). Neurological complications in infants and children with acquired immune deficiency syndrome. *Annals of Neurology*, **18**, 560–6.

Belman, A.L., Diamond, G.W., Dickinson, D., Llena, J., Lantos, G. and Rubinstein, A. (1988). Pediatric acquired immunodeficiency syndrome. *American Journal of Disorders of Childhood*, **142**, 29–35.

Beltran, E., Ostrow, D. and Joseph, J. (1993). Predictors of sexual behaviour change among men requesting their HIV-1 antibody status: the Chicago MACS of homosexual/bisexual men, 1985–1986. *AIDS Education and Prevention*, **5**, 185–95.

Bennett, L., Michie, P. and Kippax, S. (1991). Quantitative analysis of burnout and its associated factors in AIDS nursing. *AIDS Care*, **3**, 181–92.

Bernardo, M., Gatell, J. and Parellada, E. (1991). Acute exacerbation of chronic schizophrenia in a patient treated with antituberculosis drugs. *American Journal of Psychiatry*, **148**, 1402.

Bernstein, L.J., Krieger, B.Z. Novick, B., Sicklick, M.J., Rubenstein, A. et al (1985). Bacterial infection in the acquired immunodeficiency syndrome of children. *Paediatric Infectious Diseases*, **4**, 472–5.

Bernstein, L.J. and Rubinstein, A. (1986). Acquired immunodeficiency in infants and children. *Progress in Allergy*, **37**, 194–206.

Berrios, D., Hearst, N., Coates, T., Stall, R., Hudes, E., Turner, H. et al (1993). HIV antibody testing among those at risk for infection. *Journal of the American Medical Association*, **270**, 1576–80.

Bialer, P. and Wallack, J. (1990). Mixed factitious disorder presenting as AIDS. *Hospital and Community Psychiatry*, **41**, 552–3.

Bialer, P. (1992). Psychological distress in women infected with HIV. *VIIIth International Conference on AIDS*, Amsterdam, 1992.

Binder, R. (1987). AIDS antibody tests on inpatient psychiatric units. *American Journal of Psychiatry*, **144**, 176–81.

Bird, A.G. and Gore, S.M. (1993). Revised guidelines for HIV infected health care workers: we need data not dogma. *British Medical Journal*, **306**, 1013–14.

Bird, A.G., Gore, S.M., Joliffe, D. and Burns, S. (1992). Anonymous HIV surveillance in Sangleton prison, Edinburgh. *AIDS*, **6**, 725–33.

Bird, A.G., Gore, S., Burns, S. and Duggie, J. (1993). Study of infection with HIV and related risk factors in a young offenders' institution. *British Medical Journal*, **307**, 228–31.

Blackburn, I.M., Bishop, S., Glen, A., Whalley, L. and Christie, J. (1981). The efficacy of cognitive therapy in depression. *British Journal of Psychiatry*, **139**, 181–9.

Blaney, N., Millon, C., Morgan, R., Eisdorfer, C. and Szapocznic, J. (1990). Emotional distress, stress-related disruption and coping among healthy HIV positive gay males. *Psychology and Health*, **4**, 259–73.

Blaney, N., Goodkin, K., Morgan, R., Feaster, D., Millon, C., Szapocznik, J. and Eisdorfer, C. (1991). A stress-moderator model of distress in early HIV infection: concurrent analysis of life events, hardiness and social support. *Journal of Psychosomatic Research*, **35**, 297–305.

Blum, L.W., Chambers, R.A. and Schwartzman, R.S. (1985). Progressive multifocal leukoencephalopathy in AIDS. *Archives of Neurology* **42**, 137–9.

Boccellari, A., Dilley, J., Barlow, I., Hernandez, S., Haskell, W. and Steketee, M. (1991). HIV-related cognitive impairment in San francisco: associated management and residential placement problems. *VIIth International Conference on AIDS*, Florence, 1991.

Bond, T. (1991). *HIV counselling–report on national survey and consultation 1990*. British Association for Counselling, Rugby.

Booth, R.E., Watters, J.K. and Chitwood, D.D. (1993). HIV Risk-related sex behaviours among injection drug users, crack smokers, and injection drug users who smoke crack. *American Journal of Public Health*, **83**, 1144–8.

Bor, R. (1992). The impact of HIV/AIDS on the family. *AIDS Care*, **4**, 453–6.

Bor, R. (1993). Counselling patients with AIDS-associated Kaposi's sarcoma. *Counselling Psychology Quarterly*, **6**, 91–8.

Bor, R., Perry, L., Miller, R. and Jackson, J. (1989). Strategies for counselling the 'worried well' in relation to AIDS: discussion paper. *Journal of the Royal Society of Medicine*, **82**, 218–20.

Bor, R., Prior, N. and Miller, R. (1990). Complementarity in relationships of couples affected by HIV. *Counselling Psychology Quarterly*, **3**, 217–20.

Bor, R., Miller, R. and Johnson, M. (1991). A testing time for doctors: counselling patients before an HIV test. *British Medical Journal*, **303**, 905–7.

Bor, R., Miller, R. and Goldman, E. (1992). *Theory and practice of HIV counselling*. Cassell, London.

Bor, R., Elford, J., Hart, G. and Sherr, L. (1993a). The family and HIV disease. *AIDS Care*, **5**, 3–4.

Bor, R., Miller, R., Goldman, E. and Sherr, L. (1993b). The meaning of bad news in HIV disease: counselling about dreaded issues revisited. *Counselling Psychology Quarterly*, **6**, 69–80.

Bornstein, R.A., Nasrallah, H.A., Para, M.F., Fass, R.J., Whiteacre, C.C. and Rice, R.R. (1991). Rate of CD4 decline and neuropsychological performances in HIV infection. *Archives of Neurology*, **48**, 704–7.

Bornstein, R.A., Nasrallah, H.A., Para, M.F., Whitacre, C.C. and Fass, R.J. (1993). Change in neuropsychological performance in asymptomatic HIV infection: 1 year follow up. *AIDS*, **7**, 1607–11.

Bowen, D.L., Lane, H.C. and Fanci, A.S. (1986). Immunological abnormalities in the acquired immunodeficiency syndrome. *Progress in Allergy*, **37**, 207–23.

Bowlby, J. (1980). *Attachment and loss: loss, sadness and depression*. Basic Books, New York.

Boyd, K.M. (1989). Ethical Questions. In *Counselling in HIV infection and AIDS* (ed. J. Green and A. McCreaner). Blackwell, Oxford.

Boyd, K.M. (1992). HIV infection and AIDS: the ethics of medical confidentiality. *Journal of Medical Ethics*, **18**, 173–9.

Boyd, J.S., Kerr, S., Maw, R.D., Finnigan, E.A., Kilblane, P.K. (1990). Knowledge of HIV infection and AIDS, and attitudes to testing and counselling among general practitioners in Northern Ireland. *British Journal of General Practice*, **40**, 158–60.

Boyton, R. and Scambler, G. (1988). Survey of general practitioners' attitudes to AIDS in the north-west Thames and East Anglian regions. *British Medical Journal*, **296**, 539–40.

Bozzette, S.,0 Larsen, R.A., Chiu, J., Leal, M.E.A., Jacobsen, J., Rothman, P. et al (1991). A placebo-controlled trial of maintenance therapy with Fluconazole after treatment of cryptococcal meningitis in the acquired immunodeficiency syndrome. *New England Journal Medicine*, **324**, 580–84.

Brener, N. and Jadresic, D. (1992). Learning disabilities and the HIV epidemic. *Psychiatric Bulletin*, **16**, 638–9.

Breo, D.L. (1990).The slippery slope: handling HIV-infected health workers, *Journal of the American Medical Association*, **262**, 1464–6.

Brettle, R. (1991). HIV and harm reduction for injecting drug users. *AIDS*, 5, 125–36.

Brew, B.J., Evans, L. and Hurran, L. (1991). The correlation between AIDS dementia complex and the presence of macrophage tropic viruses in the cerebrospinal fluid of patients infected with HIV–1. *International Conference on the Neuroscience of HIV Infection, Padua*, 1991.

Bridge, T.P., Heseltine, P.N.R., Parker, E.S., Eaton, E., Ingraham, L.J., Gill, M. et al (1989). Improvement in AIDS patients on peptide T. *Lancet*, ii, 226–7.

British Medical Association (1993). *Complementary medicine—new approaches to good practice*. Oxford University Press, Oxford.

Britton, P., Zarski, J. and Hobfoll, S. (1993). Psychological distress and the role of significant others in a population of gay and bisexual men in the era of HIV. *AIDS Care*, **5**, 43–54.

Brockmeyer, N., Mertins, L. and Goos, M. (1989). Andrological features in HIV–1 infected patients. *Vth International Conference on AIDS*, Montreal, 1989.

Broderick, D.F., Wippold, F.J., Clifford, D.B., Kido, D. and Wilson, B.S. (1993). White matter lesions and cerebral atrophy on MR images in patients with and without AIDS dementia complex. *American Journal of Radiology*, **161**, 177–81.

Brouwers, P., Moss, H., Wolters, P., Eddy, J., Balis, F., Poplack, D.G. et al (1990). Effect of continuous-infusion zidovudine therapy on neuropsychologic functioning in children with symptomatic human immunodeficiency. *Journal of Paediatrics*, **117**, 980–5.

Brown, D. (1991). HIV infection in persons with prior mental retardation. *AIDS Care*, **3**, 165–73.

Brown, G. and Pace, J. (1989). Reduced sexual activity in HIV infected homosexual men. *Journal of the American Medical Association*, **261**, 2503.

Brown, G. and Rundell, J. (1989). Suicidal tendencies in women with HIV. *American Journal of Psychiatry*, **146**, 556–7.

Brown, G. and Rundell, J. (1990). Prospective study of psychiatric morbidity in HIV-seropositive women without AIDS. *General Hospital Psychiatry*, **12**, 30–5.

Brown, L. and DeMaio, D. (1992). The impact of secrets in haemophilia and HIV disorders. *Journal of Psychosocial Oncology*, **10**, 91–101.

Brown, G., Rundell, J., McManis, S., Kendall, S., Zachary, R. and Temoshok, L. (1992). Prevalence of psychiatric disorder in early stages of HIV infection. *Psychosomatic Medicine*, **54**, 588–601.

Brunetti, A., Berg, G.,Di Chiro, G., Cohen, R.M., Yarchoan, R. Pizzo, P.A. et al (1989). Reversal of brain metabolic abnormalities following treatment of AIDS dementia complex with 3′-azido–2′,3′-dideoxythymidine (AZT, zidovudine): a PET-FDG study. *Journal of Nuclear Medicine*, **30**, 581–90.

Buckley, N., Dawson, A., Whyte, I. and Henry, D. (1994). Greater toxicity in overdose of dothiepin than other tricyclic antidepressants. *Lancet*, **343**, 159–62.

Buckman, R. (1984). Breaking bad news: why is it still so difficult? *British Medical Journal*, **288**, 1597–9.

Buckman, R. (1993). Communications in palliative care: a practical guide. In *Oxford textbook of palliative medicine* (ed. D. Doyle, G. Hanks and N. MacDonald). Oxford University Press, Oxford.

Budka, H., Costanzi, G., Cristina, S., Lechi, A., Parravicini, C., Trabattoni, R. et al (1987). Brain pathology induced by infection with human immunodeficiency virus (HIV): a histological, immunocytochemical and electron microscopical study of 100 autopsy cases. *Acta Neuropathologica*, **75**, 185–98.

Budka, H.H. Wiley, C.A., Kleihues, P., Artigas, J., Asbury, A.K., Cho, E.S. et al (1993) HIV-associated disease of the nervous system: review of nomenclature and proposal for neuropathology-based terminology. *Brain Pathology*, **1**, 143–52.

Buehler, J., Devine, O., Berkelman, R. and Chevarley, F. (1990). Impact of HIV on mortality trends in young men in the US. *American Journal of Public Health*, **80**, 1080–6.

Buhrich, N. and Cooper, D. (1987). Request for psychiatric consultation concerning 22 patients with AIDS and ARC. *Australia and New Zealand Journal of Psychiatry*, **21**, 346–53.

Buhrich, N., Cooper, D. and Freed, E. (1988). HIV infection associated with symptoms indistinguishable from functional psychosis. British *Journal of Psychiatry*, **152**, 649–53.

Burack, J.H., Barrett, D.C., Stall, R.D., Chesney, M.A., Ekstrand, M.L., Coates, T.J. et al (1993). Depressive symptoms and CD4 lymphocyte decline among HIV-infected men. *Journal of the American Medical Association*, **270**, 2568–73.

Burgess, M. and Welch, J. (1991). Child sexual abuse and HIV infection. *British Medical Journal*, **303**, 415.

Burgess, A.P. and Riccio, M. (1992). Cognitive impairment and dementia in HIV–1 infection. *Bailliere's Clinical Neurology*, **1**, 155–74.

Burgess, C., Morris, T. and Pettingale, K. (1988). Psychological response to cancer diagnosis—II. Evidence for coping styles. *Journal of Psychosomatic Research*, **32**, 263–72.

Burgess, A.P., Dayer, M., Catalán, J., Hawkins, D.A., Gazzard and B.G. (1993). The reliability and validity of two HIV-specific health-related quality of life measures: a preliminary anlysis. *AIDS*, **7**, 1001–8.

Burgess, A.P., Riccio, M., Jadresic, D., Pugh, K., Catalán, J., Hawkins, D.A. et al. A longitudinal study of the neuropsychiatric consequences of HIV–1 infection in gay men: I—neuropsychological performance and neurological status at baseline and 12 month follow-up. *Psychological Medicine*, **24**, 885–95.

Butters, N., Grant, I., Haxby, J., Judd, L.L., Martin, A. McClelland, J. et al (1990). Assessment of AIDS-related cognitive changes: recommendations of the NIMH workshop on neuropsychological assessment approaches. *Journal of Clinical and Experimental Neuropsychology*, **12**, 963–78.

Butters, E., Higginson, I., Wade, A., Mccarthy, M., George, R. and Smits, A. (1991). Community HIV/AIDS teams. *Health Trends*, **23**, 59–62.

Buzy, J., Brenneman, D.E., Pert, C.B., Martin, A., Salazaar, A. and Ruff, M.R. (1992). Potent gp120-like neurotoxic activity in the cerebrospinal fluid of HIV-infected individuals is blocked by peptide T. *Brain Research*, **598**, 10–18.

Calabrese, L. and LaPerriere, A. (1993). HIV, exercise and athletics. *Sports Medicine*, **15**, 6–13.

Calvert, G.M., Flynn, R. and Fraser, P. (1991). Volunteers' motivation and the Terrence Higgins Trust. *British Psychological Society Conference*, London, 1991.

Cameron, D.W., Simonsenm, J.N., D'Costa, L.J., Ronald, A.R., Maitha, G.M., Eakinya, M.N. et al (1989). Female to male transmission of human immunodeficiency virus type 1: risk factors for seroconversion in men. *Lancet*, **ii**, 403–6.

Camus, A. (1948). *The plague*, (trans. S Gilbert). Penguin, London.

Campbell, A. and Baldwin, W. J. (1991). The response of American women to the threat of AIDS and other sexually transmitted diseases. *Journal of Acquired Immune Deficiency Syndromes*, **4**, 1133–40.

Campostrini, S. and McQueen, D. (1993). Sexual behaviour and exposure to HIV infection: estimates from a general-population risk index. *American Journal of Public Health*, **83**, 1139–43.

Canosa, C. (1991). HIV infection in children. *AIDS Care*, **3**, 303–9.

Cantacuzino, M. (1993). *Till break of day*. Heinemann, London.

Carlson, G., Greeman, M. and McClellan, T. (1989). Management of HIV positive patients who fail to reduce high-risk behaviour. *Hospital and Community Psychiatry*, **40**, 511–14.

Carmichael, A.J. and Paul, C.J. (1989). Idiosyncratic dapsone-induced manic depression. *British Medical Journal*, **298**, 1524.

Carr, E. (1989). Psychosocial issues of AIDS patients in hospice: case studies. *The Hospice Journal*, **5**, 135–51.

Carver, C., Scheier, M. and Weintraub, J. (1989). Assessing coping strategies: a theoretically based approach. *Journal of Personality and Social Psychology*, **56**, 267–83.

Casabona, J., Sanchez, E., Graus, F., Abos, J., Segura, A. (1991). Trends and survival for AIDS patients presenting with indicative neurological diseases. *Acta Neurologica Scandinavica*, **84**, 51–4.

Cassel, C.K. and Meier, D. (1990). Morals and moralism in the debate over euthanasia and assisted suicide. *New England Journal of Medicine*, **323**, 750–52.

Castro, F., Coates, T. and Ekstrand, M. (1989). Prevalence and predictors of depression in gay and bisexual men during the AIDS epidemic: the San Francisco Men's Health Study. *Vth International Conference on AIDS*, Montreal, 1989.

Catalán, J. (1988). Psychosocial and Neuropsychiatric aspects of HIV infection—review of their extent and implications for psychiatry. *Journal of Psychosomatic Research*, **32**, 237–48.

Catalán, J. (1990a). Psychiatric manifestations of HIV disease. Bailliére's Clinical Gastroenterology, **4**, 547–62.

Catalán, J. (1990b). HIV and AIDS-related psychiatric disorder: what can the psychiatrist do? In *Dilemmas and difficulties in the management of psychiatric patients* (ed K. Hawton and P. Cowen). Oxford Medical Publications, Oxford.

Catalán, J. (1991a). Deliberate self-harm and HIV disease. In *HIV and AIDS-related suicidal behaviour*, (ed. Beskow, Bellini, Faria and Kerkhof). Monduzzi Editore, Bologna.

Catalán, J. (1991b). Psychosocial and neuropsychiatric aspects of HIV infection in men with haemophilia. *Ist International Conference on the Biopsychosocial Aspects of HIV Infection*, Amsterdam, 1991.

Catalán, J. (1991c). Neuropsychiatric disorders and HIV-1 associated dementia: conceptual and terminological problems. *International Review of Psychiatry*, **3**, 331–42.

Catalán, J. (1992). Psychotic illnesses in HIV disease. *International Conference on the Neuroscience of HIV Infection*, Amsterdam, 1992.

Catalán, J. (1993). *HIV infection and mental health care: implications for services*. World Health Organization Regional Office for Europe, Copenhagen.

Catalán, J. and Riccio, M. (1990a). Psychiatric disorders associated with HIV disease. *AIDS Care*, **2**, 377–80.

Catalán, J. and Riccio, M. (1990b). Recognition and treatment of drug users with HIV infection. *Current Opinion in Psychiatry*, **3**, 398–402.

Catalán, J. and Riccio, M. (1990c). Response to Bow Group report. Psychiatric Bulletin, 14, 694–6.

Catalán, J. and Goos, C. (1991). European symposium on AIDS and drug misuse: providing care for HIV infected drug users. *AIDS Care*, **3**, 203–5.

Catalán, J. and Klimes, I. (1991). Psychiatric problems in HIV-infected men with haemophilia. *International Review of Psychiatry*, **3**, 373–81.

Catalán, J. and Thornton, S. (1993). Whatever happened to HIV-associated dementia?. *International Journal of STD and AIDS*, **4**, 1–4.

Catalán, J., Bradley, M., Gallwey, J. and Hawton, K. (1981). Sexual dysfunction and psychiatric morbidity in patients attending a clinic for sexually transmitted diseases. *British Journal of Psychiatry*, **138**, 292–6

Catalán, J., Day, A. and Gallwey, J. (1988). Alcohol misuse in patients attending a genitourinary clinic. *Alcohol and Alcoholism*, **23**, 421–8.

Catalán, J., Riccio, M. and Thompson, C. (1989). HIV disease and psychiatric practice. *Psychiatric Bulletin*, **13**, 316–32.

Catalán, J., Hawton, K. and Day, A. (1990). Couples referred to a sexual dysfunction clinic: psychological and physical morbidity. *British Journal of Psychiatry*, **156**, 61–7.

Catalán, J., Gath, D., Anastasiades, P., Bond, A., Day, A. and Hall, L. (1991). Evaluation of a brief psychological treatment for emotional disorders in primary care. *Psychological Medicine***21**, 1013–18.

Catalán, J., Klimes, I., Day, A., Garrod, A., Bond, A. and Gallwey, J. (1992a). The psychosocial impact of HIV infection in gay men—controlled investigation and factors associated with psychiatric morbidity. *British Journal of Psychiatry*, **161**, 774–8.

Catalán, J., Klimes, I., Bond, A., Day, A., Garrod, A. and Rizza, C. (1992b). The psychosocial impact of HIV infection in men with haemophilia—controlled investigation and factors associated with psychiatric morbidity. *Journal of Psychosomatic Research*, **161**, 409–16.

Catalán, J., Klimes, I., Day, A., Garrod, A., Bond, A. and Elcombe, S. (1992c). Factors associated with psychological morbidity in HIV positive men. *VIIIth International Conference on AIDS*, Amsterdam, 1992.

Catalán, J., Burgess, A.P., Pergami, A., Hulme, N., Gazzard, B.G. and Phillips, R. (in press). The psychological impact on staff of caring for people with serious diseases: The case of HIV infection and oncology.

Catania, J., Kegeles, S. and Coates, T. (1990a). Psychosocial predictors of people who fail to return for their HIV test results. *AIDS*, **4**, 261–2.

Catania, J., Kegeles, S. and Coates T. (1990b). Towards an understanding of risk behaviour: and AIDS risk reduction model (ARRM). *Health Education Quarterly*, **17**, 53–72.

Catania, J., Turner, H., Choi, K.H. and Coates, T. (1992a). Coping with death anxiety; help-seeking and social support among gay men with various HIV diagnosis. *AIDS*, **6**, 999–1005.

Catania, J., Coates, T., Stall, R., Turner, H., Peterson, J., Hearst, T et al (1992b). Prevalence of AIDS-related risk factors and condom use in the US. *Science*, **258**, 1101–6.

Cates, W. and Handsfield, H. (1988). HIV counseling and testing: does it work? *American Journal of Public Health*, **78**, 1533–4.

Cavanaugh, S., Clark, D. and Gibbons, R. (1983). Diagnosing depression in the hospitalized medically ill. *Psychosomatics*, **24**, 809–15.

Cazzullo, C., Gala, C., Martini, S., Pergami, A., Rossini, M. and Russo, R. (1990). Psychopathologic features amongst drug addicts and homosexuals with HIV infection. *International Journal of Psychiatry in Medicine*, **20**, 285–92.

Ceballos-Capitaine, A., Szapocznic, J., Blaney, N., Morgan, R., Millon, C. and Eisdorfer, C. (1990). Ethnicity, emotional distress, stress-related disruption and coping among HIV positive gay males. *Hispanic Journal of Behavioral Sciences*, **12**, 135–52.

Centers for Disease Control (1981). Pneumocystis pneumonia. *Morbidity and Mortality Weekly Report*, **30**, 250–52.

Centers for Disease Control (1987a). Revision of the CDC Surveillance definition for acquired immunodeficiency syndrome. *Morbidity and Mortality Weekly Report*, **36**, 15, 35–155.

Centers for Disease Control (1987b). Update: Acquired immunodeficiency syndrome—United States. *Morbidity and Mortality Weekly Report*, **35**, 595–606.

Centers for Disease Control (1988). Update: Universal precautions for prevention of transmission of human immunodeficiency virus, hepatitis B virus, and other blood-borne pathogens in health care settings. *Morbidity and Mortality Weekly Report*, **37**, 378–88.

Centers for Disease Control (1990). Public Health Service statement on management of occupational exposure to human immunodeficiency virus, including considerations regarding zidovudine postexposure use. *Morbidity and Mortality Weekly Report*, **39**, RR–1.

Centers for Disease Control (1991a). Patterns of sexual behaviour change among homosexual bisexual men selected US sites. *Morbidity and Mortality Weekly Report*, **40**, 792–4.

Centers for Disease Control (1991b). Update: transmission of HIV infection during an invasive medical procedure—Florida. *Morbidity and Mortality Weekly Report, 18th January*, **40**, 21–7.

Centers for Disease Control (1993). Revised classification system for HIV infection and expanded surveillance definition for AIDS among adolescents and adults. *Morbidity and Mortality Weekly Report*, **41**, 1–19.

Centres for Disease Control (1994a). Zidovudine for the prevention of HIV transmission from mother to infant. Morbidity and Mortality Weekly Report, 43, 285–7.

Centers for Disease Control (1994b). Strategies to reduce vertical transmission of HIV–1. *Communicable Disease Report Weekly*, **281**, 127–30.

Centers for Disease Control (1994c). Heterosexually acquired AIDS—US 1993. *Morbidity and Mortality Weekly Report*, **43**, 155–60.

Chaisson, R., Bacchetti, P. and Osmond, D. (1989). Cocaine use and HIV infection in IDU in San Francisco. *Journal of the American Medical Association*, **261**, 561–65.

Chalmers, A., Catalán, J., Nelson, M. and Day, A. (1992). Sexual dysfunction in HIV seropositive gay men. *VIIIth International Conference on AIDS*, Amsterdam, 1992

Chen, J., Brocavich, J. and Lin, A. (1992). Psychiatric disturbances associated with gancyclovir therapy. *The Annals of Pharmacotherapy*, **26**, 193–5.

Chiarello, R.J. and Cole, J.O. (1987). The use of psychostimulants in general psychiatry: a reconsideration. *Archives of General Psychiatry*, **44**, 286–95.

Chin, J. (1990). Current and Future dimensions of the HIV/AIDS pandemic in women and children. *Lancet*, **447**, 221–4.

Chiswick, A., Egan, V., Brettle, B. and Goodwin, G. (1992). The Edinburg cohort of HIV positive drug users: who are they and who cares for them. *AIDS Care*, **4**, 421–24.

Chong, W.K., Sweeney, B., Wilkinson, I.D., Paley, M., Hall-Craggs, M.A., Kendall, B.E. et al (1993). Proton spectroscopy of the brain in HIV infection: correlation with clinical immunologic and MR findings. *Radiology*, **188**, 119–24.

Chorba, T., Holman, R. and Levatt, B. (1993). Heterosexual and mother-to-child transmission of AIDS in the haemophilia community. *Public Health Reports*, **108**, 99–105.

Chrysikopoulos, H.S., Press, G.A., Grafe, M.R., Hesselink, J.R. and Wiley, C.A. (1990). Encephalitis caused by use of human immunodeficiency virus: CT and MRI imaging manifestations with clinical and pathologic correlation. *Radiology*, **175**, 185–91.

Chuang, H., Devins, G., Hunsley, J. and Gill, M. (1989). Psychosocial distress and well-being among gay and bisexual men with HIV infection. *American Journal of Psychiatry*, **146**, 876–80.

Church, J., Kocsis, A. and Green, J. (1988). Effects on lovers of caring for HIV infected individuals related to the perception of cognitive, behaviourial and personality changes. *IVth International Conference on AIDS*, Stockholm, 1988.

Church, J., Green, J., Vearnals, S. and Keogh, P. (1993). Investigation of motivational and behavioural factors influencing men who have sex with other men in public toilets (cottaging). *AIDS Care*, **5**, 337–46.

Ciesielski, C., Marianos, D., and Ou, C.Y. (1992). Transmission of human immunodeficiency virus in a dental practice. *Annals of Internal Medicine*, **116**, 798–805.

Claxton, R. and Harrison, T. (ed) (1991). *Caring for children with HIV and AIDS.* Edward Arnold, London.

Claxton, R.P.R., Burgess, A.P. and Catalán, J. (1994). Factors associated with burnout in emotional support volunteers for people living with AIDS. *IInd International Conference on the Biopsychosocial aspects of HIV infection*, Brighton, 1994.

Clayton, P.J. (1990). Bereavement and depression. *Journal of Clinical Psychiatry*, **51**, 34–8.

Clifford, D.B., Jacoby, R.G., Miller, J.P., Seyfried, W.R. and Glicksman, M. (1990). Neuropsychometric performance of asymptomatic HIV-infected subjects. *AIDS*, **4**, 767–74.

Clift, M.S., Wilkins, C.J. and Davidson, E.A.F. (1993). Impulsiveness, venturesomeness and sexual risk-taking among heterosexual GUM clinic attenders. *Personality and Individual Differences*, **15**, 403–10.

Cline, D.J. (1990). The psychosocial impact of HIV infection: what clinicians can do to help. *Journal of the American Academy of Dermatology*, **22**, 1299–1302.

Clough, A.H. (1850). The latest decalogue. Cited in *The Oxford book of quotations (3rd edn), (1979). Oxford University Press, Oxford.*

Coates, R. and Ferroni, P. (1991). Sexual dysfunction and marital disharmony as a consequence of chronic lumbar pain. Sexual and Marital Therapy, **6**, 65–9.

Coates, T.J., McKusick, L., Kuno, R. and Stites, D.P. (1989). Stress reduction training changed number of sexual partners but not immune function in men with HIV. *American Journal of Public Health* **79**, 885–7.

Cohen, S. (1991). Social supports and physical health: symptoms, health behaviours and infectious disease. In *Life-span developmental psychology: perspectives on stress and coping* (ed. E. Cummings, A. Greene and K. Karraker). Lawrence Erlbaum Associates, Hillsdale, NJ.

Cohen, S. and Wills, T.A. (1985). Stress, social support and the buffering hypothesis. *Psychological Bulletin*, **98**, 310–57.

Cohen, D., Dent, C., MacKinnon, D. and Hahn G. (1992). Condoms for men, not women. *Sexually Transmitted Diseases*, **19**, 245–51.

Cohen, S., Mermelstein, R., Kamarck, T. and Hoberman, H. (1985). Measuring the functional components of social support. In *Social support: theory, research and applications* (ed. I. Sarason and B. Sarason). Nato ASI, Nijhoff.

Cohen, S.E., Mundy, T., Karassik, B., Lieb, L., Ludwig, D.D. and Ward, J. (1991). Neuropsychological functioning in human immundodeficiency virus type 1 seropositive children infected through neonatal blood transfusion. *Pediatrics*, **88**, 58–69.

Cohen, W.A., Maravilla, K.R., Gerlach, G., Claypoole, K., Collier, A.C., Marra, C. et al (1992). Prospective cerebral MR study of HIV seropositive and seronegative men: correlation of MR findings with neurologic, neuropsychologic and cerebrospinbal fluid analysis. *American Journal of Neuroradiology*, **13,** 1231–40.

Cole, R. (1991). Medical aspects of care for the person with advanced AIDS: a palliative care perspective. *Palliative Medicine*, **5**, 96–111.

Collier, A.C., Marra, C., Coombs, R.W., Claypoole, K., Cohen, W., Longstreth, W.T. et al (1992). Central nervous system manifestations in human immunodeficieny virus infection without AIDS. *Journal of Acquired Immune Deficiency Syndromes*, **5**, 229–41.

Commissie Onderzoek Medische Praktijk inzake Euthanasie (1991). *Medische belissingen rond het levenseinde*. SDU Uitgeverij, The Hague.

Communicable Disease Surveillance Centre (1984). Surveillance of health care staff: HTLV 3. *Communicable Disease Report*, **52**(1).

Concorde Co-ordinating Committee (1994). Concorde: MRC/ANRS randomized double-blind controlled trial of immediate and deferred zidovudine in symptom-free HIV infection. *Lancet*, **343**, 871–81.

Connell, R. and Kippax, S. (1990). Sexuality in the AIDS crisis: patterns of sexual practice and pleasure in a sample of gay and bisexual Austrialian men. *Journal of Sex Research*, **27**, 167–96.

Connolly, G.M., Dryden, M.S., Shanson, D.C. and Gazzard, B.G. (1988). Cryptosporidial diarrhoea in AIDS and its treatment. *Gut*, **29**, 593–7.

Connolly, G.M., Hawkins, D.A., Harcourt-Webster, J.N., Parsons P.A., Hussain, D.A. and Gazzard B.G. (1989). Oesophageal symptoms—their causes, treatment and prognosis in patients with the acquired immunodeficiency syndrome. *Gut*, **30**, 1033–39.

Connors, M.M. (1992). Risk perception, risk taking and risk management among intravenous drug users: implications for aids prevention. *Social Science*, **34**, 591–601.

Cote, T., Biggar, R. and Dannenberg, A. (1992). Risk of suicide among persons with AIDS—a national assessment. *Journal of the American Medical Association*, **268**, 2066–68.

Cottam, S., Cuthbert, A. and Parapia, L. (1991). Malingering, AIDS and haemophilia. *European Journal of Haematology*, **46**, 125.

Coughlan, A.K. and Hollows, S.E. (1985). *The adult memory and information processing battery test manual*, available from Dr A.K. Coughlan, St James's University Hospital, Beckett Street, Leeds, LS9 7TF.

Cournos, F., Empfield, M., Horwarth, E. and Schage, H. (1990). HIV infection in state hospitals: case reports and long-term management strategies. *Hospital and Community Psychiatry*, **41**, 163–6.

Cournos, F., Empfield, M., Horwath, E., McKinnon, K., Meyer, I., Schrage, H. et al (1991). HIV seroprevalence among patients admitted to two psychiatric hospitals. *American Journal of Psychiatry*, **148**, 1225–30.

Cournos, F., Guido, J., Coomaraswamy, S. and Meyer-Bahlburg, H. (1994). Sexual activity and risk of HIV infection among patients with schizophrenia. *American Journal of Psychiatry*, **151**, 228–32.

Croxson, T., Chapman, W., Miller, L., Levit, C., Senie, R. and Zumoff, B. (1989). Changes in the hypothalamic-pituitary gonadal axis in HIV infected gay men. *Journal of Clinical Endocrinology and Metabolism*, **68**, 317–21.

Cummings, J.L. (1986). Subcortical dementia: Neuropsychology, neuropsychiatry and pathophysiology. *British Journal of Psychiatry*, **149**, 682–97.

Cummings, M.A., Rapaport, M. and Cummings, K.L. (1986). A psychiatric staff response to acquired immune deficiency syndrome. *American Journal of Psychiatry*, **143**, 682.

Curran, L., McHugh, M. and Nooney, N.(1989). HIV counselling in prisons. *Counselling Psychology Quarterly*, **2**, 33–51.

Dal Pan, G.J., McArthur, J.H., Aylward, E.H., Selnes O.A., Nance-Spronson, T.E., Kumar, A.J. et al (1992). Patterns of cerebral atrophy in HIV–1 infected individuals: results of a quantitative MRI analysis. *Neurology*, **42**, 2125–30.

Daneshmend, T. (1989). Idiosyncratic dapsone induced manic depression. *British Medical Journal*, **299**, 324.

Danis, M., Southerland, L.I., Garrett, J.M., Smith, J.L., Hielema, F., Pickard, C.G. et al (1992). A prospective study of advance directives for life-sustaining care. *New England Medical Journal*, **324**, 882–8.

D'Antonio, R.G., Winn, R.E., Taylor, J.P., Gustafson, T.L., Current, W.L., Rhodes, M. et al (1985). A waterborne outbreak of Cryptosporidiosis in normal hosts. *Annals of Internal Medicine*, **103**, 886–8.

Dauncey, K. (1988). Mania in the early stages of AIDS. *British Journal of Psychiatry*, **152**, 716–17.

Davey, T. and Green, J. (1991). The worried well: ten years of a new face for an old problem. AIDS Care, **3**, 289–93.

Davidson, R.J. (1984). Affect, cognition and hemisphere specialisation. In *Emotion, Cognition and Behaviour* (ed. C.E. Izard, J. Kagan and R. Zajonc). Cambridge University Press, New York.

Davidson, C., Hudson, C., Ades, E. and Peckham, C. (1989). Antenatal tests for HIV. *Lancet*, **2**, 1441–4.

Davies, J., Everall, I., Bell, J., Esiri, M., Lucas, S., Harrison, M. et al (1993). Does azidothymidine alter HIV associated neuropathology. *Clinical Neuropathology*, **12** (suppl.), S9.

Davies, P., Weatherburn, P., Hickson, F., McManus, T. and Coxon, A. (1992). The sexual behaviour of young gay men in England and Wales. *AIDS Care*, **4**, 259–72.

Davies, C.L., Springmeyer, S. and Gmerer, B.J. (1990). CNS side-effects of gancyclovir. *New England Journal of Medicine*, **322**, 933.

Davis, L.E., Hjelle, B.J., Miller, V.E., Palmer, D.L., Llewellyn, A.L., Merlin, T.L. et al (1992). Early viral brain invasion in iatrogenic human immunodeficiency virus infection. *Neurology*, **42**, 1736–9.

Day, S., Ward, H. and Perrotta, L., (1993). Prostitution and risk of HIV: male partners of female prostitutes. *British Medical Journal*, **307**, 359–62.

Deary, I.J. and Matthews, G. (1993). Personality traits are alive and well. *The Psychologist*, **6**, 299–310.

Defoe, D. (1966). *A journal of the plague year*. Penguin, London.

De Graaf, R., Vanwesenbeek, I., Van Zessen, G., Straver, C. and Visser J. (1992). Condom use and heterosexual prostitiution in the Netherlands. *AIDS*, **6**, 1223–6.

De Graaf, R., Vanwesenbeeck, I., Van Zessen, G., Straver, C. and Visser J. (1994). Male prostitutes and safe sex: different settings, different risks. *AIDS CARE*, **6**, 277–8.

De Gruttrola, V. and Mayer, K.H. (1988). Assessing and modelling heterosexual spread of human immunodeficiency virus in the United States. *Review of Infectious Diseases*, **10**, 138–50.

Dening, T., Klimes, I., Catalán, J., Rizza, C. and Peto, T. (1992). Major psychiatric disorder without cognitive impairment before or after the episode. *International Journal of STD and AIDS*, **3**, 132–3.

Dent, J. (1989). Obtaining informed consent for HIV testing: the decision-making process. *Counselling Psychology Quarterly*, **2**, 73–7.

Dent, J., Vergnaud, S. and Piachaud, J. (1994). HIV infection and people with learning disabilities. *Lancet*, **343**, 919.

Department of Health and Social Security (1989). *HIV infection, breast feeding and human milk banking in the UK*. HMSO, London.

Department of Health (1990). Expert Advisory Group on AIDS: *Guidance for clinical health care workers*. HMSO, London.

Department of Health (1991). *AIDS–HIV infected healthcare workers. Occupational guidance for health care workers, their physicians and employers.* Recommendations of the expert advisory group on AIDS. HMSO, London.

Department of Health (1992). *Offering voluntary named HIV antibody testing to women receiving antenatal care*. HMSO, London.

Department of Health (1992). Expert Advisory Group on AIDS: *Occupational exposure to HIV and use of zidovudine*. HMSO, London.

Department of Health (1994). Expert Advisory Group on AIDS: *AIDS/HIV infected health care workers: guidance on the management of infected health care workers.* HMSO, London.

Derix, M.M., de Gans, J., Stam, J. and Portegies, P. (1990). Mental changes in patients with AIDS. *Clinical Neurology and Neurosurgery*, **93**, 215–22.

Derogatis, L.R. (1986). The psychological adjustment to illness scale (PAIS). *Journal of Psychosomatic Research*, **30**, 77–91.

Desenclos, J.C., Papaevangelou, G., Ancelle-Park, R. (1993). Knowledge of HIV serostatus and preventive behaviors among European injecting drug users. *AIDS*, **7**, 1371–7.

Desrosiers, R.C., Wyand, N.S., Kodama, T., Ringler, D.J., Arthur, L.O., Seghal, P.K. et al (1989). Vaccine protection against simian immunodeficiency virus infection. *Proceedings of the National Academy of Sciences of the United States of America*, **86**, 6353.

Deutsch, H. (1937). Absence of grief. *Psychoanalysis Quarterly*, **6**, 12–22.

Dew, A., Ragni, M. and Nimorwicz, P. (1990). Infection with HIV and vulnerability to psychiatric distress—a study of men with haemophilia. *Archives of General Psychiatry*, **47**, 737–44.

Dew, A., Ragni, M. and Nimorwicz, P. (1991). Correlates of psychiatric distress among wives of haemophilic men with and without HIV infection. *American Journal of Psychiatry*, **148**, 1016–22.

Des Jarlais, D. (1994). Cross-national studies of AIDS among injecting drug users. *Addiction*, **89**, 383–92.

Des Jarlais, D., Friedman, S., Sotheran, J., Wenston, J., Marmor, M., Yancovitz S. et al (1994). Continuity and change within an HIV epidemic, injecting drug users in New York city, 1984 through 1992. *Journal of the American Medical Association*, **271**, 121–7.

Diagnostic and Statistical Manual of Mental Disorders (third edition, revised) (1987). The American Psychiatric Association, Washington, DC.

Diamond, G.W., Kaufman, J., Belman, A.L., Cohen, L., Cohen, H.J. and Rubinstein,

A. (1987). Characterisation of cognitive functioning in a subgroup of children with congenital HIV infection. *Archives of Clinical Neuropsychology*, **2**, 1–16.

Dickinson, G.M., Morhart, R.E., Klimas, N.G., Bandea, C.I., Laracuente, J.M. and Bisno, A. (1993). Absence of HIV transmission from an infected dentist to his patients: an epidemiologic and DNA sequence analysis. *Journal of the American Medical Association*, **269**, 1802–6.

Dilley, J., Ochitill, H., Perl, M. and Volberding, P. (1985). Findings in psychiatric consultation with patients with AIDS. *American Journal of Psychiatry*, **142**, 82–6.

Di Clememte, R. and Ponton, L. (1993). HIV-related risk behaviours among psychiatrically hospitalised adolescent and school-based adolescents. *American Journal Psychiatry*, **150**, 324–5.

Di Clemente, R., Zorn, J. and Temoshok, L. (1986). Adolescents and AIDS: a survey of knowledge, attitudes and beliefs about AIDS in San Francisco. *American Journal of Public Health* **76**, 1443–5.

Di Clemente, R., Boyer, C. and Morales, E. (1988). Minorities and AIDS: knowledge, attitudes and misconceptions among black and latino adolescents. *American Journal of Public Health* **78**, 55–7.

Di Pasquale, J. (1990). The psychological effects of support groups on individuals infected by the AIDS virus. *Cancer Nursing*, **13**, 278–85.

Di Stefano, M., Norkrans, G., Chiodi, F., Hagberg, L., Nielsen, C. and Svennerholm, B. (1993). Zidovudine-resistant variants of HIV-1 in brain. *Lancet*, **342**, 865.

Dixon, A.S. and Morely, J.S. (1992). Euthanasia. *British Medical Journal*, **305**, 1224–5.

Dixon, P., Flanigan, T., DeBuono, B., Laurie, J., DeCiantis, M., Hoy, J. et al (1993). Infection with HIV in prisons: meeting the health care challenge. *American Journal of Medicine*, **95**, 629–35.

Dobs, A., Dempsey, M., Ladenson, P. and Polk, B. (1988). Endocrine disorders in men infected with HIV. *American Journal of Medicine*, **84**, 611.

Doll, L., Byers, R., Bolan, G, Douglas, J, Moss, P, Weller, P. et al (1991). Homosexual men who engage in high-risk behaviour. *Sexually Transmitted Diseases*, **18**, 170–5.

Donchin, E., Karis, D., Bashore, T.R., Coles, M.G. and Gratton, G. (1986). Cognitive psychophysiology and human information processing. In *Psychophysiology. Systems, processes and applications* (ed. M.G. Coles, E. Donchin and S.W. Porges). Elsevier, Amsterdam, Oxford.

Dooneief, G., Bello, J., Todak, G., Mun, K., Marder, K., Malouf, R. et al (1992). A prospective study of magnetic resonance imaging of the brain in gay men and parenteral drug users with human immunodeficiency virus infection. *Archives of Neurology*, **49**, 38–43.

Douzenis, A., Brener, N., Catalán, J. and Meadows, J. (1991). Psychiatric disorder in HIV disease: description of 200 patients referred to a liaison psychiatry service. *VIIth International Conference on AIDS*, Florence, 1991.

Dow, M.G. and Knox M.D. (1991). Mental health and substance abuse staff: HIV/AIDS knowledge and attitudes. *AIDS Care*, **3**, 75–87.

Dublin, S., Rosenberh, P. and Goedert, J. (1992). Patterns and predictors of high-risk sexual behaviour in female partners of HIV-infected men with haemophilia. *AIDS*, **6**, 475–82.

Dunbar, N., Perdices, M. and Grunseit, A. (1991). The neuropsychological performance of ARC patients who progress to AIDS. *International Conference on the Neuroscience of HIV Infection*, Padua, 1991.

Dunkeld Turnball, J., Freeman, C. and Barry, F. (1987). Physical and psychological characteristics of 5 male bulimics. *British Journal of Psychiatry*, **150**, 25–9.

Dunlop, O., Bjorklund, R.A., Abdelnoor, M. and Myrvang, B. (1992). Five different tests of reaction time evaluated in HIV seropositive men. *Acta neurologica Scandinavia*, **86**, 260–6.

Dupras, A. and Morisset, R. (1993). Sexual dysfunction among HIV positive gay males. *Sexual and Marital Therapy*, **8**, 37–45.

Dursun, S. (1993). HIV infection, serotonin and sexual dysfunction. *British Journal of Psychiatry*, **162**, 570–1.

Dyer, C. (1991). Assisted Suicide: 1. America, 2. Britain. *British Medical Journal*, **303**, 431–2.

Dyer, C. (1992). Rheumatologist convicted of attempted murder. *British Medical Journal*, **305**, 731.

Eakin, J. and Taylor, R. (1990). *The psychosocial impact of AIDS on health care workers: an international annotated bibliography and review of the literature.* Federal Centre for AIDS, Health and Welfare, Canada, Montreal.

Eakin, J.M. and Taylor, K.M. (1990). The psychosocial impact of AIDS on health workers. *AIDS*, **4** (suppl.1), s257–s262.

Easterbrook, P. and Hawkins, D.A. (1993).What is the potential for a heterosexual HIV epidemic in the UK? *International Journal of STD's and AIDS*, **4**, 187–9.

Egan, V., Crawford, J.R., Brettle, R.P. and Goodwin, G.M. (1990). The Edinburgh cohort of HIV-positive drug users: current intellectual function is impaired, but not due to early AIDS dementia complex (1990). *AIDS*, **4**, 651–6.

Egan, V., Brettle, R. and Goodwin, G. (1992). The Edinburgh cohort of HIV positive drug users: patterns of cognitive impairment in relation to progression of disease. *British Journal of Psychiatry*, **161**, 522–31.

Ehrhardt, A. (1994). Gender risk behavior intervention programs for women. *IInd International Conference on the Biopsychosocial aspects of HIV infection*, Brighton, 1994.

Eickhoff, T.C. (1994). Position paper on HIV infection by the American College of Physicians and Infectious Diseases Society of America. *Annals of Internal Medicine*, **120**, 310–19.

Ekstrand, M. (1992). Safer sex maintenance among gay men: are we making any progress? *AIDS*, **6**, 875–7.

Ekstrand, M. and Coates T. (1990). Maintenance of safer sexual behaviours and predictors of risky sex: the San Francisco men's health study. *American Journal of Public Health* **80**, 973–8.

El-Bassel, N. and Schilling, R. (1992). 15 month followup of women methadone patients taught skills to reduce heterosexual HIV transmission. *Public Health Reports*, **107**, 500–4.

Elkin, C.M, Leon, E., Grenell, S.L., and Leeds, N.E. (1985). Intracranial lesions in acquired immunodeficiency syndrome. Radiological (computed tomographic) features. *Journal of the American Medical Association*, **253**, 393–6.

Ellebrock, T., Lieb, S. and Harrington, P. (1992). Heterosexually transmitted HIV infection among pregnant women in a rural Florida community. *England Journal of Medicine*, **327**, 1705–9.

Ellis, D., Collis, I. and King, M. (1994). A controlled comparison of HIV and general medical referrals to a liaison psychiatric service. *AIDS Care*, **6**, 69–76.

El-Mallakh, R.S. (1991). Mania and AIDS: clinical significance and theoretical considerations. *International Journal of Psychiatry in Medicine*, **21**, 383–91.

Elovaara, I., Saar P., Valle, S.L., Hokkanen, L., Iivanainen, M. and Lahdevirta, L. (1991). EEG in early HIV-1 infection is characterised by anterior dysrhythmicity of low maximal amplitude. *Clinical Electroencephalography*, **22**, 515–21.

Emanuel, L.L., Barry, M.J., Stoeckle, J.D., Ettelson, L.M. and Emanuel, E.J. (1991). Advance directives for medical care—a case for greater use. *New England Medical Journal*, **324**, 889–95.

Empfield, M., Cournos, F., Meyer, I., McKinnon, K., Horwarth, E., Silver, M. et al (1993). HIV seroprevalence among homeless patients admitted to a psychiatric in-patient unit. *American Journal of Psychiatry*, **150**, 47–52.

Engel, G.L. (1961). Is grief a disease? A challenge for medical research. *Psychosomatic Medicine*, **23**, 18–22.

Epstein, L.G., Sharer, L.R., Oleske, J.M., Connor, E.M., Goudsmit, J., Bagdon, L. et al (1986). Neurologic manifestations of HIV infection in children. *Paediatrics*, **78**, 678–87.

Epstein, L.G., Sharer, L.R. and Joshi, V.V. (1988). Progressive encephalopathy in children with acquired immuno-deficiency syndrome. *Annals of Neurology*, **17**, 488–96.

Esiri, M.M., Scaravelli, P.R., Millard, P.R. and Harcourt-Webster, J.N. (1990). Neuropathology of HIV infection in haemophiliacs: comparative necroscopy study. *British Medical Journal*, **299**, 1312–15.

Estebanez, P., Fitch, K. and Najera, R. (1993). HIV and female sex workers. *Bulletin of World Health Organization*, **71**, 397–412.

Esterson, A., Harris, H. and Kessinger, J. (1992). The AIDS dementia unit. *VIIIth International Conference on AIDS*, Amsterdam, 1992

Estreich, S., Forster, G. and Robinson, A. (1990). Sexually transmitted diseases in rape victims. *Genitourinary Medicine*, **66**, 433–8.

European Collaborative Study (1990). Neurologic signs in young children with human immunodeficiency virus infection. *Paediatric Infectious Diseases Journal*, **9**, 402–6.

European Collaborative Study (1994).Caesarean section and risk of vertical transmission of HIV infection. *Lancet*, **343**, 1464–7.

European Study Group (1989). Risk factors for male to female transmission of HIV. *British Medical Journal*, **298**, 411–15.

Evans, P.D. and Edgerton, N. (1991). Life events and mood as predictors of the common cold. *British Journal of Medical Psychology*, **64**, 35–44.

Evans, G., Gill, M. and Gerhart, S. (1988a). Factitious AIDS. *New England Journal of Medicine*, **319**, 1605–6.

Evans, P.D., Pitts, M.K.P. and Smith, K. (1988b). Minor infection, minor life events and the four day desirability dip. *Journal of Psychosomatic Research*, **32**, 533–9.

Evans, B., McCormack, S., Bond, R. and MacRae, K. (1991). Trends in sexual behaviour and HIV testing among women presenting at a genitourinary medicine clinic during the advent of AIDS. *Genitourinary Medicine*, **67**, 194–8.

Evans, B., Catchpole, M. and Heptonstall, J. (1993). Sexually transmitted diseases and HIV-1 infection among homosexual men in England and Wales. *British Medical Journal*, **306**, 426–8.

Everall, I. and Lantos, P.L. (1991). The neuropathology of HIV infection: a review of the first 10 years. *International Review of Psychiatry*, **3**, 307–20.

Everall, I., Luthert, P.J. and Lantos, P.L. (1991). Neuronal loss in the frontal cortex in HIV infection. *Lancet*, **337**, 1991.

Everall, I., Lutherert, P.J. and Lantos, P.L. (1993). Neuronal number and volume alterations in the neocortex of HIV infected individuals. *Journal of Neurology*, Neurosurgery and Psychiatry, **56**, 481–6.

Fairburn, C. and Cooper, P. (1982). Self-induced vomiting and bulimia nervosa: an undetected problem. *British Medical Journal*, **284**, 1153–55.

Fairburn, C., Peveler, R., Davies, B., Mann, J. and Mayou, R. (1991). Eating disorders in young adults with IDMM: a controlled study. *British Medical Journal*, **303**, 17–20.

Farthing, C.F., Henry, K.I., Shanson, D.C., Taube, M., Lawrence, A.G., Harcourt-Webster, J. et al (1986). Clinical investigations of lymphadenopathy including lymph node lymonotropic virus type III (HTLV-III). *British Journal Surgery*, **73**, 180–2.

Fawzy, F.I., Namir, S. and Wolcott, D.L. (1989). Structured group intervention model for AIDS patients. *Psychiatric Medicine*, **7**, 35–45.

Feinstein, A., du Boulay, G. and Ron, M. (1992). Psychotic illness in multiple sclerosis—a clinical and MRI study. *British Journal of Psychiatry*, **161**, 680–5.

Fell, M., Newman, S., Herns, M., Durrance, P., Manji, H., Connolly, S. et al (1993). Mood and psychiatric disturbance in HIV and AIDS: changes over time. *British Journal of Psychiatry*, **167**, 604–10.

Fennema, J., Van Ameijden, E., Coutinho, R., Van Doornum, G., Henquet, C. and Van den Hoek J. (1993). HIV prevalence among clients attending a sexually transmitted diseases clinic in Amsterdam: the potential risk for heterosexual transmission. *Genitourinary Medicine*, **69**, 23–8.

Fernandez, F. and Levy, J. (1990). Psychiatric diagnosis and pharmacotherapy of patients with HIV infection. *Review of Psychiatry*, **9**, 614–30.

Fernandez, F., Adams, F., Levy, J., Holmes, V., Neidhart, M. and Mansell, P. (1988). Cognitive impairment due to ARC and its response to psychostimulants. *Psychosomatics*, **29**, 38–46.

Fernandez, F., Levy, J. and Mansell, P. (1989a). Management of delirium in terminally ill AIDS patients. *International Journal of Psychiatry in Medicine*, **19**, 165–72.

Fernandez, F., Holmes, V., Levy, J. and Ruiz, P. (1989b). Consultation-liaison psychiatry and HIV-related disorders. *Hospital and Community Psychiatry*, **40**, 146–53.

Fernandez, F., Levy, J. and Mansell, P. (1989c). Response to antidepressant treatment in depressed persons with advanced HIV infection. *Vth International Conference on AIDS*, Montreal, 1989

Ferro, S. and Salit, I. (1992). HIV infection in patients over 55 years of age. *Journal of AIDS*, **5**, 348–55.

Fischl, M.A., Richman, D.D., Grieco, M.H. Gottleib M.S., Volberding P.A., Laskin D.L. et al (1987). The efficacy of azidothymidine (AZT) in the treatment of patients with AIDS and AIDS related complex: a double blind placebo controlled trial. *New England Journal of Medicine*, **317**, 185–91.

Fischl, M.A., Richman, D.D., Hansen N., Collier A.C., Carey J.T., Para, M.F. et al (1990a). The safety and efficacy of zidovudine (AZT) in the treatment of subjects with mildly symptomatic human immunodeficiency virus type 1 (HIV) infection. A double-blind, placebo-controlled trial. The AIDS Clinical Trials Group. *Annals of Internal Medicine*, **112**, 727–37.

Fischl, M.A., Parker, C.B., Pettinelli, C., Wulfsohn M., Hirsch, M.S., Collier, A.C. et al (1990b). A randomised controlled trial of a reduced daily dose of zidovudine in patients with the acquired immunodeficiency syndrome. The AIDS Clinical Trials Group. *New England Journal Medicine*, **323**, 1009–14.

Fitzgibbon, M.L., Cella, D.F., Humfleet, G. and Sheridan, K. (1989). Motor slowing in asymptomatic HIV infection. *Perceptual and Motor Skills*, **68**, 1331–8.

Fitzpatrick, R., McLean, J., Dawson, J., Boulton, M. and Hart, G. (1990). Factors influencing condom use in a sample of homosexually active men. *Genitourinary Medicine*, **66**, 346–50.

Flavin, D., Franklin, J. and Frances, R. (1986). AIDS and suicidal behaviour in alcohol-dependent homosexual men. *American Journal of Psychiatry*, **143**, 1440–2.

Florence, M. (1994). Noah's Ark-Red Cross Foundation: a Swedish model. *AIDS Care*, **5**, 467–70.
Flowers, K.A. and Roberstson, C. (1987). The effects of Parkinson's disease on the ability to maintain mental set. *Journal of Neurology, Neurosurgery and Psychiatry*, **48**, 517–29.
Forstein, M. (1984). AIDS anxiety in the worried well. In *psychiatric implications of AIDS* (ed S. Nichols and D. Ostrow). American Psychiatric Press Inc., Washington, DC.
Forster, G. (1992). Rape and sexually transmitted diseases. *British Journal of Hospital Medicine*, **47**, 94–5.
Forster, G. (1994). STDs and the sexual abuse of children. *British Journal of Hospital Medicine*, **51**, 206–8.
Fox, B.H., Stanek, E.J., Boyd, S.C. and Flannery, J.T. (1982). Suicide rates among cancer patients in Connecticut. *Journal of Chronic Diseases*, **35**, 85–100.
Fox, L., Bailey, P., Clarke-Martinez, K., Coello, M., Ordonez F. and Barahona, F. (1993). Condom use among high-risk women in Honduras: evaluation of an AIDS prevention program. *AIDS Education and Prevention*, **5**, 1–10.
Frances, R., Wikstrom, T. and Alcena, V. (1985). Contracting AIDS as a means of committing suicide. *American Journal of Psychiatry*, **142**, 656.
Frank, J. (1986). What is psychotherapy? In *An introduction to the psychotherapies* (ed. S. Bloch) (2nd edn). Oxford University Press, Oxford.
Franke, G., Jager, H., Thomann, B. and Beyer, B. (1992). Assessment and evaluation of psychological distress in HIV-infected women. *Psychology and Health*, **6**, 297–312.
Freud, S. (1917). Mourning and melancholia. *Standard edition of the complete psychological works of Sigmund Freud*. Hogarth Press, London.
Friedland, G.N. and Klein, R.S. (1987). Transmission of human immunodeficiency virus. *New England Journal of Medicine*, **317**, 1125–35.
Frierson, R. (1990). The psychotic fear of AIDS. *Psychosomatics*, **31**, 217–9.
Frischer, M., Bloor, M., Green, S., Goldberg, D., Covell R., McKeganey, N. et al (1992). Reduction in needle sharing among community wide samples of injecting drug users. *International Journal of STD and AIDS*, **3**, 288–90.
Frost, D. (1985). Recognition of hypochondriasis in a clinic for sexually transmitted diseases. *Genitourinary Medicine*, **61**, 133–7.
Frumkin, L. and Victoroff, J. (1990). Chronic factitious disorder with symptoms of AIDS. *American Journal of Medicine*, **88**, 694–5.
Fuller, G.N., Gill, S.K., Guiloff, R.J., Kapoor, R., Lucas, D.B., Sinclair, E. et al (1990) Ganciclovir for lumbosacral polyradiculopathy in AIDS. *Lancet*, **335**, 48–9.
Fullilove, R., Fullilove, M., Bowser, B. and Gross S. (1990). Risk of sexually transmitted disease among black adolescent crack users in Oakland and San Francisco, California. *Journal of the American Medical Association*, **263**, 851–5.
Gabel, R., Barnard, N., Norko, M. and O'Connell, R. (1986). AIDS presenting as mania. *Comprehensive Psychiatry*, **27**, 251–4.
Gabuzda, D.H., Levy, S.R. and Chiappa, K.H. (1988). Electroencephalography in AIDS and AIDS-related Complex. *Clinical Electroencephalography*, **19**, 1–6.
Gague, R. W. and Wilson-Jones, E. (1978). Kaposi's sarcoma and immunosuppressive therapy—a reappraisal. *Clinical and Experimental Dermatology*, **3**, 135–46.
Gala, C., Pergami, A., Catalán, J., Riccio, M., Durbano, F., Musicco, M. et al (1992a). Risk of deliberate self-harm and factors associated with suicidal behaviour among asymptomatic individuals with HIV infection. *Acta Psychiatrica Scandinavica*, **86**, 70–5.
Gala, C., Pergami, A., Catalán, J., Riccio, M., Durbano, F., Zanello, D. et al (1992b).

Factors associated with psychological help-seeking in HIV disease. *Journal of Psychosomatic Research*, **36**, 667–76.

Gala, C., Pergami, A., Catalán, J., Riccio, M., Durbano, F., Baldeweg, T. et al (1993). The psychosocial impact of HIV infection in gay men, drug users and heterosexuals—a controlled investigation. *British Journal of Psychiatry*, **163**, 651–9.

Gallop, R.M., Taerk, G., Lancee, W.J., Coates, R.A. and Fanning, M. (1992). A randomized trial of group interventions for hospital staff caring for persons with AIDS. *AIDS Care*, **4**, 177–85.

Ganz, P.A., Schag, C.A.C., Kahn, B., Peterson, L. and Hirij, K. (1993). Describing the health-related quality of life impact of HIV infection: findings from a study using the HIV Overview of problems-evaluations systems (HOPES). *Quality of Life Research*, **2**, 109–20.

Garrett, A.S. and Corcos, A.S. (1952). Dapsone treatment of leprosy. *Leprosy Review*, **23**, 106–8.

Gattari, P., Rezza, G., Zaccarelli, M., Valenzi, C. and Tirelli, U. (1991). HIV-infected drug using transvestites and transexuals. *European Journal of Epidemiology*, **7**, 711–12.

Gattari, P., Spizzichino, L., Valenzi, C., Zaccarelli, M., Rezza, G. (1992). Behaviour patterns and HIV infection among drug using transvestites practising prostitution in Rome. *AIDS Care*, **4**, 83–7.

Gawkrodger, D. (1989). Manic depression induced by dapsone in patient with dermatitis herpetiformis. *British Medical Journal*, **299**, 860–1.

Gawlitza, M. and Reuter, P. (1988). Schizophrenia-like psychosis in patients with HIV infection. *AIDS-FORSCHUNG (AIFO)*, **3**, 150–4.

Gelder, M., Gath, D. and Mayou, R. (1989). *Oxford textbook of psychiatry* (2nd edn). Oxford University Press, Oxford.

Gellert, G., Durfee, M., Berkowitz, C., Higgins, K. and Tubiolo, V. (1993). Situational and sociodemographic characteristics of children infected with HIV from pediatric sexual abuse. *Pediatrics*, **91**, 39–44.

General Medical Council (1988). *HIV infection and AIDS: the ethical considerations*. General Medical Council, London.

General Medical Council (1993). *HIV infection and AIDS: the ethical considerations*. General Medical Council, London.

George, H. (1990). Sexual and relationship problems among people affected by AIDS: three case studies. *Counselling Psychology Quarterly*, **3**, 389–99.

George, R. (1991). Palliation in AIDS—where do we draw the line? *Genitourinary Medicine*, **67**, 85–6.

George, R. (1992). Coping with death anxiety—trying to make sense of it all? AIDS, 6, 1037–8.

George, L., Blazer, D., Hughes, D. and Fowler, N. (1989). Social support and the outcome of major depression. *British Journal of Psychiatry*, **154**, 478–85.

Gerberding, J.L. (1991). Surgery and AIDS—reducing the risk. *Journal of American Medical Association*, **265**, 1572–3.

Gerbert, B. (1987). AIDS and infection control in dental practice: dentists' attitudes, knowledge, and behavior. *Journal of American Dental Association*, **114**, 311–14.

Gerbert, B. (1989). The impact of AIDS on dental practice—update 1989. *Abstracts of the 18th Annual Session of the American Association for Dental Research*, San Francisco, March 15–9.

Gerbert, B., Maguire, B.T., Badner, V., Greenspan, D., Greenspan, J., Barnes, D. et al (1988a). Changing dentists' knowledge, attitudes, and behaviors relating to AIDS: a controlled educational intervention. *Journal of the American Dental Association*, **116**, 851–4.

Gerbert, B., Maguire, B., Badner, V., Altman, D. and Stone, G. (1988b). Why fear persists: Health care professionals and AIDS. *Journal of the American Medical Association*, **260**, 3481–3.

Gerbert, B., Sumser, J., Chamberlin, K., Maguire, B.T., Greenblatt, R.M. and McMaster, J.R. (1989). Dental care experience of HIV-positive patients. *Journal of the American Dental Association*, **119**, 601–3.

Giaquinto, C., Giacomet, V., Pagliaro, A., Ruga, E., Cozzani, S., D'Elia, R. et al (1992). Social care of children born to HIV infected parents. *Lancet*, **339**, 189–90.

Gibb, D.M. (1991). *HIV infection in children. Hospital Update*, **April**, 267–81.

Gibb, D., Duggan, C. and Lwin R (1991). The family and HIV. *Genitourinary Medicine*, **67**, 363–6.

Gibb D. and Newell M.L. (1992). *HIV infection in children: epidemiological and diagnostic aspects. International Journal of STD and AIDS*, **3**, 235–8.

Gibson, B. and Aggleton, P. (1993). *Young homeless men selling sex in central London identify their HIV/AIDS educational needs*. London Streetwise Youth, London.

Giesecke, J., Ramstedt, K., Granath, F., Ripa, T., Rado, G. and Westrell, M. (1991). Efficacy of partner notification for HIV infection. *Lancet*, **338**, 1096–100.

Ginzburg, H. and Hanlon, S. (1990). HIV-infected children and the school system. *Pediatric AIDS and HIV infection*, **1**, 15–20.

Giraldo, G., Beth, E. and Huang, E.S. et al (1980). Kaposi's sarcoma and its relationship to cytomegalovirus III. CMV DNA and CMV early antigens in Kaposi's sarcoma. *International Journal of Cancer*, **26**, 23–9.

Glass, R. (1988). AIDS and suicide. *Journal of the American Medical Association*, **259**, 1369–70.

Glass, J. D., Wesselingh, S. L., Selnes, D. A., and McArthur, J. C. (1993). Clinical-neuropathologic correlation in HIV associated dementia. *Neurology*, **43**, 2230–7.

Glazer, G. and Dudley, H. (1985). AIDS and the health professions. *Lancet*, **1**, 852–3.

GMHC (Gay mens' health crisis) (1993/94). *Treatment issues*, **7**, 1–32.

Goedert, J.J., Eyster, M.E. and Biggar, R.J. (1987). Heterosexual transmission of human immunodeficiency virus. Association with severe depletion of T-helper lymphocytes in men with haemophilia. *AIDS Research and Human Retrovirus*, **3**, 355–61.

Goethe, K.E., Mitchell, J.E., Marshall, D.W., Brey, R.L., Cahill, W.T., Leger, G.D. et al (1989). Neuropsychological and neurological function of human immunodeficiency virus seropositive asymptomatyic individuals. *Archives of Neurology*, **46**, 129–33.

Gold, R. and Skinner, M. (1992). Situational factors and thought processes associated with unprotected intercourse in young gay men. *AIDS*, **6**, 1021–30.

Gold, R., Skinner, M., Grant, P. and Plummer, D. (1991). Situational factors and thought processes associated with unprotected intercourse in gay men. *Psychological Health*, **5**, 259–78.

Gold, R., Smith, A., Skinner, M. and Morton, J. (1992). Situational factors and thought processes associated with unprotected intercourse in heterosexual students. *AIDS Care*, **4**, 305–23.

Goldberg, D. (1972). *The detection of psychiatric illness by questionnaire*. Oxford University Press, Oxford.

Goldberg, D., Cooper, B., Eastwood, M., Kenward, H. and Shepherd, D. (1970). A standardized psychiatric interview for use in community surveys. *British Journal of Preventive and Social Medicine*, **24**, 18–23.

Goldberg, D. and Hillier, V.F. (1979). A scaled version of the General Health Questionnaire. *Psychological Medicine*, **9**, 139–45.

Goldberg, D. and Huxley, P. (1992). *Common mental disorders: a bio-social model.* Tavistock Routledge, London.

Goldberg, D., Bridges, K., Cook, D., Evans, B. and Grayson, D. (1990). The influence of social factors on common mental disorders: destabilization and restitution. *British Journal of Psychiatry*, **156**, 704–13.

Goldman, J. (1987). An elective seminar to teach first-year students the social and medical aspects of AIDS. *Journal of Medical Education*, **62**, 557–61.

Goldman, E., Miller, R. and Lee, C. (1992). Counselling HIV positive haemophilic men who wish to have children. *British Medical Journal*, **304**, 829–30.

Goldman, E., Lee, C., Miller, R., Kernoff, P., Morris-Smith, J. and Taylor, B. (1993a). Children of HIV haemophilic men. *Archives of Disease in Childhood*, **68**, 133–4.

Goldman, E., Miller, R. and Lee, C. (1993b). A family with HIV and haemophilia. *AIDS Care*, **5**, 79–85.

Goldstone, I. (1992). Trends in hospital utilization in AIDS care 1987–1991: implications for palliative care. *Journal of Palliative Care*, **8**, 22–9.

Goodin, D.S., Aminoff, M.J., Chernoff, D.N. and Hollander, H. (1990). Long latency event related potentials in patients infected with human immunodeficiency virus. *Annals of Neurology*, **27**, 414–41.

Goodkin, K., Blaney, N.T., Feaster, D., Fletcher, M.A., Baum, M.A., Mantero-Atrenza, A. et al (1992a). Active coping style is associated with natural killer cell cytotoxicity in asymptomatic HIV–1 seropositive homosexual men. *Journal of Psychosomatic Research*, **36**, 635–50.

Goodkin, K., Fuchs, I., Feaster, D., Leeka, J., Dickson-Rishel, D., Fletcher, M.A. et al (1992b). Life stressors and coping style are associated with immune function in HIV–1 infection: a preliminary report. *International Journal of Psychiatry and Medicine*, **22**, 155–72.

Goodkin, K., Mulder, C.L., Blaney, N.T., Ironson, N.T., Kumar, M. et al (1994). Psychoneuroimmunology and human immunodeficiency virus type 1 infection revisited. *Archives of General Psychiatry*, **51**, 246–7.

Goodwin, G. (1994). Drug treatment in mania. *Prescribers' Journal*, **34**, 19–26.

Goodwin, G.M., Chiswick, A., Egan, V., St Clair, D. and Brettle, R.P. (1990). The Edinburgh cohort of HIV-positive drug users: auditory event-related potentials show progressive slowing in patients with centres for disease control stage IV disease. *AIDS*, **4**, 1243–50.

Gordin, F.M., Willboghby, A.D., Levine, L.A., Gurel, L. and Neill K.M. (1987). Knowledge of AIDS among hospital workers: behavioral correlates and consequences. *AIDS*, **1**, 183–8.

Gordon, J.H., Ulrich, C., Feeley, M. and Pollack, S. (1993). Staff distress among haemophilia nurses. *AIDS Care*, **5(3)**, 359–67.

Gore, S.M. and Bird, G.A. (1993). No escape: HIV transmission in jail. *British Medical Journal*, **307**, 147–8.

Gorman, J.M. and Kertzner, R. (1990). Psychoneuroimmunology and HIV infection. *Journal of Neuropsychiatry*, **2**, 241–52.

Gorman, J., Kertzner, R., Todak, G., Goetz, R., Williams, J., Rabkin J. et al (1991). Multidisciplinary baseline assessment of homosexual men with HIV infection—i: overview of study design. *Archives of General Psychiatry*, **48**, 120–3.

Gorton, G., Benjamin, R. and Hauptman, S. (1989). Malingering in AIDS. *Lancet*, **ii**, 1522.

Gostin, L. (1991). The HIV-infected health care professional: public policy, discrimination and patient safety, *Archives of Internal Medicine*, **151**, 663–5.

Government response to the report of the select committee on medical ethics (Cm 2553). (1994). HMSO, London.

Grady, C.L., Haxby, J.V., Horwitz, B., Sundaram, M., Berg, G., Shapiro, M. et al (1988). Longitudinal study of the early neuropsychological and cerebral metabolic changes in dementia of the Alzheimer type. *Journal of Clinical and Experimental Neuropsychology*, **10**, 576–96.

Grafe, M.R., Press, G.A., Berthoty, D.P., Hesselink, J.R. and Wiley, C.A. (1990). Abnormalities of the brains in AIDS patients: correlation of postmortem MR findings with neuropathology. *American Journal of Neuroradiology*, **11**, 905–11.

Grant, I., Atkinson, J., Hesselink, J., Kennedy, C., Richman, D., Spector, S. et al (1987). Evidence for early central nervous system involvement in the acquired immunodeficiency syndrome (AIDS). and other human immunodeficiency virus (HIV). infections. *Annals of Internal Medicine*, **107**, 828–36.

Grassi, M., Clerici, F., Zocchetti, C., Cargnel, A. and Mangoni, A. (1993). Neuropsychological performance in HIV-1 infected drug abusers. *Acta Neurologica Scandinavica*, **88**, 119–22.

Gray, A., (1991). *Economic aspects of AIDS and HIV infection in the UK*. Department of Public Health and Policy, London School of Hygiene and Tropical Medicine, London.

Gray, F., Geny, C., Dournon, E., Fenelon, G., Lionnet, F. and Gheradi, R. (1991). Neuropathological evidence that zidovudine reduces the incidence of HIV infection of brain. *Lancet*, **337**, 852–3.

Gray, F., Lescs, M., Keohane, C., Paraire, F., Marc, B., Durigon, M. et al (1992). Early brain changes in HIV infection: neuropathological study of 11 HIV seropositive, non-AIDS cases. *Journal of Neuropathology and Experimental Neurology*, **51**, 177–85.

Gray, F., Belec, L., Keohane, C., de Truchis, P. and Clair, B. (1994). Zidovudine therapy and HIV encephalitis: a 10 year neuropathological survey. *AIDS*, **8**, 489–93.

Green, J. and Kocsis, A. (1988). Counselling patients with AIDS-related encephalopathy. *Journal of the Royal College of Physicians of London*, **22**, 166–8.

Green, J. and McCreaner, A. (1989). *Counselling in HIV infection and AIDS*. Blackwell Scientific Publications, Oxford.

Greenblat, C., Katz, S., Gagnon, J. and Shannon, D. (1989). An innovative programme of counselling family members and friends of seropositive haemophiliacs. *AIDS Care*, **1**, 67–75.

Greenblatt, R.M., Holander, H., McMaster, J.R. and Henke, C.J. (1991). Polypharmacy among patient attending and AIDS clinic: utilization of prescribes, unorthodox, and investigational treatments. *Journal of AIDS*, **4**, 136–43.

Greenspan, D., Greenspan, J.S., Conant, M., Peterson, V., Silverman, S., de Souza, Y. et al (1984). Oral hairy leucoplakia in male homosexuals: evidence of association with both papillomavirus and a herpes group virus. *Lancet*, **ii**, 831–4.

Greer, S., Moorey, S., Baruch, J., Watson, M., Robertson, B., Mason, A. et al (1992). Adjuvant psychological therapy for patients with cancer: a prospective randomised trial. *British Medical Journal*, **304**, 675–80.

Grimshaw, J. (1987). Being HIV antibody positive. *British Medical Journal*, **295**, 256–7.

Grinstead, O. (1994). HIV vaccine trials and behavioural are not seperate roads to ending the HIV epidemic. *IInd International Conference on the Biopsychosocial aspects of HIV infection*, Brighton, 1994.

Gruer, L. and Ssembatya-Lule, G. (1993). Sexual behaviour and use of the condom by men attending gay bars and clubs in Glasglow and Edinburgh. *International Journal of STD and AIDS*, **4**, 95–8.

Gruer, L., Cameron, J. and Elliott, L. (1993). Building a city-wide service for exchanging needles and syringes. *British Medical Journal*, **306**, 1394–7.

Grunseit, A., Perdices, M., Dunbar, D., Craven, A. and Cooper, D.A. (1991). The Effects of zidovudine on neuropsychological performance in patients with asymptomatic HIV infection. *VIIth International Conference on AIDS*, Florence, 1991.

Guinan, J.J., McCallum, L.W., Painter, L., Dykes, J. and Gold, J. (1991). Stressors and rewards of being an AIDS emotional-support volunteer: a scale for use by care-givers for people with AIDS. *AIDS Care*, **3**, 137–50.

Gunnell, D. and Frankel, S. (1994). Preventing suicide: aspirations and evidence. *British Medical Journal*, **308**, 1227–32.

Guthrie, E., Creed, F., Dawson, D. and Tomenson, B. (1993). A randomized controlled trial of psychotherapy in patients with refractory irritable bowel syndrome. *British Journal of Psychiatry*, **163**, 315–21.

Gutman, L., St Claire, K., Weedy, C., Herman-Giddens, M., Lane, B., Niemeyer, J. et al (1991). HIV transmission by child sexual abuse. *American Journal of Childhood Diseases*, **145**, 137–41.

Gutman, L., St Claire, K., Weedy, C., Herman-Giddens, M. and McKinney, R. (1992). Sexual abuse of HIV positive children. *American Journal of Childhood Diseases*, **146**, 1185–9.

Gutman, L., Herman-Giddens, M. and McKinney, R. (1993). Paediatric AIDS: barriers to recognizing the role of child sexual abuse. *American Journal of Diseases of Childhood*, **147**, 775–80.

Gwede, C. and McDermott, R. (1992). ADIS in sub-Saharan Africa: implications for health education. *AIDS Education and Prevention*, **4**, 350–61.

Gwirtsman, H., Roy-Byrne, P. and Lerner, L. (1984). Bulimia in men: report of three cases with neuroendocrine findings. *Journal of Clinical Psychiatry*, **45**, 78–81.

Halevie-Goldman, B., Potkin, S. and Poyourow, P. (1987). AIDS-related complex presenting as psychosis. *American Journal of Psychiatry*, **144**, 964.

Hall, H.H. (1983). Hypnosis and the immune system: a review with implications for cancer and the psychology of healing. *American Journal of Clinical Hypnosis*, **25**, 92–103.

Hall, R., Popkin, M., Devaul, R., Faillace, L. and Stickney, S. (1978). Physical illness presenting as psychiatric disease. *Archives of General Psychiatry*, **35**, 1315–20.

Hall, P., Crosby, P., Talwatte, B. and Logan, C. (1990). HIV/AIDS and mental handicap. *Psychiatric Bulletin*, **14**, 171–8.

Halman, M.H., Worth, J., Sanders, K., Renshaw, P. and Murray, G. (1993). Anticonvulsant use in the treatment of manic syndromes in patients with HIV–1 infection. *Journal of Neuropsychiatry and Clinical Neuroscience*, **5**, 430–4.

Halstead, S., Riccio, M., Harlow, P., Oretti, R. and Thompson, C. (1988). Psychosis associated with HIV infection. *British Journal of Psychiatry*, **153**, 618–23.

Halttunen, A., Henriksson, M. and Lonnqvist, J. (1991). Completed suicide with fear of having contracted AIDS: a study of 28 cases. In *HIV and AIDS-related suicidal behaviour* (ed. Beskow, Bellini, Faria, Kerkhof). Monduzzi Editore, Bologna.

Hamel, M.A., DiMeco, P. and Lamping, D.L. (1991a). HIV seropositive caregivers: physical and psychological well-being. *VIIth International Conference on AIDS*, Florence, 1991.

Hamel, M., Ryan, B., DiMeco, P. and Lamping, D. (1991b). Determinants of well-being in HIV caregivers. *Ist International Conference on the Biopsychosocial aspects of HIV infection*, Amsterdam, 1991.

Hammond, J.S., Eckes, J.M., Gomez, G.A. and Cunningham, D.N. (1990). HIV, trauma, and infection control: universal precautions are universally ignored. *The Journal of Trauma*, **30**, 555–8.

Hankins, C. and Handley, M. (1992). HIV disease and AIDS in women: current knowledge and a research agenda. *Journal of AIDS*, **5**, 957–71.

Harden, C.L., Daras, M., Tuchman, A.J. and Koppel, B.S. (1993). Low amplitude EEGs in demented AIDS patients. *Electroencephalography and clinical neurophysiology*, **87**, 54–6.

Harding, T. (1990). *HIV infection and AIDS in the prison environment: a test case for the respect of human rights. In AIDS and drug misuse* (ed. J. Strang and G. Stimson). Routledge, London.

Harris, T.O. and Brown, G.W. (1989). The LEDS findings in the context of other research: an overview. In *Life events and illness* (ed. G.W. Brown and T.O. Harris). Hyman Unwin, London.

Harris, M.J., Jeste, D., Gleghorn, A. and Sewell, D. (1991). New-onset psychosis in HIV-infected patients. *Journal of Clinical Psychiatry*, **52**, 369–76.

Hart, G. and Whittaker, D. (1994). Sex workers and HIV. *AIDS Care*, **6**, 267–8.

Hartgers, C., van den Hoek, J.A.R., Coutinho, R.A. and van der Plight, J. (1992). Psychopathology, stress and HIV-risk injecting behaviour among drug users. *British Journal of Addiction*, **87**, 857–65.

Hawton, K. (1992). By their own hand. *British Medical Journal*, **304**, 1000.

Hawton, K. and Catalán, J. (1987). *Attempted suicide—a practical guide to its assessment and management*. Oxford University Press, Oxford.

Hawton, K. and Kirk, J. (1989). Problem-solving. In *Cognitive behaviour therapy for psychiatric problems: a practical guide* (ed. K. Hawton K, P. Salkovskis, J. Kirk and D. Clark). Oxford University Press, Oxford.

Hawton, K., Salkovskis, P., Kirk, J. and Clark, D. (eds) (1989). *Cognitive behaviour therapy for psychiatric problems: a practical guide*. Oxford University Press, Oxford.

Hays, R., Chauncey, S. and Tobey, L. (1990a). The social support networks of gay men with AIDS. *Journal of Community Psychiatry*, **18**, 374–85.

Hays, R., Kegeles, S. and Coates, T. (1990b). High HIV risk taking among young gay men. *AIDS*, **4**, 901–7.

Hays, R., Kegeles, S. and Coates, T. (1992). Changes in peer norms and sexual enjoyment predict changes in sexual risk-taking among young gay men. *VIIIth International Conference on AIDS*, Amsterdam, 1992

Hedge, B., Sherr, L. and Green, J. (1991). To take or not to take antiretrovirals: psychological sequelae of the decision-making process. *VIIth International Conference on AIDS*, Florence, 1991.

Hedge, B., Petrak, J., Sherr, L., Sichel, T., Glover, L. and Slaughter, J. (1992). Psychological crisis in HIV infection. *VIIIth International Conference on AIDS*, Amsterdam, 1992.

Heim, E., Augustiny, K., Schaffner, L. and Valach, L. (1993). Coping with breast cancer over time and situation. *Journal of Psychosomatic Research*, **37**, 523–42.

Heimer, R., Kaplan, E., Khoshnood, K., Jariwala, B. and Cadman, E. (1993). Needle exchange decreases the prevalence of HIV–1 proviral DNA in returned syringes in New Haven, Connecticut. *American Journal of Medicine*, **95**, 214–20.

Helme, T. (1992). Euthanasia around the world. *British Medical Journal*, **304**, 717.

Hencke, D. and Veitch, A. (1987). Family doctors ducking duty to AIDS patients, The Guardian, 26th February 1987.

Henry, K., Willenbrig, K. and Crossley K. (1988). Human immunodeficiency virus antibody testing: a description of practices and policies at US infectious disease-teaching hospitals and Minnesota hospitals. *Journal of the American Medical Association*, **259**, 1819–22.

Henry, K., Campbell, S. and Willenbring, K. (1990). A cross-sectional analysis of variables impacting on AIDS-related knowledge, attitudes, and behaviors among employees of a Minnesota teaching hospital. *AIDS Education and Prevention*, **2**, 36–47.

Henry, K., Collier, P., O'Boyle-Williams, C. and Campbell, S. (1991). Observed and self-reported compliance with universal precautions among emergency department personnel at two suburban community hospitals. *VIIIth International Conference on AIDS*, Amsterdam, 1992

Heptonstall, J., Gill, O.N., Porter, K., Black, M.B. and Gilbart, V.L. (1993). Health care workers and HIV: surveillance of occupationally acquired infection in the United Kingdom. *Communicable Disease Report Review*, **11**, 147–53.

Herth, K. (1990). Fostering hope in terminally ill people. *Journal of Advanced Nursing*, **15**, 1250–9.

Herzlich, B.C. and Schiano, T.D. (1993). Reversal of apparent AIDS dementia complex following treatment with vitamin B_{12}. *Journal of Internal Medicine*, **233**, 495–7.

Herzog, D., Norman, D. and Gordon, C. (1984). Sexual conflict and eating disorder in 27 males. *American Journal of Psychiatry*, **141**, 989–90.

Hestad, K., McArthur, J.H., Dal Pan, G.J., Selnes, O.A., Nance-Spronson, T.E., Aylward, E. et al (1993). Regional brain atrophy in HIV–1 infection: association with specific neuropsychological test performance. *Acta Neurologia Scandinavia*, **88**, 112–18.

Heyes, M.P., Brew, B.J., Martin, A., Price, R.W., Salazar, A.M., Sidtis, J.J. et al (1991). Quinolinic acid in cerebrospinal fluid and serum in HIV–1 infection: relationship to clinical and neurological status. *Annals of Neurology*, **29**, 202–9.

Heyman, I. and Fahy, T. (1992). Koro-like symptoms in a man infected with HIV. *British Journal of Psychiatry*, **160**, 119–21.

Heyward, W., Batter, V., Malulu, M., Nbuyi, N., Mbu, L., StLoud, M. et al (1993). Impact of HIV counselling and testing among child-bearing women in Kinshasa, Zaire. *AIDS*, **7**, 1633–7.

Higgins, D., Galavotti, C., O'Reilly, K., Schnell, D., Moore, M. et al (1991). Evidence for the effects of HIV antibody testing and counseling on risk behaviours. *Journal of the American Medical Association*, **266**, 2419–29.

Higginson, I. (1993). Pallative care: a review of past changes and future trends. *Journal of Public Health Medicine*, **15**, 3–8.

Higginson, I., Wade, A. and McCarthy, M. (1990). Palliative care: views of patients and their families. *British Medical Journal*, **301**, 277–81.

Hillier, R. (1988). Palliative medicine: a new specialty. *British Medical Journal*, **297**, 874–5.

Hockings, J. (1989). AIDS counselling in the context of the Terrence Higgins Trust. *Counselling Psychology Quarterly*, **2**, 83–7.

Ho, D.D., Rota, T.R., Schooley, R.T., Kaplan, J.C., Allan, J.D., Groopman, J.E. et al (1985). Isolation of HTLV-III from cerebrospinal fluid and neural tissues of patients with neurologic syndromes related to acquired immune deficiency syndrome. *New England Journal of Medicine*, **313**, 1493–7.

Hollander, H., Golden, J., Mendelson, T. and Cortland, D. (1985). Extrapyramidal symptoms in AIDS patients given low-dose metochlopramide or chlorpromazine. *Lancet*, **ii**, 1186.

Holman, B.L. and Johnson, K.A. (1991). HIV encephalopathy: on the road to a useful diagnostic test? *Journal of Nuclear Medicine*, **32**, 1475–7.

Holman, B.L., Garada, B., Johnson, K.A., Mendelson, J., Hallgring, E., Teoh, S.K. et al (1992). A comparison of SPECT im cocaine abuse and AIDS dementia complex. *Journal of Nuclear Medicine*, **33**, 1312–15.

Holmes, V., Fernandez, F. and Levy, J. (1989). Psychostimulant response in AIDS-related complex patients. *Journal of Clinical Psychiatry*, **50**, 5–8.

Holtgrave, D., Valdiserri, R., Gerber, R. and Hinman, J. (1993). Human immunodeficiency virus counseling, testing, referral , and partner notification services. *Archives of Internal Medicine*, **153**, 1225–30.

Holzemer, W.L., Bakken, H.S., Stewart, A. and Janson-Bjerklie, S. (1993). The HIV quality audit marker (HIV-QAM): an outcome measure for hospitalised AIDS patients. *Quality of Life research*, **2**, 99–108.

Hoover, D., Saah, A., Bacellar, H., Murphy, R., Visscher, B., Anderson, R. et al (1993). Signs and symptoms of asymptomatic HIV–1 infection in homosexual men. *Journal of AIDS*, **6**, 66–71.

Horn, J. and Chetwynd, J. (1989). *Changing sexual practices among homosexual men in response to AIDS: who as changed, who hasn't and why?* New Zealand Department of Health, Auckland.

Horton, B. (1991). Sexual outcomes arising from the diagnosis and treatment of cervical cancer and cervical intra-epithelial neoplasia: a review of the literature. *Sexual and Marital Therapy*, **6**, 29–39.

House, A. (1988). Mood disorders in the physically ill: problems of definition and measurement. *Journal of Psychosomatic Research*, **32**, 345–53.

Howlett, W.P., Nkya, V.M., Nmuni, K.A. and Missalele, W.R. (1989). Neurological disorders in AIDS and HIV disease in the northern zone of Tanzania. *AIDS*, **3**, 289–96.

Hriso, E., Kuhn, T., Masdeu, J. and Grundman, M. (1991). Extrapyramidal symptoms due to dopamine-blocking agents in patients with AIDS encephalopathy. *American Journal of Psychiatry*, **148**, 1558–61.

Huang, K., Watters, J. and Case, P. (1988). Psychological assessment and AIDS research with intravenous drug users: challenges in measurement. *Journal of Psychoactive Drugs*, **20**, 191–5.

Hudson, C. (1992). HIV infection in pregnancy: the position in the United Kingdom and Europe. *Australian and New Zealand Journal of Obstetrics and Gynaecology*, **32**, 91–4.

Hull, H., Sewell, C., Wilson, J. and McFeeley, P. (1988). The risk of suicide in persons with AIDS. *Journal of the American Medical Association*, **260**, 29–30.

Hunt, S.M., McKenna, S.P., McEwan, J., Williams, J. and Papp, E. (1981). The Nottingham Health Profile: subjective health status and medical consultations. *Social Science and Medicine*, **15A**, 221.

Hunt, A., Davies, P. and McManus, T. (1992). HIV infection in a cohort of homosexual and bisexual men. *British Medical Journal*, **305**, 561–2.

Hunt, A., Weatherburn, P., Hickson, F., Davies, P., McManus, T. and Coxon, A. (1993). Changes in condom use by gay men. *AIDS Care*, **5**, 439–48.

Hunter, S. (1990). Orphans as a window on the AIDS epidemic in sub-Saharan Africa. Social Science and Medicine, **31**, 681–90.

Ippolito, G., Puro, V., De Carli, G. and the Italian Study Group on Occupational Risk of HIV Infection (1993). The risk of occupational human immunodeficiency virus infection in health care workers. *Archives of International Medicine*, **153**, 1451–8.

Ironson, G., LaPerriere, A., Antoni, M., O'Hearn, P. and Schneiderman, N. (1990).

Changes in immune and psychological measures as a function of anticipation and reaction to news of HIV–1 antibody status. *Psychosomatic Medicine*, **52**, 247–70.

Jabbari, B., Coats, M., Salazar, A., Martin, A., Scherokman, B. and Laws, W.A. (1993). Longitudinal study of EEG and evoked potentials in neurologically asymptomatic HIV infected subjects. *Electroencephalography and Clinical Neurophysiology*, **86**, 145–51.

Jacob, K., John, J., Verghesse, A. and John, T. (1987). AIDS-phobia. *British Journal of Psychiatry*, **150**, 412.

Jacobs, S.C. (1993). *Pathologic Grief: maladaptation to loss*. American Psychiatric Press, Inc., Washington, DC.

Jacobs, S.C., Hansen, F.F. and Berkman, L. (1989). Depressions of bereavement. *Comprehensive Psychiatry*, **30**, 218–24.

Jacobs, S.C., Hansen, F.F. and Kasl, S.V. (1990). Anxiety disorders during acute bereavement: risk and risk factors. *Journal of Clinical Psychiatry*, **51**, 269–74.

Jakobsen, J., Smith, T., Gaub, J., Helweg-Larsen, S. and Trojaborg, W. (1989). Progressive neurological dysfunbction during latent HIV infection. *British Medical Journal*, **299**, 225–8.

James, M. (1988). HIV seropositivity diagnosed during pregnancy. *General Hospital Psychiatry*, **10**, 309–16.

James, N., Gillies, P. and Bignell, C. (1991). AIDS-related risk perception and sexual behaviour among sexually transmitted diseases clinic attenders. *International Journal of STD and AIDS*, **2**, 264–71.

Janssen, R.S., Saykin, A., Cannon, L., Campbell, J., Pinsky, P., Hessol, N. et al (1989). Neurological and Neuropsychological Manifestations of HIV–1 Infection: Association with AIDS-related Complex but not Asymptomatic HIV–1 Infection. *Annals of Neurology*, **26**, 592–600.

Janssen, R.S., Nwanyanwu, O.C., Selik, R.M. and Stehr-Green, J.K. (1990). Epidemiology of human immunodeficiency virus encephalopathy in the US. *Neurology*, **42**, 1472–6.

Jekot, W. and Purdy, D. (1993). Treating HIV/AIDS patients with anabolic steroids: a retrospective study. *AIDS Patient Care*, **7**, 68–74.

Jemmott, J.B., Jemmott, L.S. and Fong, G. (1992). Reduction in HIV risk-assessment behaviour among black male adolescents: effects of an AIDS prevention intervention. *American Journal of Public Health* **82**, 372–7.

Jenike, M. and Pato, C. (1986). Disabling fear of AIDS responsive to imipramine. *Psychosomatics*, **27**, 143–4.

Jennet, B. and Dyer, C. (1991). Persistent vegetative state and the right to die: the United States and Britain. *British Medical Journal*, **302**, 1256–8.

Jenny, C., Hooton, T., Bowers, A., Bowers, A., Copass, M., Krieger, J. et al (1990). Sexually transmitted diseases in victims of rape. *New England Journal of Medicine*, **322**, 713–16.

Johnson, A. (1993). Tougher HIV rules issued for health staff. *The Guardian*, 6th April, 1993.

Johnstone, F., Brettle, R., MacCallan, L., Mok, J., Peutherer, J., Burns S. et al (1990). Women's knowledge of their HIV antibody state: its effect on their decision whether to continue the pregnancy. *British Medical Journal*, **300**, 23–4.

Johnstone, F., Brettle, R., Burns, S., Peutherer, J., Mok, J., Robertson, J. et al (1994). HIV testing and prevalence in pregnency in Edinburgh. *International Journal of STD and AIDS*, **5**, 101–4.

Jones, G., Kelly, C. and Davies, J. (1987). HIV and onset of schizophrenia. *Lancet*, **i**, 1982.

Jones, J., Wykoff, R., Hollis, S., Longshore, S., Gamble, W. and Gunn, R. (1990). Partner acceptance of health department notification of HIV exposure, South Carolina. *Journal of the American Medical Association*, **264**, 1284–6.

Joseph, J., Caumartin, S., Tal, M., Kirscht, J., Kessler, R., Ostrow, D. et al (1990). Psychological functioning in a cohort of gay men at risk of AIDS: a three year descriptive study. *Journal of Nervous and Mental Disorders*, **178**, 607–15.

Kalichman, S. and Hunter, T. (1992). The disclosure of celebrity HIV infection: its effects on public attitudes. *American Journal of Public Health* **82**, 1374–6.

Kalichman, S., Keely, J., Johnson, J. and Bulto, M. (1994). Factors associated with risk for HIV infection among chronic mentally ill adults. *American Journal Psychiatry*, **151**, 221–7.

Kamlana, S. and Gray, P. (1988). Fear of AIDS. *British Journal of Psychiatry*, **153**, 129.

Kang, D., Davidson, R.J., Coe, C.L., Wheeler, R.E., Tormarken, A.J., Ershler, W.B. et al (1991). Frontal brain asymmetry and immune function. *Behavioural Neuroscience*105, 860–9.

Kaplan, R.M. and Anderson, J.P. (1988). The quality of well being scale: rationale for a single quality of life index. In *Quality of life: assessment and applications* (ed. C.S. Walker). London, MTP Press.

Kaplan, J., Spira, T. and Fishbain, D. (1988). Reasons for decrease in sexual activity amongst homosexual men with HIV infection. *Journal of the American Medical Association*, **260**, 2836–7.

Kappel, S., Vogt, R., Brozicevic, M. and Kutzko, D. (1989). AIDS knowledge and attitudes among adults in Vermont. *Public Health Reports*, **104**, 388–91.

Karlsen, R.V., Reinvang, I. and Froland, S.S. (1992). Slowed reaction time in asymptomatic HIV-positive patients. *Acta Neurologica Scandinavica*, **86**, 242–6.

Karnofsky, D.A. and Burchenal, J.H. (1949). The clinical evaluation of chemotherapeutic agents in cancer. In *Evaluation of chemotherapeutic agents* (ed. C.M. McLeod). Columbia University Press, New York.

Kassler, W., Zenilman, J., Erickson, B., Fox, R., Peterman, T. and Hook, E. (1994). Seroconversion in patients attending sexually transmitted disease clinics. *AIDS*, **8**, 351–5.

Kastner, T., Kickman, M. and Bellehumeur, D. (1989). The provision of services to persons with mental retardation and subsequent infection with HIV. *American Journal of Public Health* 79, 4914.

Katz, M. (1992). Coping with HIV: why people delay care. *Annals of Internal Medicine*, **117**, 797.

Kavalier, F. (1989). Munchausen AIDS. *Lancet*, **i**, 852.

Keene, J., Stimson, G. and Jones, S. (1993). Evaluation of syringe-exchange for HIV prevention among injecting drug users in rural and urban areas of Wales. *Addiction*, **88**, 1063–70.

Keenlyside, R. (1991). HIV testing, counselling and partner notification. *AIDS Care*, **3(4)**, 413–17.

Kegeles, S., Adler, N. and Irwin, C. (1988). Sexually active adolescents and condoms: changes over one year in knowledge, attitudes and use. *American Journal of Public Health* **78**, 460–1.

Kelen, G.D., Chan, D.W., Green, G.B., Siverston, K.T. and Quinn, T.C. (1991). Seroprevalence of HIV, HTLV, HCV and HBV among emergency department patients and potential risk to health care workers. *VIIth International Conference on AIDS*, Florence, 1991.

Keller, M. (1993). Why don't young adults protect themselves against sexual transmission of HIV? possible answers to a complex question. *AIDS Education and Prevention*, **5**, 220–33.

Kelly, J.A., (1994). HIV/AIDS prevention: strategies that work. *IInd International Conference on the Biopsychosocial aspects of HIV infection*, Brighton, 1994.

Kelly, J.A. and St Lawrence, J. (1990). The impact of community-based groups to help persons reduce HIV infection risk behaviours. *AIDS Care*, **2**, 25–36.

Kelly, J.A., St Lawrence, J.S., Smith, S., Hood, H.V. and Cook, D.J. (1987). Stigmatization of AIDS patients by physicians. *American Journal of Public Health* **77**, 789–91.

Kelly, J.A., Murphy, D., Roffman, R., Soloman, L., Winett, R., Stevenson, L.Y. et al (1989). Behavioural intervention to reduce AIDS risk activities. *Journal of Consulting and Clinical Psychology*, **57**, 60–7.

Kelly, J.A., St Lawrence, J., Brasfield, T., Lemke, A., Amidei, T. and Roffman, R. (1990). Psychological factors that predict AIDS high-risk versus AIDS precautionary behaviour. *Journal of Consultant Clinical Psychology*, **58**, 117–20.

Kelly, B., Dunne, M., Raphael, B., Buckham, C., Zournazi, A., Smith, S. et al (1991a). Relationships between mental adjustment to HIV diagnosis, psychological morbidity and sexual behaviour. *British Journal of Clinical Psychology*, **30**, 370–2.

Kelly, J.A., St Lawrence, J. and Brasfield, T. (1991b). Predictors of vulnerability to AIDS risk behaviour relapse. *Journal of Consulting and Clinical Psychology*, **59**, 163–6.

Kelly, J.A., Brasfield, T., Kalichman, S., Smith, J. and Andrew, M. (1991c). HIV risk behaviour reduction following intervention with key opinion leaders of population: an experimental analysis. *American Journal of Public Health* **81**, 168–71.

Kelly, J.A., Murphy D., Bahr, G.R., Brasfield, T., Davis, D., Hauth, A., Morgan, M., Stevenson. L.Y., and Eilers. M.K. (1992a). AIDS/HIV risk behaviours among the chronic mentally ill. *American Journal of Psychiatry*, **149**, 886–9.

Kelly, J.A., St Lawrence, J., Diaz, Y., Stevenson, L., Hauth, A., Steiner, K. et al (1992b). Acquired immunodeficiency syndrome/human immunodeficiency virus risk behaviour among gay men in small cities. *Archives of Internal Medicine*, **152**, 2293–7.

Kelly, J.A., St Lawrence, J., Stevenson, L. (1992c). Community AIDS/HIV risk reduction: the effects of endorsement by popular people in three cities. *American Journal of Public Health* **82**, 1483–9.

Kelly, J.A., Murphy, D., Bahr, R., Koob, J., Morgan, M., Kalichman, L. et al (1993a). Factors associated with severity of depression and high-risk sexual behaviour among persons diagnosed with human immunodeficiency virus (HIV) infection. *Health Psychology*, **12**, 215–19.

Kelly, J.A., Murphy, D., Bahr, G., Kalichman, S., Morgan, M., Stevenson, Y. et al (1993b). Outcome of cognitive-behaviourial and support brief therapies for depressed HIV infected persons. *American Journal of Psychiatry*, **150**, 1679–86.

Kemeny, M.E., Weiner, H., Taylor, S.E., Schneider, S., Visscher, B., Fahey, J.L. et al (1994). Repeated bereavement, depressed mood and immune parameters in HIV seropositive and seronegative gay men. *Health Psychology*, **13**, 14–24.

Kempainnen, J., St Lawrence, J.S., Irizarry, A., Weidema, D.R., Benne, C., Fredericks, C.D. et al (1991). Nurses' willingness to perform AIDS patient care: differences between staff nurses in high, moderate and low AIDS prevalence hospitals. *VIIth International Conference on AIDS*, Florence, 1991.

Kermani, E., Borod, J., Brown, P. and Tunnell, G. (1985). New psychopathological findings in AIDS: case report. *Journal of Clinical Psychiatry*, **46**, 240–1.

Kerwin, R.W. (1994). The new atypical antipsychotics. *British Journal of Psychiatry*, **164**, 141–8.

Kessler, R., O'Brien, K., Joseph, J., Ostrow, D., Phair, J., Chimiel, J. et al (1988). Effects of HIV infection, perceived health and clinical status on a cohort at risk of AIDS. *Social Science and Medicine*, **27**, 569–78.

Kessler, R.C., Foster, C., Joseph, J., Ostrow, D., Wortman, C., Phair, J. et al (1991). Stressful life events and symptom onset in HIV infection. *American Journal of Psychiatry*, **148**, 733–8.

Ketzler, S., Weis, S., Haug, H. and Budka, H. (1990). Loss of neurones in the frontal cortex in AIDS brains. *Acta Neuropathologica*, **80**, 92–4.

Kertzner, R.M., Goetz, R., Todak, G., Cooper, T., and Lin, S. (1993). Cortisol levels, immune status and mood in homosexual men with and without HIV infection. *American Journal of Psychiatry*, **150**, 1674–8.

Kieburtz, K.D., Ketonen, L., Zettelmaier, A.E., Kido, D., Caine, E.D. and Simon, J.H. (1990). Magnetic resonance imaging findings in HIV cognitive impairment. Archives of Neurology, **47**, 643–5.

Kieburtz, K.D., Giang, D.W., Schiffer, R.B. and Vakil, N. (1991a). Abnormal vitamin B12 metabolism in human immuno-deficiency virus infection. *Archives of Neurology*, **48**, 312–4.

Kieburtz, K.D., Zettelmaier, A., Ketonen, L., Tuite, M. and Caine, E. (1991b). Manic syndrome in AIDS. *American Journal of Psychiatry*, **148**, 1068–70.

Kieburtz, K.D. and Caine, E. (1992). Mania and AIDS. *American Journal of Psychiatry*, **149**, 583–4.

Kiecolt-Glaser, J.K., Glaser, R., Wiiliger, D., Stout, J. and Messick, G. (1985). Psychosocial enhancement of immunocompetence in a geriatric population. *Health psychology*, **4**, 25–41.

Kiecolt-Glaser, J.K., Glaser, R., Strain, E.C., Stout, J.C. and Tarr, K.L. (1986). Modulation of cellular immunity in medical students. *Journal of Behavioural Medicine*, **9**, 5–21.

King, M. (1988). AIDS and the GP: views of patients with HIV infection and AIDS. *British Medical Journal*, **297**, 182–8.

King, M. (1989a). Psychosocial status of 192 out-patients with HIV infection and AIDS. *British Journal of Psychiatry*, **154**, 237–42.

King, M. (1989b). Prejudice and AIDS: the views and experiences of people with HIV infection. *AIDS Care*, **1**, 137–43.

King, M. (1989c). London general practitioner' involvement with HIV infection. *Journal of the Royal College of General Practitioners*, **39**, 280–3.

King, M. (1989d). Psychological and social problems in HIV infection: interviews with general practitioners in London. *British Medical Journal*, **299**, 713–17.

King, E. (1993a). *Safety in numbers*. Cassell, London.

King, M. (1993b). *AIDS, HIV and mental health*. Cambridge Univerity Press, Cambridge.

Kingsley, L.A., Delels, R., Kaslow, R., Polk, B.F., Rinaldo, C.R. and Chimel, J. (1987). Risk factors for seroconversion to human immunodeficiency virus among male homosexuals. *Lancet*, **i**, 345–8.

Kirby, D., Barth, R.P., Leland, N. and Fetro, J.V. (1991). Reducing the risk: impact of a new curriculum on sexual risk-taking. *Family Planning*, **23**, 253–63.

Kirkpatrick, W. (1993). *AIDS: sharing the pain*. Darton, Longman and Todd, London.

Kirkpatrick, W. (1994). *Cry love, cry hope*. Darton, Longman and Todd Ltd, London.

Kizer, K., Green, M., Perkins, C., Doebbert, G. and Hughes, M. (1988). AIDS and suicide in California. *Journal of the American Medical Association*, **260**, 1881.

Klauke, S., Falkenbach, A., Schmidt, K., Staszewski, S., Helm, E.B., Althoff, P. et al (1990). Hypogonadism in male patients with AIDS. *VIth International Conference on AIDS*, San Francisco 1990.

Klee, H. (1992). A new target for behaviourial research—amphetamine misuse. *British Journal of Addiction*, **87**, 439–46.

Klein, S. and Fletcher, W. (1987). Gay grief: an examination of its uniqueness brought to light by the AIDS crisis. *Journal of Psychosocial Oncology*, **4**, 15–25.

Klein, R.S., Harris, C.A., Small, C.B., Moll, B., Lesser, M. and Friedland, G.H. (1984). Oral candidiasis in high-risk patients as the initial manifestation of the acquired immunodeficiency syndrome. *New England Journal Medicine*, **311**, 354–8.

Klimes, I., Catalán, J., Bond, A. and Day, A. (1989). Knowledge and attitudes of health care staff about HIV infection in a health district with low HIV prevalence. *AIDS Care*, **1**, 313–17.

Klimes, I., Catalán, J. and Hodges, S. (1990). Neuropsychological functioning of men with haemophilia and HIV infection. *International Conference on the Neuroscience of HIV Infection*, Monterey, 1990.

Klimes, I., Elcombe, S., Hodges, S., Catalán, J., Day, A., Garrod, A. et al (1991). Neuropsychological status of men with haemophilia and HIV infection: a controlled investigation—one year follow-up. Published abstract. *VIIth International Conference on AIDS*, Florence, 1991.

Klimes, I., Catalán, J., Garrod, A., Day, A., Bond, A. and Rizza, C. (1992). Partners of men with HIV infection and hamophilia: controlled investigation and factors associated with psychological morbidity. *AIDS Care*, **4**, 149–56.

Klonoff, A.E. and Ewers, D. (1990). Care of AIDS patients as a source of stress to nursing staff. *AIDS Education and Prevention*, **2**, 338–48.

Kochen, M., Hasford, J., Jager, H., Zippel, S., L'Age, M., Rosendahl, C. et al (1991). How do patients with HIV perceive their GP? *British Medical Journal*, **303**, 365–8.

Kocsis, A. (1989). Counselling those with AIDS dementia. In *Counselling in HIV infection and AIDS* (ed. J. Green J and A. McCreaner). Blackwell Scientific Publications, Oxford.

Kocsis, A.E., Helbert, M., Peters, B., Mann, J. and Church, J. (1989). Study of cognitive functioning in AIDS and ARC patients receiving AZT. In *Current approaches to neuropsychiatric aspects of AIDS* (ed. C. Thompson C and M. Page). Duphar, London.

Kopelman, L. and Moskop, J. (1981). The holistic health movement: a survey and critique. *Journal of Medicine and Philosophy*, **6**, 209–35.

Koralnik, I.J., Beaumanoir, A., Hausler, R., Kohler, A., Safran, A.B., Delacroix, R. et al (1991a). A controlled study of early neurologic abnormalities in men with asymptomatic human immunodeficieny virus infection. *The New England Journal of Medicine*, **323**, 864–70.

Koralnik, I.J., Mayer, E. and Hirschel, B. (1991b). Correspondence: Early neurologic abnormalities in HIV infection. *The New England Journal of Medicine*, **44**, 324.

Kotler, D.P. (1989). Malnutrition in HIV infection and AIDS. *AIDS*, **3**, 175–80.

Krajeski, J.P. (1990). Public policy, legal, and ethical issues. *Review of Psychiatry*, **9**, 656–73.

Krasnik, A., Fouchard, J.R., Bayer, T. and Keiding, N. (1990). Health workers and AIDS: knowledge, attitudes and experiences as determinants of anxiety. *Scandinavian Journal of Social Medicine*, **18**, 103–13.

Krieger, J., Coombs, R., Collier, A., Koehler, J., Ross, S., Chaloupka, K. et al (1991). Fertility parameters in men infected with HIV. *Journal of Infectious Diseases*, **164**, 464–9.

Krikorian, R. and Wrobel, A.J. (1991). Cognitive impairment in HIV infection. *AIDS*, **5**, 501–7.

Ku, L., Sonensen, F.L. and Pleck, J. (1993). Young men's risk behaviour for HIV infection and sexually transmitted diseases, 1988 through 1991. *American Journal of Public Health* **83**, 1609–15.

Kubler-Ross, E. (1970). *On death and dying*. Tavistock, London.

Kuni, C.C., Rhame, F.S., Meier, M.J., Foehse, M.C., Loewenson, R.B., Lee, B.C. et al (1991). Quantitative I–123-IMP brain SPECT and neuropsychological testing in AIDS dementia. *Clinical Nuclear Medicine*, **16**, 174–7.

Kurdek, L. and Siesky, G. (1990). The nature and correlates of psychological adjustment in gay men with AIDS-related conditions. *Journal of Applied Social Psychology*, **20**, 846–60.

Kuykendall, J. (1991). Aspects of psychological support for families and children affected by HIV. In *Caring for children with HIV and AIDS* (ed. R. Claxton and T. Harrison). Edward Arnold, London.

Laane, H.M. (1993). Euthanasia on out-patient AIDS patients in Amsterdam. *IXth International Conference on AIDS*, Berlin, 1993.

Lackner, J., Joseph, J., Ostrow, D. and Eshleman, S. (1993). The effects of social support on Hopkins Symptom Checklist-assessed depression and distress in a cohort of HIV positive and negative gay men. *The Journal of Nervous and Mental Disease*, **181**, 632–8.

LaFrance, N.D., Pearlson, G., Schaerf, F., McArthur, J.C., Bascom, M.J., Kumar, A.J. et al (1988). SPECT imaging with I–123 isopropyl amphetamine in asymptomatic HIV seropositive persons. Published Abstract. *Journal of Nuclear Medicine*, **29**, 742–8.

Lamping, D.L., Sewitch, M., Clark, E., Ryan, B., Gilmore, N., Grover, S.A. et al (1991). HIV-related mental health distress in persons with HIV infection, caregivers, and family members/significant others: results of a cross-Canada survey. *VIIth International Conference on AIDS*, Florence, 1991.

Lamping, D.L., Gilmore, N., Grover, S., Tsoukas, C., Falutz, J., Hamel, M. et al (1992). Social support and health-related outcomes in persons with HIV infection. *VIIIth International Conference on AIDS*, Amsterdam, 1992.

Lamping, D.L., Abrahamowicz, M., Gilmore, N., Edgar, L., Grover, S., Tsoukas, C. et al (1993). A randomized controlled trial to evaluate a psychosocial intervention to improve quality of life in HIV infection. *IXth International Conference on AIDS*, Berlin, 1993.

Lancet (1984). Needlestick transmission of HTLV-III from a patient infected in Africa. *Lancet*, **ii**, 1376–7.

Lancet (1990). Ziodovudine for symptomless HIV infection. *Lancet*, **335**, 821–2.

Landesman, S., Minkoff, H., Holman, S., McCalla, S. and Sijin, O. (1987). Seropositivity of HIV infection in parturients. *Journal of American Medical Association*, **258**, 2701–3.

Landis, P., Schoebach, V.J., Weber, D.J., Mittal, M., Krishan, B., Lewis, K. et al (1992). Results of a randomised trial of partner notification in cases of HIV infection in North Carolina. *New England Journal of Medicine*, **326**, 101–6.

Lantos, P.L., McLaughlkin, J.E., Scholtz, C.L., Berry, C.L. and Tighe, J.R. (1989). Neuropathology of the brain in HIV infection. *Lancet*, **i**, 309–11.

LaPerriere, A.R., Antoni, M.H., Schneiderman, N., Ironson, G., Klimas, N.G., Canalis, P. et al (1990). Exercise intervention attenuates emotional distress and natural killer cell decrements following notification of positive serologic status for HIV–1. *Biofeedback and Self Regulation*, **15**, 229–42.

LaPerriere, A., Fletcher, M.A., Antoni, M.H., Klimas, N.G. and Ironson, G. (1991). Aerobic exercise training in an AIDS risk group. *Intentional Journal of Sports Medicine*, **12** (suppl.). S53-S57.

Larder, B.A., Darby, G. and Richman, D.D. (1989). HIV with reduced sensitivity to zidovudine (AZT). isolated during prolonged therapy. *Science*, **243**, 1731–4.

Larsson, M., Hagberg, L. and Norkrans, G. (1989). Indoleamine deficiency in blood and CSF from patients with HIV. *Journal of Neuroscience Research*, **23**, 441–6.

Lau, R., Jenkins, P., Caun, K., Forster, S., Weber, J., McManus, T. et al (1992). Trends in sexual behaviour in a cohort of homosexual men: a 7 year prospective study. *International Journal of STD and AIDS*, **3**, 267–72.

Lauer-Listhaus, B. and Watterson, J. (1988). A psychoeducational group for HIV positive patients on a psychiatric service. *Hospital and Community Psychiatry*, **39**, 776–7.

Laughon, B.E., Druckman D.A., Vernon, A., Quinn, T.C., Polk B.F., Modlin, J. F. et al (1989). Prevalence of enteric pathogens in homosexual men with and without acquired immunodeficiency syndrome. *Gastroenterology*, **94**, 984–93.

Lawlor, B. and Stewart, J. (1987). AIDS delusions: a symptom of our times. *American Journal of Psychiatry*, **144**, 1244.

Lazare, A. (1979). Unresolved grief. In *Outpatient psychiatry: Diagnosis and treatment* (ed. A. Lazare). Williams and Wilkens, Baltimore.

Learner, M. (1980). *The belief in a just world: a fundamental delusion*. Plenum Press, New York.

Lefrere, J.J., Laplanche, J.L., Vittecoq, D., Villette, J.M., Fiet, J., Modai, J. et al (1988). Hypogonadism in AIDS. *AIDS*, **2**, 135–43.

Leighton, K., Sonestein, F. and Pleck, J. (1993). Young men's risk behaviours for HIV infection and sexually transmitted diseases, 1988 through 1991. *American Journal of Public Health* **83**, 1609–15.

Lenhardt, T.M., Super, M.A. and Wiley, C.A. (1988). Neuropathological changes in an asymptomatic HIV seropositive man. *Annals of Neurology*, **23**, 209–10.

Lennon, M, Martin, J and Dean, L. (1990). The influence of social support on AIDS-related grief among gay men. *Social Science and Medicine*, **4**, 477–84.

Lerton, D. (1983). AIDS: hospital guidelines, clinical clues. *American Medical News*, **26**, 1.

Leserman, J., Perkins, D. and Evans, D. (1992). Coping with the threat of AIDS: the role of social support. *American Journal of Psychiatry*, **149**, 1514–20.

Levin, B., Berger, J.R. and Kumar, M. (1991). Cerebrospinal fluid dopamine levels in HIV–1 infection: correlation with immune function and neuropsychological profile. *International Conference on the Neuroscience of HIV Infection*, Padua, 1991.

Levy, R., Rosenbloom, S. and Perret, L. (1986). Neuroradiologic findings in AIDS: a review of 200 cases. *American Journal of Radiology*, **147**, 977–83.

Levy, R., Mills, C., Posin, J., Moore, S., Rosenblum, M. and Bredesen, D. (1990). The efficacy and clinical impact of brain imaging in neurologically asymptomatic AIDS patients: a prospective CT/MRI study. *Journal of AIDS*, **3**, 461–71.

Lewin, C. and Williams, R. (1988). Fear of AIDS: impact of public anxiety in young people. *British Journal of Psychiatry*, **153**, 823–4.

Lewis, C.E., Freeman, H.E. and Corey, C.R. (1987). AIDS-related competence of California's primary care physicians. *American Journal of Public Health* **77**, 795–9.

Lindeman, E. (1944). Symptomatology and management of acute grief. *American Journal of Psychiatry*, **101**, 141–8.

Lipowski, Z. (1990). *Delirium: acute confusional states*. Oxford University Press, New York.

Lippmann, S., James, W. and Frierson, R. (1993). AIDS and the family: implications for counselling. *AIDS Care*, **5**, 71–8.

Lipton, S.A. (1992). Models of neuronal injury in AIDS: another role for the NMDA receptor? *Trends in Neuroscience*, **15**, 75–9.

Livingstone, M. (1994). Benzodiazepine dependence. *British Journal of Hospital Medicine*, **51**, 281–6.

Lloyd, G.G. (1991). Textbook of general hospital psychiatry. Churchill Livingstone, Edinburgh.

Loft, J., Marder, W., Bresolin, L. and Rinaldi, R. (1994). HIV preventive practices of primary-care physicians, US, 1992. *Morbidity and Mortality Weekly Report*, **42**, 988–92.

Logan, F., MacLean, A., Howie, C., Gibson, B., Hann, I. and Parry-Jones, W. (1990). Psychological disturbance in children with haemophilia, British Medical Journal, **301**, 1253–6.

Logsdail, S., Lovell, K., Warwick, H. and Marks, I. (1991). Behavioural treatment of AIDS-focused illness phobia. *British Journal of Psychiatry*, **1599**, 422–5.

Louhivuori, K.A. and Hakama, M. (1979). Risk of suicide among cancer patients. *American Journal of Epidemiology*, **109**, 59–65.

Lovejoy, N., Paul, S., Freeman, E. and Christianson, B. (1991). Potential correlates of self-care and symptom distress in homosexual and bisexual men who are HIV positive. *Oncology Nursing Forum*, **18**, 1175–85.

Lovett, E., Pugh, K., Baldeweg, T., Catalán, J., Riccio, M., Burgess, A.P. et al (1993). Psychological morbidity in a cohort of gay men with HIV infection: role of disease stage, coping strategies and life events. *IXth International Conference on AIDS*, Berlin, 1993.

Luft, B.J. and Remington J.S. (1983). Toxoplasmosis. In *Infectious Diseases* (3rd edn) (ed. P.D. Hoeprich). Harper and Row, Philadelphia.

Lunn, S., Skydsbjerg, M., Schulsinger, H., Parnas, J., Pederson, C. and Mathiesen L. (1991). A preliminary report on the neuropsychologic sequelae of human immunodeficiency virus. *Archives of General Psychiatry*, **48**, 139–42.

Lurie, P., Bishaw, M., Chesney, M., Cooke, M., Fernandes, M., Hearst, N. et al (1994). Ethical, behavioural, and social aspects of HIV vaccine trials in developping countries. *Journal of the American Medical Association*, **271**, 295–301.

Lyketsos, C., Hanson, A., Fishman, M., Rosenblatt, A., McHugh, P. and Treisman, G. (1993a). Manic syndrome early and late in the course of HIV. *American Journal of Psychiatry*, **150**, 326–7.

Lyketsos, C.G., Hoover, D.R., Guccione, M., Senterfitt, W., Dew, M.A., Wesch, J. et al (1993b). Depressive symptoms as predictors of medical outcomes in HIV infection. *Journal of the American Medical Association*, **270**, 2563–7.

Lyons, J., Larson, D., Anderson, R. and Bilheimer, L. (1989). Psychosocial services for AIDS patients in the general hospital. *International Journal of Psychiatry in Medicine*, **19**, 385–92.

Maccario, M. and Scharre, D. (1987). HIV and acute onset psychosis. *Lancet*, **ii**, 342.

MacDiarmond-Gordon, A.R., O'Connor, M., Beaman, M. and Ackrill, P. (1992). Neurotoxicity associated with oral acyclovir in patient undergoing dialysis. *Nephron*, **62**, 280–3.

Maddocks, I. (1990). Changing concepts in palliative care. *The Medical Journal of Australia*, **152**, 535–9.

Maehlen, J., Dunlop, O., Dobloug, J.H., Liestol, K. and Torvik, A. (1993). Brain lesions in AIDS patients in Norway 1983–1992. Unexplained changes with time and opposing effects of length of survival and azidothymidine treatment. *Clinical neuropathology*, **12** (suppl.), S12.

Magura, S., Shapiro, J., Siddiqui, Q. and Lipton, D. (1990). Variables influencing condom use among intravenous drug users. *American Journal of Public Health* **80**, 82–4.

Magura, S., Kang, S., Shapiro, J. and O'Day, J. (1993). HIV risk among women injecting drug users who are in jail. *Addiction*, **88**, 1351–60.

Mahorney, S. and Cavenar, J. (1988). A new and timely delusion: the complaint of having AIDS. *American Journal of Psychiatry*, **145**, 1130–2.

Mail, P. and Matheny, S. (1989). Social services for people with AIDS: needs and approaches. *AIDS*, **3**, 273–7.

Maj, M. (1991). Psychological problems of families and health workers dealing with people infected with HIV–1. *Acta Psychiatrica Scandinavica*, **83**, 161–8.

Maj, M., Janssen, R. and Satz, P. (1991). The World Health Organisation's Cross Cultural Study on Neuropsychiatric Aspects of Infection with the Human Immunodeficiency Virus (HIV–1): Preparation and Pilot Phase. *British Journal of Psychiatry*, **159**, 351–6.

Maj, M., Janssen, R., Starace, F., Zaudig, M., Satz, P., Sughondhabirom, B. et al (1994a). WHO Neuropsychiatric AIDS study—cross-sectional phase I. *Archives of General Psychiatry* **51**, 39–49.

Maj, M., Satz, P., Janssesn, R., Zaudig, M., Starace, F., D'Elia, L. et al (1994b). WHO neuropsychiatric AIDS study–cross-sectional phase I. Neuropsychological and neurological findings. *Archives of General Psychiatry* **51**, 51–61.

Malcolm, J. and Sutherland, D. (1992). AIDS palliative care demands a new model. *Medical Journal of Australia*, **157**, 572–3.

Malow, R., West, J., Corrigan, S., Pena, J. and Cunningham, S. (1994). Outcome of psychoeducation for HIV risk reduction. *AIDS Education and Prevention*, **6**, 113–25.

Mandal, B., Clarke, K.R. and Dunbar, E.M. (1991). Health care of HIV patients: survey of patients' views. *VIIth International Conference on AIDS*, Florence, 1991.

Manji, H., Connolly, S., McAllister, R., Valentien, A.R. and Kendall, B.E. (1994). Serial MRI of the brain in asymptomatic patients infected with HIV: results from the UCMSM/Medical Research Council neurology cohort. *Journal of Neurology*, Neurosurgery and Psychiatry, **57**, 144–9.

Mann, J., Tarantola, D. and Netter, T. (ed.) (1992). *A global report: AIDS in the world*. Harvard University Press, Cambridge, Mass.

Manning, D., Jacobsberg, L. and Erhart, S. (1990). The efficacy of imipramine in the treatment of HIV-related depression. *VIth International Conference on AIDS*, San Francisco 1990.

Mansfield, S. and Singh, S. (1989). The GP and HIV: an insight into patients' attitudes. *Journal of the Royal College of General Practitioners*, **39**, 104–5.

Mansfield, S., Barter, G. and Singh, S. (1992). AIDS and palliative care. *International Journal of STD and AIDS*, **3**, 248–50.

Mansfield, S. and Singh, S. (1993). Who should fill the gap in HIV disease? *Lancet*, **342**, 726–8.

Mansson, S. (1990). Psycho-social aspects of HIV testing—the Swedish case. *AIDS Care*, **2**, 5–6.

Marazzi, M., Palombi, L., Mancinelli, S., Liotta, G. and Pana, A. (1994). Care requirements of people with ARC/AIDS in Rome: non-hospital services. *AIDS Care*, **6**, 95–103.

Marcus, R. and The CDC Cooperative Needlestock Surveillance Group (1988). Surveillance of health care workers exposed to blood from patients infected with the human immunodeficiency virus. *New England Journal of Medicine*, **319**, 1118–23.

Marimsky, O., Reider-Groswasser, I.R., Inbor, M. and Chaitchik, S. (1990). Interferon-related mental deterioration and behavioural changes in patients with renal cell carcinoma. *European Journal of Cancer*, **26**, 596–600.

Markowitz, J., Rabkin, J. and Perry, S. (1994). Treating depression in HIV patients. *AIDS*, **8**, 403–12.

Marmar, C., Horowitz, M. and Weiss, D. (1988). A controlled trial of brief psychotherapy and mutual help group treatment of conjugal bereavement. *American Journal of Psychiatry*, **145**, 203–9.

Martelli, L., Peltz, F. and Messina, W. (1987). *When someone you know has AIDS*. Crown Publishers Inc., New York.

Martin, J.P. (1991). Issues in the current treatment of hospice patients with HIV disease. *Hospice Journal*, **7**, 31–40.

Martin, G., Serpelloni, G., Galvan, U., Rizzetto, A., Gomma, M., Morgante, S. et al (1990). Behavioural change in drug users: evaluation of an HIV/AIDS education programme. *AIDS Care*, **2**, 275–9.

Martin, E.M., Sorensen, D.J., Edelstein, H.E. and Robertson, L.C. (1992). Decision making speed in HIV–1 infection: a preliminary report. *AIDS*, **6**, 109–13.

Marzuk, P. (1991). Suicidal behaviour and HIV illness. International Review of Psychiatry, **3**, 365–71.

Marzuk, P. and Perry, S. (1993). Suicide and HIV: researchers and clinicians beware. *AIDS Care*, **5**, 387–9.

Marzuk, P., Tierney, H., Tardiff, K., Gross, E., Morgan, E., Hsu, M.A. et al (1988). Increased risk of suicide in persons with AIDS. *Journal of the American Medical Association*, **259**, 1333–37.

Masdeu, J., Yudd, A., van Heertum, R.L., Grundum, M., Hriso, E., O'Connell, R.A. et al (1991). Single photon emission tomography in human immunodeficiency virus encephalopathy: a preliminary report. *Journal of Nuclear Medicine*, **32**, 1475–7.

Maslach, C.H. (1982). Burnout: a social psychological analysis. In The burnout syndrome: current research, theory and interventions (ed. J.W. Jones). London House Press, Park Ridge, Ill.

Maslanka, H. (1992). Social support and volunteering. *VIIIth International Conference on AIDS*, Amsterdam, 1992

Matta, H., Thompson, A.M. and Rainey, J.B. (1988). Does the wearing of two pairs of gloves protect operating theatre staff from skin contamination? *British Medical Journal*, **297**, 597–8.

Matthews, C. and Klove, H. (1964). Instruction manual for the adult neuropsychology test battery. University of Wisconsin Medical School, Madison, Wisconsin.

Mauri, M., Sinforiani, E., Muratori, S., Zerboni, R. and Bono, G. (1993). Three year follow-up in a selected group of HIV-infected homosexual/bisexual men. *AIDS*, **7**, 241–5.

Mawson, D., Marks, I. and Ramm, L. (1981). Guided mourning for morbid grief: a controlled study. *British Journal of Psychiatry*, **138**, 185–93.

Maxwell, S., Scheftner, W., Kessler, H. and Busch, K. (1988). Manic syndrome associated with zidovudine treatment. *Journal of the American Medical Association*, **259**, 3406–7.

Mayeux, R., Stern, Y., Tang, M., Todak, G., Marder, K., Sano, M. et al (1993). Mortality risk in gay men with HIV infection and cognitive impairment. *Neurology*, **43**, 176–82.

Mayfield, D., McLeod, G. and Hall, P. (1974). The CAGE questionnaire: validity of a new alcohol screening instrument. *American Journal of Psychiatry*, **131**, 1121–3.

Mayou, R. (1987). Burnout. *British Medical Journal*, **295**, 284–5.

Mayou, R. and Huyse, F. (1991). Consultation-liaison psychiatry in Western Europe. *General Hospital Psychiatry*, **13**, 188–208.

Mays, V. and Cochran, S. (1987). AIDS and black Americans: special psychosocial issues. *Public Health Reports*, **102**, 224–31.

McAllister, R.H., Herns, M.V., Harrison, M.J., Newman, S.P. and Connolly, S. (1992). Neurological and neuropsychological performance in HIV seropositive men without symptoms. *Journal of Neurology Neurosurgery and Psychiatry*, **55**, 143–8.

McArthur, J.C. (1987). Neurologic Manifestations of AIDS. Medicine, **66**, 407–37.

McArthur, J.C., Cohen, B., Selnes, O.A., Kumar, A., Cooper, K., McArthur, J.H. et al (1989). Low prevalence of neurological and neuropsychological abnormalities in otherwise healthy HIV–1 infected individuals: results from the multicenter AIDS cohort study. *Annals of Neurology*, **26**, 601–11.

McArthur, J.C., Kumar, A.J., Johnson, D.W., Selnes, O.A. and Becker, J.T. (1990a). Incidental white matter hyperintensities on magnetic resonance imaging in HIV–1 infection. Multi-center AIDS cohort study. *Journal of Acquired Immune Deficiency Syndromes*, **3**, 252–9.

McArthur, J.C., Miller, E.N., Selnes, O.A., Becker, J.T., Cohen, B.A., Starkey, D. et al (1990b). Effects of longterm zidovudine use on neuropsychological performance in the multicentre AIDS cohort study. *International Conference on the Neuroscience of HIV Infection*, Monterey, 1990.

McArthur, J.C., Nance-Spronson, T.E., Griffin, D.E., Hoover, D., Selnes, O.A., Miller, E.N. et al (1992). The diagnostic utility of elevation in cerebrospinal fluid ß2-microglobulin in HIV–1 dementia. *Neurology*, **42**, 1707–12.

McArthur, J.C., Hoover, D.R., Bacellar, H., Miller, E.N., Cohen, B.A., Becker, J.T. et al (1993). Dementia in AIDS patients: incidence and risk factors. *Neurology*, **43**, 2245–52.

McCann, L. and Pearlman, L.A. (1990). Vicarious traumatization: a framework for understanding the psychological effects of working with victims. *Journal of Trauma and Stress*, **3**, 131–46.

McCann, K. and Wadsworth, E. (1991). The experience of having a positive HIV test. *AIDS Care*, **3**, 43–53.

McCann, K. and Wadsworth, E. (1992). The role of informal carers in supporting gay men who have HIV-related illness: what do they do and what are their needs?. *AIDS Care*, **4**, 25–34.

McCarthy, M. (1990). Hospice patients: a pilot study in 12 services. *Palliative Medicine*, **4**, 93–104.

McCarthy, M. and Rooney, M. (1991). *Conference report: HIV and people with learning difficulties*. HIV Project, North West Thames Regional Health Authority, London.

McCrae, R.R. and Costa, P.T. (1986). Personality, coping and coping effectiveness in an adult sample. *Journal of Personality*, **54**, 385–405.

McCue, J.D. and Zandt, J.R. (1991). Acute psychosis associated with the use of ciprofloxacine and trimethoprin-sulphamethoxazole. *American Journal of Medicine*, **90**, 528–9.

McCullum, L.W., Dykes, J., Painter, L. and Gold, J. (1989). The Ankali project: a model for the use of volunteers to provide emotional support in terminal illness. *The Medical Journal of Australia*, **151**, 33–8.

McCusker, J., Stoddard, A., Zapka, J., Zorn, M. and Mayer, K. (1989). Predictors of AIDS-preventive behaviour among homosexually active men: a longitudinal study. *AIDS*, **3**, 443–8.

McEwan, R., McCallum, A., Bhopal, R. and Mdhok, R. (1992). Sex and the risk of HIV infection: the role of alcohol. *British Journal of Addiction*, **87**, 577–84.

McGowan, I., Potter, M., George, R., Michaels, L., Sinclair, E., Scaravilli, F. et al

(1991). HIV-encephalopathy presenting as hypomania. *Genitourinary Medicine*, **67**, 420–4.

McGrath, J., Ankrah, E.M., Schumann, D., Nkumbi, S. and Lubega, M. (1993). AIDS and the urban family: its impact in Kampala, Uganda. *AIDS Care*, **5**, 55–70.

McKeganey, N. and Barnard, M. (1992). Selling sex: female street prostitution and HIV risk behviour in Glasgow. *AIDS Care*, **4**, 395–407.

McKegney, F.P. and O'Dowd, M.A. (1992). Suicidality and HIV status. *American Journal of Psychiatry*, **149**, 396–8.

McKegney, F.P., O'Dowd, M.A., Feiner, C., Selwyn, P., Drucker, E. and Friedland, G.H. (1990). A prospective comparison of neuropsychologic function in HIV-seropositive and seronegative methadone-maintained patients. *AIDS*, **4**, 565–9.

McKinnon, M.D., Gooch, C.D. and Cockroft, A. (1990). Knowledge and attitudes of health care workers about AIDS and HIV infection before and after distribution of an educational booklet. *Journal of Social and Occupational Medicine*, **40**, 15–18.

McKusick, L. and Horstman, W. (1986). The impact of AIDS on the physician. In *What to do about AIDS?* (ed. L. McKusick and W. Horstman). University of California Press, Berkeley, Ca.

McKusick, L., Coates, T., Morin, S., Pollack, L. and Hoff, C. (1990). Logitudinal predictors of reductions in unprotected anal intercourse among gay men in San Francisco. *American Journal of Public Health* **80**, 978–83.

McKusker, J., Westenhouse, J., Stoddard, A., Zapka, J., Zorn, M. and Mayer, K. (1990). Use of drugs and alcohol by homosexually active men in relation to sexual practices. *Journal of Acquired Immune Deficiency Syndromes*, **3**, 729–36.

McNair, D. and Lorr, M. (1964). An analysis of mood in neurotics. *Journal of Abnormal and Social Psychology*, **69**, 620–7.

Meadows. J, Catalán, J. and Gazzard, B.G. (1993a). I plan to have the HIV test: predictors of testing intention in women attending a London ante-natal clinic. *AIDS Care*, **5**, 141–8.

Meadows, J., Catalán, J. and Gazzard, B.G. (1993b). HIV antibody testing in the antenatal clinic. *Midwifery*, **9**, 17–27.

Meadows, J., Catalán, J. and Gazzard, B.G. (1993c). HIV antibody testing in the antenatal clinic: the views of the consumers. *Midwifery*, **9**, 63–9.

Meadows, J., Catalán, J., Singh, A.N. and Burgess, A.P. (1993d). Prevalence of HIV associated dementia (HAD) in a central London Health District in 1991. *IXth International Conference on AIDS*, Berlin, 1993.

Melbye, M., Goedert, J.J., Grossman, R.J., Goederl, J.J., Eyster, M.M. and Biggan, R.J. (1987). Risk of AIDS after herpes zoster. *Lancet*, **i**, 728–30.

Mellers, J., Smith, J., Harris, J. and King, M. (1991). Case control study of psychosocial status in HIV positive women. *VIIth International Conference on AIDS*, Florence, 1991.

Melnick, S., Jefferey, R.W., Burke, G.L., Gilbertson, D.T. and Perkins, L.A. (1993). Changes in sexual behaviour by young urban heterosexual adults in response to the AIDS epidemic. *Public Health Reports*, **108**, 582–9.

Melvin, D. and Sherr, L. (1993). The child in the family – responding to AIDS and HIV. *AIDS Care*, **5**, 35–42.

Messenheimer, J.A., Robertson, K.R., Wilkins, J.W., Kalkowski, J.C. and Hall, C.D. (1992). Event-related potentials in human immunodeficiency virus infection: a prospective study. *Archives of Neurology*, **49**, 396–400.

Metzger, D.S., Woody, G.E., McLellan, A.T., O'Brien, C.P., Druely, P., Navaline, H. et al (1993). Human immunodeficiency virus seroconversion among intravenous drug users in and out of treatment: an 18 month prosepective follow-up. *Journal of Acquired Immune Deficiency Syndromes*, **6**, 1049–56.

Meyer, G. (1993). Occupational infection in health care: the century-old lessons from syphilis. *Archives of International Medicine*, **153**, 2439–47.

Meyerhoff, D.J., Mackay, S., Bachman, L., Poole, N., Dillon, W.P. et al (1993). Reduced brain N-acetylaspartate suggests neuronal loss in cognitively impaired human immunodeficiency virus-seropositive individuals: in vivo 1H magnetic resonance spectroscopic imaging. *Neurology*, **43**, 509–15.

Michaels, D. and Levine, C. (1992). Estimates of the number of motherless youth orphaned by AIDS in the US. *Journal of the American Medical Association*, **268**, 3456–61.

Milgrom, H. and Bender, B. (1993). Psychologic side-effects of therapy with corticosteroids. *Annual Review of Respiratory Diseases*, **147**, 471–3.

Miller, D. (1986). The worried well. In *The management of AIDS patients* (ed. D. Miller, J. Weber and J. Green). Macmillan, London.

Miller, D. (1987). *Living with AIDS and HIV*. Macmillan Education, London.

Miller, D. (1988). HIV and social psychiatry. *British Medical Bulletin*, **44**, 130–48.

Miller, R. (1991). Some notes on the impact of treating AIDS patients in hospices. *Hospice Journal*, **7**, 1–12.

Miller, D. and Pinching, A. (1989). HIV tests and counselling: current issues. *AIDS*, **3** (suppl. 1), S187-S193.

Miller, D. and Riccio, M. (1990). Non-organic psychiatric and psychological syndromes associated with HIV–1 infection and disease. *AIDS*, **4**, 381–8.

Miller, R. and Bor, R. (1992). Pre-HIV antibody testing—too much fuss? *Genitourinary Medicine*, **68**, 9–10.

Miller, D., Green, J., Farmer, R. and Carroll, G. (1985). A pseudo-AIDS syndrome following from a fear of AIDS. *British Journal of Psychiatry*, **146**, 550–2.

Miller, D., Weber, J. and Green, J. (eds.) (1986a). *The management of AIDS patients*. Macmillan. London.

Miller, D., Jeffries, D., Green, J., Harris, J.W. and Pinching, A. (1986b). HTLV-III: should testing ever be routine? *British Medical Journal*, **292**, 941–3.

Miller, F., Weiden, P., Sacks, M. and Wozniak, J. (1986c). Two cases of factitious AIDS. *American Journal of Psychiatry*, **143**, 1483.

Miller, D., Acton, T. and Hedge, B. (1988). The worried well: their identification and management. *Journal of the Royal College of Physicians of London*, **22**, 158–65.

Miller, R., Goldman, E., Bor, R. and Kerkoff, P. (1989). Counselling children and adults about HIV/AIDS: the ripple effect on haemophilia care settings. *Counselling Psychology Quarterly*, **2**, 65–72.

Miller, E.N., Selnes, O.A., McArthur, J.C., Satz, P., Becker, J.T., Cohen, B. et al (1990). Neuropsychological performance in HIV–1-infected homosexual men: The multicenter AIDS cohort study (MACS). *Neurology*, **40**, 197–203.

Miller, E.N., Satz, P. and Visscher, B. (1991a). Computerised and conventional neuropsychological assessment of HIV-1 infected homosexual men. *Neurology*, **41**, 1608–1616.

Miller, R., Bor, R., Salt, H. and Murray, D. (1991b). Counselling patients with HIV infection about laboratory test with predictive value. *AIDS Care*, **2**, 159–64.

Miller, E.N., Satz, P., Bing, E.G. and van Gorp, W.G. (1992). Methodological issues in the assessment of human immunodeficiency virus-related syndrome-related cognitive impairment. *Archives of General Psychiatry* **49**, 586–7.

Milner, G. (1989). Organic reaction in AIDS. *British Journal of Psychiatry*, **154**, 255–7.

Mishu, B. and Schaffner, W. (1993). HIV-infected surgeons and dentists: looking back and looking forward. *Journal of the American Medical Association*, **269**, 1843–4.

Mitchell, J.E., Marshall, D.W., Goethe, E., Leger, D. and Boswell, R.N. (1989). Human immunodeficiency virus (HIV): immune system and neuropsychological functioning. *Neurology*, **39** (suppl.), 199.

Modan, B., Goldschmidt, R., Rubinstein, E., Vonsover, A., Zinn, M., Golan, R. et al (1992). Prevalence of HIV antibodies in transsexual and female prostitutes. *American Journal of Public Health* **82**, 590–92.

Mok, J.Q., Giaquinto, C., De Rossi, A., Grosch-Worner, I., Ades, A.E. and Peckham, C.S. (1990). Infants born to mothers seropositive for human immunodeficiency virus. Preliminary findings from a multicentre European study. *Lancet*, **1**, 1164–8.

Monroe, S., Bromet, E., Connell, M. and Steiner, S. (1986). Social support, life events and depressive symptoms: a 1 year prospective study. *Journal of Consulting and Clinical Psychology*, **54**, 424–31.

Morgan, M. and Jones, J. (1993). Intentional self-infection with HIV by long-term partners of HIV positive homosexual men. *AIDS Patient Care*, **7**, 10–15.

Morin, S., Charles, K. and Malyon, A. (1984). The psychological impact of AIDS on gay men. *American Psychologist*, **39**, 1288–93.

Morris, M. (1991). American legislation on AIDS. *British Medical Journal*, **303**, 325–6.

Morissette, M. (1990). AIDS and palliative care. *Journal of Palliative Care*, **6**, 26–31.

Moss, A.R., Osmond, D., Bachetti, J.C., Chermann, J.C., Barre-Sinoussi, F. and Carlson, J. et al (1988). Risk factors for AIDS and HIV seropositivity in homosexual men. *American Journal of Epidemiology*, **125**, 1035–47.

Moss, V. (1988). The Mildmay approach. *Journal of Palliative Care, 4, 102–6.*

Moss, V. (1990). Palliative care in advanced HIV disease: presentation, problems and palliation. AIDS, **4** (suppl. 1), S235-S242.

Mulleady, G. (1992). *Counselling drug users about HIV and AIDS*. Blackwell Scientific Publications, Oxford.

Mulleady, G., Riccio, M. and Hogarth, S. (1989). HIV infection and drug users: setting up support groups. *Counselling psychology Quarterly*, **2**, 53–7.

Munckhof, W. and Jenkins, K. (1993). Factitious AIDS, Australian and New Zealand Journal of Medicine, **23**, 524.

Mundinger, A., Adam, T., Ott, D., Dinkel, E., Beck, A., Peter H.H. et al (1991). CT and MRI: prognostic tools in patients with AIDS. *Neuroradiology*, **35**, 75–8.

Murphie-Corb, M., Martin, L.N., Davison-Fairburn, B., Montelaro R.C., Miller, M., West, M. et al (1989). A formalin-inactivated whole SIV vaccine confers protection in macaques. *Science*, **246**, 1293–7.

Murphy, S. (1990). Rape, sexually transmitted diseases and HIV infection. *International Journal of STD and AIDS*, 1, 79–82.

Murphy, S., Kitchen, V., Harris, J. and Forster, S. (1989). Rape and subsequent seroconversion to HIV. *British Medical Journal*, **299**, 718.

Murphy, D., Kelly, J., Brasfield, T., Koob, J., Bahr, R. and Lawrence, J. (1991). Predictors of depression among persons with HIV infection. *VIIth International Conference on AIDS*, Florence, 1991.

Myers, T., Rowe, C. and Tudiver, F. (1992). HIV, substance use and related behaviour of gay and bisexual men: an examination of the talking sex project cohort. *British Journal of Addiction*, **87**, 207–14.

Nashman, H.W., Hoare, C.H. and Heddesheimer, J.C. (1990). Stress and satisfaction among professionals who care for AIDS patients: an exploratory study. *Hospital Topics*, **68**, 22–8.

Navia, B.A. and Price, R.W. (1987). The acquired immunodeficiency syndrome dementia complex as the presenting or sole manifestation of human immunodeficiency virus infection. *Archives of Neurology*, **44**, 65–9.

Navia, B.A., Jordan B.D. and Price, R.W. (1986a). The AIDS dementia complex: I clinical features. *Annals of Neurology*, **19**, 517–14.

Navia, B.A., Cho E., Petito C.K. and Price, R.W. (1986b). The AIDS dementia complex: II neuropathology. *Annals of Neurology*, **19**, 525–35.

Nelson, M.R., Bower, M., Smith, D., Reed, C., Shanson, D. and Gazzard, B.G. (1990). The value of serum cryptococcal antigen in the diagnosis of cryptococcal infection in patients infected with the human immunodeficiency virus. *Journal of Infection*, **21**, 175–81.

Nelson, J.A., Wiley, C.A., Reynolds-Kohler, C., Reese, C.E., Margaretten, W. and Levy, J.A. (1988). Human immunodeficiency virus detected in bowel epithelium from patients with gastrointestinal symptoms. *Lancet*, **i**, 259–62.

Neugebauer, R., Rabkin, J., Williams, J., Remien, R., Goetz, R. and Gorman, J. (1992). Bereavement reactions among homosexual men experiencing multiple losses in the AIDS epidemic. *American Journal of Psychiatry*, **149**, 1374–9.

Nevou, P.J., Taghzouti, K., Dantzer, R., Simon, H. and Le Moal, M. (1986). Modulation of mitogen-induced lymphoproliferation by cerebral neocortex. *Life Sciences*, **38**, 1907–13.

Nickoloff, S., Neppe, V. and Ries, R. (1989). Factitious AIDS. *Psychosomatics*, **30**, 342–5.

Nicoll, A., McGarrigle, C., Heptonstall, J., Parry, J., Mahoney, A., Nicholas, S. et al (1994). Prevalence of HIV infection in pregnant women in London and elsewhere in England. *British Medical Journal*, **309**, 376–7.

Nicolosi, A., Molinari, S., Musicco, M., Saracco, A., Ziliani, N. and Lazzarin, A. (1991). Positive modification of injecting behaviours among intravenous heroin users from Milan and Northern Italy 1987–1989. *British Journal of Addiction*, **86**, 91–102.

Nicolosi, A., Leite, M., Molinari, S., Musicco, M., Saracco, A. and Lazzarin, A. (1992). Incidence and prevalence trends of HIV infection in intravenous drug usrs attending treatment centres in Milan and Northern Italy, 1986–1990. *Journal of Acquired Immune Deficiency Syndromes, 5, 365–73.*

Noh, S., Chandarana, P., Field, V. and Posthuma, B. (1990). AIDS epidemic, emotional stress, coping and psychological distress in homosexual men. AIDS Education and Prevention, **2**, 272–83.

Nokes, K.M. and Kendrew, J. (1990). Loneliness in veterans with AIDS and its relationship to the development of infections. *Archives of Psychiatric Nursing*, **4**, 271–7.

North, R. and Rothenberg K. (1993). Partner notification and the threat of domestic violence against women with HIV infection. *New England Journal of Medicine*, **329**, 1194–6.

Novick, B.E and Rubinstein, A. (1987). AIDS—the paediatric perspective. *AIDS*, **1**, 3–7

Nurnberg, H., Prudic, J., Fiori, M. and Freedman, E. (1984). Psychopathology complicating AIDS. *American Journal of Psychiatry*, **141**, 95–6.

Nuwer, M.R., Miller, E.N., Visscher, B.R. and Satz, P. (1991). Correspondence: early neurologic abnormalities in HIV infection. *The New England Journal of Medicine*, **14**, 324.

Nuwer, M.R., Miller, E.-N., Visscher, B.R., Njedermeyes, E., Packwood, J.N., Carlson, L.G., et al (1992). Asymptomasic HIV infection does not cause ECG abnormalities: results from the Multi-center AIDS cohort study (MACS). *Neurology*, **92**, 42, 1214–19.

O'Brien, K., Wortman, C., Kesler, R. and Joseph, J. (1993). Social relationships of men at risk of AIDS. *Social Science and Medicine*, **30**, 1161–7.
O'Donnell, I., Catalán, J. and Farmer, R. (1992). Suicidal behaviour and HIV disease—a case report. *Counselling Psychology Quarterly*, **5**, 411–15.
O'Dowd, M.A. (1988). Psychosocial issues in HIV infection. *AIDS*, **2**, (suppl. 1), S201–S205.
O'Dowd, M.A. and McKegney, F.P. (1988). Manic syndrome associated with zidovudine. *Journal of the American Medical Association*, **260**, 3587.
O'Dowd, M.A. and McKegney, F.P. (1990). AIDS patients compared with others seen in psychiatric consultation. *General Hospital Psychiatry*, **12**, 50–5.
O'Dowd, M.A., Kaplan, I., Freedman, J., Bernstein, G. and McKegney, F.P. (1992). Characteristics of HIV patients who attempt suicide while attending a psychiatric clinic. *VIIIth International Conference on AIDS*, Amsterdam, 1992
Ollo, C., Johnson, R. and Grafman, J. (1991). Signs of cognitive change in HIV disease: an event-related brain potential study. *Neurology*, **41**, 109–215.
Olsen, W.L., Longo, F.M., Mills, C.M. and Norman, D. (1988). White matter disease in AIDS: findings at MR imaging. *Radiology*, **169**, 445–8.
Omoto, A.M. and Snyder, M. (1990). Basic research in action: volunteerism and society's response to AIDS. *Personality and Social Psychology Bulletin*, **16**, 152–65.
Orenstein, J.M., Chiang, J., Steinberg, W., Smith, P.D., Rotterdam, H. and Kotler, D.P. (1990). Intestinal microsporidiosis as a cause of diarrhoea in human immunodeficiency virus-infected patients: a report of 20 cases. *Human Pathology*, **21**, 475–81.
Orr, D. and Langefeld, C. (1993). Factors associated with condom use by sexually active male adolescents at risk for sexually transmitted disease. *Peadiatrics*, **91**, 873–9.
Orth, J., Ollivier, B., Vinti, H. and Cassuto, J. (1991). Occurrence of acute mania in two patients during ddI treatment at a dose of 750 mg/24h. *VIIth International Conference on AIDS*, Florence, 1991.
Ostrow, D.G. (ed.) (1990). *Behaviourial aspects of AIDS*. Plenum Medical Books Company, New York.
Ostrow, D.G., Joseph, J., Monjan, A., Kessler, R., Emmons, C., Phair, J. et al (1986). Psychosocial aspects of AIDS risk. *Psychopharmacology Bulletin*, **22**, 678–83.
Ostrow, D.G., Grant, I. and Atkinson, J.H. (1988). Assessment and management of the AIDS patient with neuropsychiatric disturbance. *Journal of Clinical Psychiatry*, **49**, 14–22.
Ostrow, D.G., Joseph, J., Kessler, R., Soucy, J., Tal, M., Eller, M. et al (1989a). Disclosure of HIV antibody status: behavioral and mental correlates. *AIDS Education and Prevention*, **1**, 1–11.
Ostrow, D.G., Monjan, A., Joseph, J., van Raden, M., Fox, R., Kingsley, L. et al (1989b). HIV-related symptoms and psychological factors in a cohort of homosexual men. *American Journal of Psychiatry*, **146**, 737–42.
Ostrow, D.G., Van Raden, M., Fos, R., Kingsley, L., Dudley J. and Kaslow R. (1990). Recreational drug use and sexual behaviour in a cohort of homosexual men. *AIDS*, **4**, 759–65.
Ostrow, D.G., Whitaker, R., Frasier, K., Cohen, C., Wan, J., Frank, C. et al (1991). Racial differences in social support and mental health in men with HIV infection: a pilot study. *AIDS Care*, **3**, 55–62.
Ostrow, D.G., Harris, H. and Mill, K. (1992). Assessing a new model: inpatient subacute care for HIV-related dementia. *VIIIth International Conference on AIDS*, Amsterdam, 1992
Otten, M.W., Zaidi, A.A., Wroten, J., Witte, K. and Peterman, T. (1993). Changes in

sexually transmitted disease rates after HIV testing and post-test counselling, Miami, 1988 to 1989. *American Journal of Public Health* **83**, 529–33.

Ou, C.Y., Ciesielski, C.A., Myers, G., Bandea, C.I., Luo, C.C., Korber, B.J. et al (1993). Molecular epidemiology of HIV transmission in a dental practice. *Science*, **256**, 1165–71

Pace, J., Brown, G., Rundell, J., Paolucci, S., Drexler, K. and McManis, S. (1990). Prevalence of psychiatric disorders in a mandatory screening program for HIV: a pilot study. *Military Medicine*, **155**, 76–80.

Padian, N., O'Brien, T., Chang, Y., Glass, S. and Francis, D. (1993). Prevention of heterosexual transmission of HIV through couple counselling. *Journal of AIDS*, **6**, 1043–8.

Paepe, M. de and Waxman, M. (1989). Testicular atrophy in AIDS: a study of 57 autopsy cases. *Human Pathology*, **20**, 210–14

Paine S.L. and Briggs, D. (1988). Knowledge and attitudes of Victorian medical practitioners in relation to acquired immunodeficiency syndrome. *Medical Journal of Australia*, **148**, 221–5.

Pakesch, G., Loimer, N., Grunberger, J., Pfersmann, D., Linzmeyer, L. and Mayerhofer, S. (1992). Neuropsychological and psychiatric symptoms in HIV–1 infected and non-infected drug users. *Psychiatry Research*, **41**, 163–77.

Palestine A.G., Rodrigues M.M., Macher, A.M., Chan, C.C., Lane, H.C., Fauci, S. et al (1984). Ophthalmic involvement in acquired immunodeficiency syndrome. *Opthalmology*, **91**, 1092–9.

Pang, H., Pugh, K. and Catalán, J. (1994). Gender identity disorder and HIV disease. *International Journal of STD and AIDS*, **5**, 130–2.

Papathomopoulos, E. (1989). Intentional infection with the AIDS virus as a means of suicide. *Counselling Psychology Quarterly*, **2**, 79–81.

Papavasilou, A., Aronis, S. and Stamboulis, E. (1991). Involvement of central and peripheral nervous system of HIV infected haemophiliac children. *International Conference on the Neuroscience of HIV Infection*, Padua, 1991.

Parish, K., Mandel, J., Thomas, J., Gomperts, E., Steinhart, B. and Addiego, J. (1989). Psychosocial and sexual adjustment to AIDS risk among persons with haemophilia. *Vth International Conference on AIDS*, Montreal, 1989.

Parisi, A., Strosselli, M. and di Perri, G. (1988a). Electroencephalography in the early diagnosis of HIV-related subacute encephalitis: analysis of 185 patients. *Clinical Electroencephalography*, **20**, 1–5.

Parisi, A., di Perri, G., Strosselli, M., Sandrini, G., Cairoli, S., Minoli, L. et al (1988b). Instrumental evidence of zidovudine effectiveness in the treatment of HIV-associated subacute encephalitis (letter). *AIDS*, **2**, 482–3.

Parisi, A., di Perri, G. and Strosselli, M. (1989). Usefulness of computerised electro-encephalography in diagnosing, staging and monitoring AIDS-dementia complex. *AIDS*, **3**, 209–13.

Parkes, C.M. (1986). Care of the dying: the role of the psychiatrist. *British Journal of Hospital Medicine*, **36**, 250–5.

Parkes, C.M. (1970). The first year of bereavement: a longitudinal study of the reaction of London widows to the death of husbands. *Psychiatry*, **33**, 444–67.

Parkes, C.M. (1972). *Bereavement studies of grief in adult life*. International Universities Press, New York.

Parmar, M., Boag, F., Jayasuriya, P. and Catalán, J. (1990). Feigned HIV disease. *International Journal of STS and AIDS*, **1**, 447–9.

Pascal, S., Resnick, L., Barker, W., Loewenstein, D., Yoshito, F., Change, J. et al

(1991). Metabolic asymmetries in asymptomatic HIV–1 seropositive subjects: relationship to disease onset and MRI findings. *Journal of Nuclear Medicine*, **32**, 1725–9.

Pasqual-Marsettin, E., Ciavarella, N., Ghirardini, A., Di Cagno, V., Lobaccaro, C., Moscatello, A. et al (1992). HIV negative haemophiliacs are more anxious and depressed in comparison with HIV positives: 2 year follow-up. *XXth International Congress of the World Federation of Haemophilia*, Athens, 1992.

Pattman, R. and Gould, E., (1993). Partner notification for HIV infection in the United Kingdom: a look back on seven years experience in Newcastle Upon Tyne. *Genitourinary Medicine*, **69**, 94–7.

Peacock, C.S., Blanshard, C., Tovey, D.G., Ellis, D.S. and Gazzard, B.G. (1991). Histological diagnosis of intestinal microsporidiosis in patiehts with AIDS. *Journal of Clinical Pathology*, **44**, 558–63.

Pederson, C., Thomsen, C., Arlien-Sorborg, J., Praestholm, H., Kjoer, L., Boesen, F. et al, (1991). Central nervous system involvement in human immunodeficiency virus disease. *Danish Medical Bulletin*, **738**, 374–9.

Perdices, M. and Cooper, D.A. (1989). Simple and choice reaction time in patients with human immuno-deficiency virus infection. *Annals of Neurology*, **25**, 460–7.

Perdices, M. and Cooper, D.A. (1990). Neuropsychological investigation of patients with AIDS and ARC. *Journal of Acquired Immune Deficiency Syndromes*, **3**, 555–64.

Perdices, M., Dunbar, N., Grunseit, A. and Cooper, D.A. (1991). Neuropsychological changes in asymptomatic HIV-positive subjects following progression to AIDS-related complex. *International Conference on the Neuroscience of HIV Infection*, Padua, 1991.

Perera, S. (1987). Archbishop attacks Chief Constable for dangerous crusade on AIDS. *The Guardian*, 7th January 1987.

Pergami, A., Gala, C., Durbano, F., Zanello, D., Burgess, A.P., Riccio, M. et al (1993). The psychological impact of HIV infection in women: controlled investigation. *Journal of Psychosomatic Research*, **37**, 687–96.

Pergami, A., Catalán, J., Hulme, N., Burgess, A.P. and Gazzard, B.G. (1994a). How should a positive test result be given?: the patients' view. *AIDS Care*, **6**, 21–7.

Pergami, A., Gala, C., Burgess, A.P., Invernizzi, G. and Catalán, J. (1994b). Heterosexuals with HIV infection: a controlled investigation of factors associated with psychiatric morbidity. *Journal of Psychosomatic Research*, **38**, 305–13.

Pergami, A., Catalán, J., Hulme, N., Burgess, A.P. and Gazzard, B.G. (1994c). How should an AIDS diagnosis be given? *International Journal of STD and AIDS*, **5**, 21–4.

Perkins, D., Davidson, E., Leserman, J., Liao, D. and Evans, D. (1993a). Personality disorder in patients infected with HIV: a controlled study with implications for clinical care. *American Journal of Psychiatry*, **150**, 309–15.

Perkins, D., Leserman, J., Murphy, C. and Evans, D. (1993b). Psychosocial predictors of high-risk sexual behaviour among HIV-negative homosexual men. *AIDS Education and Prevention*, **5**, 141–52.

Perkins, D., Stern, R., Golden, R., Murphy, C., Naftolowitz, D. and Evans, D. (1994). Mood disorder in HIV infection: prevalence and risk factors in a non-epicentre of the AIDS epidemic. *American Journal of Psychiatry*, **151**, 233–6.

Perriens, J.H., Mussa, M., Luabeya, M.K., Kayembe, K., Kapita, B., Brown, C. et al (1992). Neurological complications of HIV–1 seropositive internal medicine patients in Kinshasa, Zaire. *Journal of Acquired Immune Deficiency Syndromes*, **5**, 333–40.

Perry, S. (1990). Organic mental disorders caused by HIV: update on early diagnosis and treatment. *American Journal of Psychiatry*, **147**, 696–710.

Perry, S. (1993). Psychiatric treatment of adults with HIV infection. In *Current Psychiatric Treatment* (ed. D. Dunner). Saunders and Co, Philadelphia.

Perry, S. and Tross, S. (1984). Psychiatric problems of AIDS in-patients at the New York Hospital: preliminary report. *Public Health Reports*, **99**, 201–5.

Perry, S. and Jacobsen, P. (1986). Neuropsychiatric manifestations of AIDS-spectrum disorders. *Hospital and Community Psychiatry*, **37**, 135–42.

Perry, S. and Markowitz, J. (1986). Psychiatric interventions fo AIDS-spectrum disorders. *Hospital and Community Psychology*, **37**, 1001–6.

Perry, S. and Markowitz, J. (1988). Counselling for HIV testing. *Hospital and Community Psychiatry*, **39**, 731–9.

Perry, S., Belsky-Barr, B., Barr, W.B. and Jacobsberg, L. (1989). Neuropsychological function in physically asymptomatic HIV seropositive men. *Journal of Neuropsychiatry and Clinical Neuroscience*, **1**, 296–302.

Perry, S., Jacobsberg, L., Fishman, B., Frances, A., Bobo, J., Jacobsberg, B. et al (1990a). Psychiatric diagnosis before serological testing for HIV. *American Journal of Psychiatry*, **147**, 89–93.

Perry, S., Jacobsberg, L. and Fishman, B. (1990b). Suicidal ideation and HIV testing. *Journal of the American Medical Association*, **263**, 679–82.

Perry, S., Fishman, B., Jacobsberg, L., Young, J., Frances, A. (1991). Effectiveness of psycho-educational intervention in reducing emotional distress after HIV antibody testing. *Archives of General Psychiatry* **48**, 143–7.

Perry, S. Fishman, B., Jacobsberg, L. and Frances, A. (1992). Relationships over 1 year between lymphocyte subsets and psychosocial variables among adults with infection by human immunodeficiency syndrome. *Archives of General Psychiatry* **49**, 396–401.

Perry, S., Jacobsberg, L., Card, C., Ashman, T., Frances, A. and Fishman, B. (1993). Severity of psychiatric symptoms after HIV testing. *American Journal of Psychiatry*, **150**, 775–9.

Peters, A., Reid, M. and Griffin S. (1994). Edinburgh drug users: are they injecting and sharing less? *AIDS*, **8**, 521–8.

Peterson, J., Coates, T., Catania, J., Middleton, L., Hilliard, J. and Hearst N. (1992). High-risk sexual behaviour and condom use among gay and bisexual African-American men. *American Journal of Public Health* **82**, 1490–4.

Petito, C.K., Navia, B.A., Cho, E.S., Jordan, B.D., George, G.C., Price, R.C. et al (1985). Vacuolar myelopathy pathologically resembling subacute combination degeneration in patients with acquired immunodeficiency syndrome. *New England Journal Medicine*, **314**, 874–9.

Petito, C.K., Cho, E.S., Lemann, W., Navia, B.A. and Price, R.C. (1986). Neuropathology of AIDS: an autopsy review. *Journal of Neuropathology and Experimental Neurology*, **45**, 643–6.

Peveler, R., Fairburn, C., Boller, I. and Dunger, D. (1992). Eating disorders in adolescents with IDDM. *Diabetes Care*, **15**, 1356–60.

Pierce, C. (1987). Underscore urgency of HIV counselling: several suicides follow positive test. *Clinical Psychiatry News*, **1**, 29.

Pillans, P.I. (1985). Hyponatraemia and confusion in a patient taking ketoconazole. *Lancet*, **1**, 821–2.

Pilowsky, L., Ring, H., Shine, P., Battersby, M. and Lader, M. (1992). Rapid tranquillization: a survey of emergency prescribing in a general hospital. *British Journal of Psychiatry*, **160**, 831–5.

Piot, P., Laga, M., Ryder, R. (1990). The global epidemiology of HIV-1 infection: continuity, heterogenity and change. *Journal of AIDS*, **3**, 403–12.

Pizzo, P.A., Eddy, J., Falloon, J., Balis, F.M., Murphy, R.F., Moss, H. et al (1988).

Effect of continuous intravenous infusion of zidovudine (AZT) in children with symptomatic HIV infection. *New England Journal of Medicine*, **319**, 889–96.

Platt, S. (1991). HIV, AIDS and suicide behaviour. *Newslink*, **17**, 8–9.

Plott, R., Benton, S. and Winslade, W. (1989). Suicide of AIDS patients in Texas: a preliminary report. *Texas Medicine*, **85**, 40–3.

Pohl, P., Vogl, G., Fill, H., Rossler, H., Zangerle, R. and Gertenbrand, F. (1988). Single photon emission tomography in AIDS dementia complex. *Journal of Nuclear Medicine*, **29**, 1382–6.

Polan, H.J., Hellerstein, D. and Amchin J. (1985). Impact of AIDS-related cases on an inpatient therapeutic milieu. *Hospital and Community Psychiatry*, **36**, 173–6.

Pomerance, L.M. and Shields, J.J. (1988). Hospital workers and AIDS: understanding the importance of contact, transmission knowledge, death anxiety and homophobic attitudes. *IVth International Conference on AIDS*, Stockholm, 1988.

Portegies, P., de Gans, J., Lange, J.M., Derix, M.A.M., Speelman, H., Bakker, M. et al (1989). Declining incidence of AIDS dementia complex after introduction of zidovudine treatment. *British Medical Journal*, **299**, 819–21.

Posner, M.I. and Mitchell, R.F. (1967). Chronometric analysis of classification. *Psychological Review*, **, 74**, 392–409.

Post, M.J.D., Tate, L.G., Quencer, R.M., Hensley, G.T., Berger, J.R., Sheremata, W.A. et al (1988). CT, MR and pathology in HIV encephalitis. *American Journal of Radiology*, **9**, 469–76.

Post, M.J.D., Berger, J.R. and Quencer, R.M. (1991). Asymptomatic and neurologically symptomatic HIV-seropositive individuals: prospective evaluation with cranial MR imaging. *Radiology*, **178**, 131–9.

Post, M.J.D., Berger, J.R., Duncan, R., Quencer, R.M., Pall, L. and Winfield, D. (1993). Asymptomatic and neurologically symptomatic HIV-seropositive subjects: results of long-term MR imaging and clinical follow-up. *Radiology*, **188**, 727–33.

Potterat, J., Mehus, A. and Gallwey, J., (1991). Partner notification: operational considerations. *International Journal of STD and AIDS*, **2**, 411–15.

Prasad, S., Waters, B., Hill, P.B., Portera, F.A. and Riely, C. (1992). Psychiatric side-effects of interferon alpha in patient treated for hepatitis C. *Clinical Research*, **40**, 840.

Price, R.W. and Brew, B.J. (1988). AIDS commentary: the AIDS dementia complex. *Journal of Infectious Diseases*, **158**: 1079–83.

Price, R.W., Brew, B. and Sidtis, J.J. (1988). The brain in AIDS: central nervous system HIV–1 infection and AIDS dementia complex. *Science*, **239**, 586–91.

Puentes, A. (1992). A personal perspective on living and dying with AIDS. In *Living and dying with AIDS* (ed. P. Ahmed). Plenum Press, New York.

Pugh, K., O'Donnell, I. and Catalán, J. (1993). Suicide in HIV disease. *AIDS Care*, **4**, 391–9.

Pugh, K., Riccio, M., Jadresic, D., Burgess, A.P., Baldeweg, T., Catalán, J. et al (1994). A longitudinal study of the neuropsychiatric consequences of HIV–1 infection in gay men: II psychosocial and health status at baseline and 12 month follow-up. *Psychological Medicine*, **24**, 897–904.

Quill, T.E. (1991). Death and dignity: a case of individualised decision making. *New England Journal of Medicine*, **324**, 691–4.

Rabkin, J.G. and Harrison, W.M. (1990). Effect of imipramine on depression and immune status in a sample of men with HIV infection. *American Journal of Psychiatry*, **147**, 495–7.

Rabkin, J., Williams, J., Neugebauer, R., Remien, R. and Goetz, R. (1990a). Maintenance of hope in HIV-spectrum homosexual men. *American Journal of Psychiatry*, **147**, 1322–226.

Rabkin, J.G., Williams, R.B.W., Remien, R.H., Goetz, R.R., Ketzner, R. and Gorman, J.M. (1990b). Depression, lymphocyte subsets and human immunodeficiency virus symptoms on two occasions in HIV-positive homosexual men. *Archives of General Psychiatry* **48**, 111–19.

Rabkin, J., Remien, R., Katoff, L. and Williams, J. (1993). Suicidality in AIDS long-term survivors: what is the evidence? *AIDS Care*, **5**, 401–11.

Rabkin, J.G., Rabkin, R., Harrison, W. and Wagner, G. (1994). Imipramine effects on mood in depressed patientswith HIV illness. *American Journal of Psychiatry*, **151**, 516–23.

Ragazzoni, A., Grippo, A., Ghidini, P., Schiavone, V., Lolli, F., Mazzotta, F. et al (1993). Electrophysiological study of neurologically asymptomatic HIV1 seropositive patients. *Acta Neurologia Scandinavia*, **87**, 47–51.

Raininko, R., Elovaara, I., Virta, A., Valanne, L., Haltia, M. and Valle, S.L. (1992). Radiological study of the brain at various stages of human immunodeficiency virus infection: early development of brain atrophy. *Neuroradiology*, **42**, 190–6.

Rajs, J. and Fugelstad, A. (1992). Suicide related to HIV infection in Stockholm. *Acta Psychiatrica Scandinavica*, **85**, 234–9.

Ramsay, N. (1992). Referral to a liaison psychiatrist from a palliative care unit. *Palliative Medicine*, **6**, 54–60.

Ramsay, N., Catalán, J. and Gazzard, B.G. (1992). Eating disorders in men with HIV infection. *British Journal of Psychiatry*, **160**, 404–7.

Rapaport, S. and Braff, D. (1985). AIDS and homosexual panic. *American Journal of Psychiatry*, **142**, 1516.

Raphael, B. (1975). The mangement of pathological grief. *Australian and New Zealand Journal of Psychiatry*, **9**, 173–80.

Raphael, B. (1977a). *The anatomy of bereavement: a handbook for the caring professions*. Unwin Hyman, Boston.

Raphael, B. (1977b). Preventive intervention with the recently bereaved. *Archives of General Psychiatry* **34**, 1450–4.

Ratigan, B. (1993). Psychoanalytic psychotherapy in treatment of patients with border-line or narcissistic personality disorders affected by HIV infection. *IXth International Conference on AIDS*, Berlin, 1993.

Reboli, A. and Mandler, H. (1992). Encephalopathy and psychosis associated with sulfadiazine in two patients with AIDS and CNS xoplasmosis. *Clinical Infectious Diseases*, **15**, 556–7.

Reeves, R.R. (1992). Ciprofloxacine-induced psychosis. *Annals of Pharmacotherapy*, **26**, 930–1.

Reidel, R.R., Helmstaedter, C., Bulau, P., Durwen, H.F., Bracjman, H., Fimmers, R. et al (1991). Early signs of cognitive deficits among human immunodeficiency virus-positive hemophiliacs. *Acta Psychiatrica Scandinavia*, **85**, 321–26.

Reidy, M., Taggart, M.E. and Asselin, L. (1991). Psychological needs expressed by the natural caregivers of HIV infected children. *AIDS Care*, **3**, 331–43.

Reitan, R. (1958). Validity of the trail making test as an indication of organic brain damage. *Perceptual and Motor Skills*, **8**, 271–6.

Remacha, A.F., Riera, A., Cadafalch, J. and Gimferrer, E. (1991). Vitamin B12 abnorm-alities in HIV–1 infected patients. *European Journal of Haematology*, **47**, 60–4.

Remien, R., Rabkin, J. and Williams, J. (1992). Coping strategies and health beliefs of AIDS long-term survivors. *Psychology and Health*, **6**, 335–45.

Renoux, G., Biziere, K., Renoux, R., Guillaumin, J. and Degenne, D. (1983). A balanced brain asymmetry modulates T-cell-mediated events. *Journal of Neuroimmunology*, **5**, 227–38.

Reyes, M., Faraldi, F., Senseng, C., Flowers, C. and Fariello, R. (1991). Nigral degeneration in AIDS. *Acta Neuropathologica*, **82**, 39–44.

Rhodes, T., Donoghue, M., Hunter, G. and Stimson G. (1993). Sexual behaviour of drug injectors in London; implications for HIV transmission and HIV prevention. *British Journal of Addiction*, **88**, 1553–60.

Ricci, S., Francisci, D., Longo, V. and del Favero, A. (1988). CNS side-effects of antiretroviral drugs. *International Journal of Clinical Pharmacology, Therapy and Toxicity*, **26**, 400–8.

Riccio, M. and Thompson, C. (1987). Pseudo-AIDS, AIDS panic or AIDS phobia? British Journal of Psychiatry, **151**, 863.

Riccio, M., Burgess, A.P., Hawkins, D.A., Wilson, B. and Thompson, C. (1990). Neuropsychological and psychiatric changes following treatment of ARC patients with zidovudine. *International Journal of STD and AIDS*, **1**, 435–7.

Riccio, M., Pugh, K., Jadresic, D., Burgess, A.P., Thompson, C, Wilson, B. et al (1993). Neuropsychiatric aspects of HIV–1 infection in gay men: controlled investigation of psychiatric, neuropsychological and neurological status. *Journal of Psychosomatic Research*, **37**, 819–30.

Riccio, M. et al (submitted). The efficacy of zidovudine in preventing or limiting the severity of HIV associated CNS dysfunction: prospective controlled investigation of neuropsychological and neurophysiological function in asymptomatic HIV seropositive men taking part in the concorde trial.

Richards, T. (1986). Don't tell me on a Friday. *British Medical Journal*, **292**, 943.

Robert, L., Chamberland, M. and Marcus, R. (1993). HIV-infected health care workers (HCW): look back investigation update. *Abstracts of the Society for Hospital Epidemiology of America, Chicago, Ill.*

Roberts, J. (1992). US Congress bypasses peer review system. British Medical Journal, **305**, 1179.

Roberts, J. (1994). Decisions in US say that doctors can assist suicides. *British Medical Journal*, **308**, 1255.

Robertson, J., Bucknall, A. and Welsby, P. (1986). Epidemic of AIDS-related infection among intravenous drug users. *British Medical Journal*, **292**, 527–9.

Robertson, P., Bhate, S. and Bhate, M. (1991). AIDS: education and adults with a mental handicap. *Journal of Mental Deficiency Research*, **35**, 475–80.

Robertson, K.R., Stern, R.A., Hall, C.D., Perkins, D.O., Wilkins, J.W., Gortner, D.T. et al (1993). Vitamin B_{12} deficiency and nervous system disease in HIV infection. Archives of Neurology, **50**, 807–11.

Robins, E., Gassner, S., Kayes, J., Wilkinson, R.H. and Murphy, G.E. (1959). The communication of suicide intent: a study of 134 successful (completed) suicides. *American Journal of Psychiatry*, **115**, 724–33.

Robins, L., Helzer, J., Crougan, J. and Ratcliff, S. (1981). National Institute of Mental Health diagnostic interview schedule. *Archives of General Psychiatry* **38**, 381–89.

Robins, L., Helzer, J., Weissman, M., Orvaschel, H., Gruenberg, E., Burke, J. et al (1984). Lifetime prevalence of specific disorders in three sites. *Archives of General Psychiatry* **41**, 949–58.

Robinson, P. and Holden, N. (1986). Bulimia nervosa in the male: a report of 9 cases. *Psychological Medicine*, **16**, 795–803.

Robinson, E. and Latham, R. (1987). A factitious case of AIDS. *Sexually Transmitted Diseases*, **14**, 54–7.

Rodin, G., Craven, J. and Littlefield, C. (1991). *Depression in the medically ill: an integrated approach*. Brunner/Mazel Publishers, New York.

Rogers, C. and Klatt, E. (1988). Pathology of the testis in AIDS. *Histopathology*, **12**, 659–65.

Rogers, D. (1992). *Motor disorder in psychiatry: towards a neurological psychiatry*. John Wiley and Sons, Chichester.

Rogers, A.S., Froggart, J.W., Townsend, T., Gordon, T., Leigh Brown, A.J. et al (1993). Investigation of potential transmission to patients of an HIV infected surgeon. *Journal of the American Medical Association*, **269**, 1795–1801.

Ronald, P., Robertson, J., Duncan, B. and Thompson, A. (1993). Chidren of parents infected with HIV in Lothian. *British Medical Journal*, **306**, 649–50.

Ronchi, D. de, Faranca, I., Volterra, V., Lazzari, C. and Chiodo, F. (1992). Psychosis in patients with HIV infection. *Abstracts of World Psychiatric Association and Italian Psychiatric Association Regional Symposium*, 202, Palermo.

Rosci, M.A., Pigorini, F., Bernabel, A., Pau, F.M., Merigliano, D.E., Meligrana M.F. et al (1992). Methods for detecting early signs of AIDS dementia complex in asymptomatic HIV-1-infected subjects. *AIDS*, **6**, 1309–16.

Rose, N. (ed.) (1994). Essential Psychiatry (2nd edn). Blackwell Scientific Publications, Oxford.

Rosen, M. (1992). Euthanasia. *British Medical Journal*, **305**, 951.

Rosengren, A., Orth-Gomer, K., Wedel, H. and Wilhelmsen, L. (1993). Stressful life events, social support and mortality in men born in 1933. *British Medical Journal*, **307**, 1102–5.

Ross, H., Glasser, F. and Germanson, T. (1988). The prevalence of psychiatric disease in patients with alcohol and other drug problems. *Archives of General Psychiatry* **45**, 1023–31.

Ross, M.W. and Seeger, V. (1988). Determinants of reported burnout in health professionals associated with the care of patients with AIDS. *AIDS*, **2**, 395–7.

Ross, J. and Scott G. (1993). The association between HIV media campaigns and number of patients coming forward for HIV antibody testing. *Genitourinary Medicine*, **69**, 193–5.

Ross, M.W., Stowe, A., Wodak, A., Miller, M.E. and Gold J. (1993). A comparison of drug use and HIV infection risk behaviour between injecting drug users currently in treatment, previously in treatment and never in treatment. *Journal of Acquired Immune Deficiency Syndromes*, **6**, 518–28.

Rosse, R.B. (1985). Reactions of psychiatric staff to an AIDS patient, *American Journal of Psychiatry*, **142**, 523.

Rotheram-Borus, M.J., Koopman, C. and Haignere, C. (1991). Reducing HIV sexual risk behaviour among runaway adolescents. *Journal of the American Medical Association*, **266**, 1237–41.

Rottenberg, D.A., Moeller, J.R., Strother, S.C., Sidtis, J.J., Navia, B.A., Dhawan, D. et al (1987). The metabolic pathology of the AIDS dementia complex. *Annals of Neurology*, **22**, 700–6.

Routy, J., Prajs, E., Blanc, A., Drony, S., Moriceau, M., Sarrazin, C. et al (1989). Seizure after zidovudine overdose. *Lancet*, **i**, 384–5.

Routy, J.P., Blanc, A.P., Rodriguez, E., Escoffier, M., Joliot, Y., Kiegel, P. et al (1990). Intrathecal zidovudine for AIDS dementia. *Lancet*, **336**, 248

Royal, W. III, Updike, M., Selnes, O.A., Proctor, T.V., Nance-Spronson, L., Solomon,

L. et al (1991). HIV–1 infection and nervous system abnormalities among a cohort of intravenous drug users. *Neurology*, **41**, 1905–10.

Rubinow, D.R. , Berrettini, C.H. and Brouwers, P. (1988). Neuropsychiatric consequences of AIDS. *Annals of Neurology*, **23** (suppl.), S24–S26.

Rubinstein, A., Monnecki, R., Silverman, B., Rharytan, M. Zion Krieger B., Andiman, W. et al (1986). Pulmonary disease in children with acquired immunodeficiency syndrome and AIDS-related complex. *Journal of Paediatrics*, **108**, 498–503.

Rundell, J., Thomason, J., Zajac, R. and Beatty, R. (1988). Psychiatric diagnosis and attempted suicide in HIV infected USAF personnel. *IVth International Conference on AIDS*, Stockholm, 1988.

Russell, G. (1979). Bulimia nervosa: an ominous variant of anorexia nervosa. *Psychological Medicine*, **9**, 429–48.

Sacks, M., Dermatis, H., Looser-Ott, S., Burton, W. and Perry, S. (1992). Undetected HIV infection among ill psychiatric patients. *American Journal of Psychiatry*, **149**, 544–5.

Salkovskis, P. and Warwick, H. (1986). Morbid preoccupations, health anxiety and reassurance: a cognitive-behaviourial approach to hypochondriasis. *Behaviour Research and Therapy*, **24**, 597–602.

Santana, R.T., Monzon, O., Hearst, N., Mandel, J. and Hall, T. (1991). A randomized controlled intervention trial to improve AIDS-related attitudes and professional competence of health care workers in Metro Manila hospitals *VIIth International Conference on AIDS*, Florence, 1991.

Satz, P. (1993). Brain reserve capacity on symptom onset after brain injury: a formulation and review of evidence for threshold theory. *Neuropsychology*, **7**, 273–95.

Satz, P., Morgernstern, H., Miller, E.N., Selnes, O.A., McArthur, J.C., Cohen, B. et al (1993). Low education as a possible risk factor for cognitive abnormalities in HIV–1: findings from the multicenter AIDS cohort study (MACS). *Journal of Acquired Immune Deficiency Syndromes*, **6**, 503–11.

Saunders, P. (1994). GP facilitators and HIV infection. *British Medical Journal*, **308**, 2–3.

Saykin, A., Janssen, R., Sprehn, G., Kaplan, J., Spira, T. and O'Connor, B. (1992). Longitudinal evaluation of neuropsychological function in homosexual men with HIV infection: 18 month follow-up. *Journal of Neuropsychiatry and Clinical Neuroscience*, **3**, 286–98.

Schaerf, F., Miller, R., Pearlson, G., Kaminsky, M. and Weaver, D. (1988). Manic syndrome associated with zidovudine. *Journal of the American Medical Association*, **260**, 3587–8.

Schaerf, F., Miller, R., Lipsey, J. and McPherson, R. (1989). ECT and major depression in patients with HIV. *American Journal of Psychiatry*, **146**, 782–4.

Schechter, M., Hogg, R., Aylward, B., Craib, K., Le, T. and Montaner, J. (1994). Higher socioeconomic status is associated with slower progression of HIV infection independent of access to health care. *Journal of Clinical Epidemiology*, **47**, 59–67.

Schielke, E., Tatsch, K., Pfister, H.W., Trenkwalder, C., Leinsinger, G., Kirsch, C.M. et al (1990). Reduced cerebral blood flow in early stages of HIV infection. *Archives of Neurology*, **47**, 1342–5.

Schietinger, H., Almedal, C., Marianne, B.N., Jacqueline, R.K. and Raven, B. (1993). Teaching Rwandan families to care for people with AIDS at home. *The Hospice Journal*, **9**, 33–52.

Schleifer, S., Keller, S., Franflin, J., La Farge, S. and Miller, S. (1990). HIV seropositivity in inner-city alcoholics. *Hospital and Community Psychiatry*, **41**, 248–9.

Schmidt, U. and Miller, D. (1988). Two cases of hypomania in AIDS. *British Journal of Psychiatry*, **152**, 839–42.

Schmitt, F.A., Bigley, J.W., McKinnis, R., Logue, P.E., Evans, R.W., Drucker, J.L. et al (1988). Neuropsychological outcome of zidovudine (AZT) treatment of patients with AIDS and AIDS-related complex. *New England Journal of Medicine*, **319**, 1573–8.

Schneider, S., Taylor, S., Hammen, C., Kemeny, M. and Dudley, J. (1991a). Factors influencing suicide intent in gay and bisexual suicide ideation. *Journal of Personality and Social Psychology*, **61**, 776–88.

Schneider, S., Taylor, S., Kemeny, M. and Hammen, C. (1991b). AIDS-related factors predictive of suicidal ideation of low and high intent among gay and bisexual men. *Suicide and Life Threatening Behaviour*, **21**, 313–28.

Schofferman, J. (1987). Hospice care of the patient with AIDS. *The Hospice Journal*, **3**, 51–74.

Scurlock, H., Singh, A. and Catalán, J. (1994). Use of remoxipride in the treatment of manic syndromes in HIV–1 infection. *IInd International Conference on the Biopsychosocial aspects of HIV infection*, Brighton, 1994.

Searle, E.S. (1987). Knowledge, attitudes and behaviour of health professionals in relation to AIDS. *Lancet*, **1**, 26–9.

Segal, M. (1988). Pseudo-AIDS, AIDS panic, or AIDS phobia. *British Journal of Psychiatry*, **152**, 424–5.

Seidl, O., and Goebel, F.D. (1984). Psychosomatic reactions of homosexuals and drug addicts to the knowledge of a positive HIV test result. *AIDS-Forschung (AIFO)*, **4**, 181–7.

Seidman, S. and Rieder, R. (1994). A review of sexual behaviour in the United States. *American Journal of Psychiatry*, **151**, 330–41.

Selnes, O.A., Miller, E.N., McArthur, J.C., Gordon, B., Muñoz, A., Sheridan, K. et al (1990). HIV–1 infection: no evidence of cognitive decline during the asymptomatic stages. *Neurology*, **40**, 204–8.

Selnes, O.A., McArthur, J.C., McArthur, J.H. and Saah, A. (1991). Incident HIV dementia in the multicenter AIDS cohort study: patterns of cognitive decline. *International Conference on the Neuroscience of HIV Infection, Padua*, 1991.

Selnes, O.A., McArthur, J.C., Royal III, W., Updike, M.L., Nance-Spronson, T., Concha, M. et al (1992). HIV–1 infection and intravenous drug use: longitudinal neuropsychological evaluation of asymptomatic subjects. *Neurology*, **42**, 1924–9.

Selwyn, P., Carter, R., Shoenbaume, E., Robertson, V., Klein R. and Rogers M. (1989). Knowledge of HIV status and decisions to continue or terminate pregnancy among intravenous drug users. *Journal of the American Medical Association*, **261**, 3567–71.

Selzer, M.L. (1971). The Michigan alcohol screening test: the quest for a new diagnostic instrument. *American Journal of Psychiatry*, **127**, 1653–8.

Semprini, A., Levi-Setti, P., Bozzo, M., Ravizza, M., Taglioretti, A., Sulpizio, P. et al (1992). Insemination of HIV negative women with processed semen of HIV positive partners. *The Lancet*, **340**, 1317–19.

Sensky, T. (1990). Patients' reactions to illness. *British Medical Journal*, **300**, 622–3.

Serrano, Y., Faruque, S., Lauffer, H. and Clatts, M. (1993). Assessment of street outreach for HIV prevention in selected sites. *Morbidity and Mortality Weekly Report*, **42**, 873–80.

Seth, R., Granville-Grossman, K., Goldmeier, D. and Lynch, S. (1991). Psychiatric illness in patients with HIV infection and AIDS referred to the liaison psychiatrist. *British Journal of Psychiatry*, **159**, 347–50.

Sewell, D., Jeste, D., Atkinson, J.H., Heaton, R., Hesselink, J., Wiley, C. et al (1994).

HIV-associated psychosis: a study of 20 cases. *American Journal of Psychiatry*, **151**, 237–42.

Shapiro, M.F., Hayward, R.A., Guillemot, D. and Jayle, D. (1992). Residents' experiences in, and attitudes toward, the care of persons with AIDS in Canada, France, and the United States. *Journal of the American Medical Association*, **268**, 510–5.

Sharpe, M., Peveler, R. and Mayou, R. (1992). The psychological treatment of patients with functional somatic symptoms: a practical guide. *Journal of Psychosomatic Research*, **36**, 515–29.

Sherr, L. (1990). Fear arousal and AIDS: do shock tactics work? *AIDS*, **4**, 361–4.

Sherr, L. (1991). *HIV and AIDS in mothers and babies*. Blackwell Scientific Publications, Oxford.

Sherr, L. and Strong, C. (1992). Safe sex and women. *Genitourinary Medicine*, **68**, 32–5.

Sherr, L., Hedge, B., Steinhart, K., Davey, T. and Petrack, J. (1992). Unique patterns of bereavement in HIV: implications for counselling. *Genitourinary Medicine*, **68**, 378–81.

Sherr, L., Petrak, J., Melvin, D., Davey, T., Glover, L. and Hedge, B. (1993). Psychological trauma associated with HIV infection in women. *Counselling Psychology Quarterly*, **6**, 99–108.

Sherrard, J., Bingham, J. and Onen, T. (1993). Clinical management of HIV disease in intravenous drug users. *International Journal of STD and AIDS*, **4**, 254–60.

Shilts, R. (1987). *And the band played on: politics, people and the AIDS epidemic*. Viking, London.

Ship, J., Wolff, A. and Selik, R. (1991). Epidemiology of AIDS in persons aged 50 years or older. *Journal of AIDS*, **4**, 84–8.

Shuff, I., Horne, A., Westberg, N., Mooney, S. and Mitchell, C. (1991). Volunteers under threat: AIDS hospice volunteers compared to volunteers in a traditional hospice. Hospice Journal, **7**, 85–107.

Sibbald, B. and Freeling, P. (1988). AIDS and the future general practitioner. *Journal of the Royal College of General Practitioners*, **38**, 500–2.

Sidtis, J.J. and Price, R.W. (1990). Early HIV–1 infection and the AIDS dementia complex, *Neurology*, **40**, 323–6.

Sidtis, J.J., Gatsonis, C., Price, R.W., Singer, E.J., Collier, A.C., Richman, D.D. et al (1993). Zidovudine treatment of the AIDS dementia complex: results of a placebo-controlled trial. *Annals of Neurology*, **33**, 343–9.

Sieghart, P. (1989). *AIDS and human rights: a UK perspective*. British Medical Association, London.

Silberman, E.K. and Weingartner, H. (1986). Hemispheric lateralisation of functions related to emotion. *Brain and Cognition*, **5**, 322–53.

Silberstein, C., McKegney, P., O'Dowd, M., Selwyn, P., Schoenbaum, E. et al (1987). A prospective longitudinal study of neuropsychological and psychosocial factors in asymptomatic individuals at risk of HTLV-III infection in methadone programs. *International Journal of Neuroscience*, **32**, 669–76.

Silberstein, C.H. O'Dowd, M.A., Chartock, P., Schoenbaum E.E., Friedland, P. et al (1994). A prospective four-year follow-up of neuropsychological function in HIV seropositive and seronegative methadone-maintained patients. *General Hospital Psychiatry*, **15**, 351–9.

Silverman, D.C. (1993). Psychosocial impact of HIV-related caregiving on health providers: a review of recommendations for the role of psychiatry, *American Journal of Psychiatry*, **150:5**, 705–12.

Simpson, D., Knight, K. and Ray, S. (1993). Psychosocial correlates of AIDS-risk drug use and sexual behaviours. *AIDS Education and Prevention*, **5**, 121–30.

Sims, R. and Moss, V. (1991). *Terminal care for people with AIDS*. Edward Arnold, London.

Sinforiani, E., Mauri, M., Bono, G., Muratori, S., Alessi, E. and Minoli, L. (1991). Cognitive abnormalities and disease progression in a selected population of asymptomatic HIV-positive subjects. *AIDS*, **5**, 1117–20.

Singh, A. and Catalán, J. (1993). The use of SSRIs for the treatment of depression in patients with AIDS. *IXth International Conference on AIDS*, Berlin, 1993.

Singh, S., Hawkins, D.A., Connolly, M. and Gazzard, B.G. (1991). Models of care for the hospital treatment of individuals with HIV infection. *Health Trends*, **23**, 55–9.

Singh, S., Mansfield, S. and King, M. (1993). Primary care and HIV infection in the 1990s. *British Journal of General Practice*, **43**, 182–3.

Singh, A., Burgess, A.P. and Catalán, J. (1994). Pharmacological treatment of depression in patients with AIDS. *IInd International Conference on the Biopsychosocial aspects of HIV infection*, Brighton, 1994.

Skinner, K. (1991). Social care for families affected by HIV infection. In *Caring for chidren with HIV and AIDS* (ed. R. Claxton R and T. Harrison). Edward Arnold, London.

Sladyk, K. (1989). Teaching safe sex practice to psychiatric patients. *American Journal of Occupational Therapy*, **44**, 284–6.

Slome, L., Moulton, J., Huffine, C., Gorter, R. and Abrams, D. (1992). Physicians' attitudes toward assisted suicide in AIDS. *Journal of Acquired Immune Deficiency Syndromes*, **5**, 712–18.

Smith, J. (1990). Manic psychosis as a neuropsychiatric complication of HIV infection. *International Conference on the Neuroscience of HIV Infection*, Monterey, 1990.

Smith, R. (1992). Euthanasia: time for a royal commission. *British Medical Journal*, **305**, 728–9.

Smith, T., Jakobsen, J., Gaub, J., Helweg-Larsen, F. and Trojaborg, W. (1988). Clinical and electrophysiological studies of human immunodeficiency virus-seropositive men without AIDS. *Annals of Neurology*, **23**, 295–7.

Smith, J., Forster, G., Kitchen, V., Hooi, Y., Munday, P., Paintin, D. et al (1991). Infertility management in HIV positive: a dilemma. *British Medical Journal*, **302**, 1447–50.

Smyser, M.S., Bryce, J. and Joseph, J.G. (1990). AIDS-related knowledge, attitudes, and precautionary behaviors among emergency medical professionals. *Public Health Reports*, **105**, 496–504.

Snider, W.D., Simpson, D.M., Nielson, S., Gold, J.W.M., Metroka, C.E. and Posner, J.B. (1983). Neurological complications of acquired immune deficiency syndrome: analysis of 50 patients. *Annals of Neurology*, **14**, 403–18.

Sno, H., Storosum, J. and Swinkels, J. (1989). HIV infection: psychiatric findings in the Netherlands. *British Journal of Psychiatry*, **155**, 814–17.

Soderlund, N., Lavis, J., Broomberg, J. and Mills A. (1993). The costs of HIV prevention strategies in developing countries. *World Health Organisation*, **71**, 595–604.

Solano, L., Costa, M., Salvati, S., Coda, R., Aiuti, F., Mezzaroma, I. et al (1993). Psychosocial factors and clinical evolution in HIV-1 infection: a longitudinal study. *Journal of Psychosomatic Research*, **37**, 39–51.

Somma-Mauvais, H., Regis, H., Gastut, J.L., Gastaut, J.A. and Farnarier, G. (1990). Potentiels evoques multimodaux dans l'infection par le virus de l'immunodeficience humaine. *Revue Neurologique*, **146**, 196–204.

Song, F., Freemantle, N., Sheldon, T., House, A., Watson, P., Long, A. and Mason, J. (1993). Selective serotonin re-uptake inhibitors: meta-analysis of efficacy and acceptability. *British Medical Journal*, **306**, 683–7.

Soni, S. and Windgassen, E. (1991). AIDS panic: effects of mass media publicity. *Acta Psychiatrica Scandinavica*, **84**, 121–24.

Sontag, S. (1988). *AIDS and its metaphors*. Penguin, London.

Sorensen, J., London, J., Heitzmann, C., Gibson, D., Morales, E., Dumontet, R. and Acree, M. (1994). Psychoeducational group approach: HIV risk reduction in drug users. *AIDS Education and Prevention*, **6**, 95–112.

Spear, J., Kessler, H., Lehrman, S. and Miranda, P. (1988). Zidovudine overdosage. *Annals of Internal Medicine*, **109**, 76–7.

Spencer, N., Hoffman, R., Rausky, C., Wolf, F. and Vernon, T. (1993). Partner notification for HIV infection in Colorado: results accross index case groups and costs. *International Journal of STD and AIDS*, **4**, 26–32.

Spielberger, C., Gorsuch, R., Luchene, R., Vagg, P. and Jacobs, G. (1983). *Manual for the State-Trait Anxiety inventory*. Consulting Psychologists Press, Palo Alto, Ca.

Squire, S., Elford, J., Bor, R., Tilsed, G., Salt, H., Bagdades, E. et al (1991). Open access clinic providing HIV-1 results on day of testing: the first twelve months. *British Medical Journal*, **302**, 1383–6.

Stafford, R.S., Janseen, R.S., StLouis, M.E., Petersen, L.R. and Dondero, T.J. (1991). Estimate of HIV-1 infection among US hospital patients. *VIIth International Conference on AIDS*, Florence, 1991.

Stall, R., Ekstrand, M., Pollack, L., McKusick, L. and Coates, T. (1990). Relapse from safer sex: the next challenge for AIDS prevention efforts. *Journal of Acquired Immune Deficiency Syndromes*, **3**, 1181–7.

Stanford, J. (1988). Knowledge and attitudes to AIDS. *Nursing Times*, **84**, 47–50.

Stedeford, A. (1984). *Facing death*. Heinemann Medical, London.

Stein, M., Miller, A.H., and Trestman, R.L. (1991). Depression, the immune system, and health and illness. *Archives of General Psychiatry* **48**, 171–7.

Stern, R. and Fernandez, M. (1991). Group cognitive and behavioural treatment for hypochondriasis. *British Medical Journal*, **303**, 1229–31.

Stern, Y., Marder, K., Bell, K., Chen, J., Doonief, G., Goldstein, S. et al (1991). Multidisciplinary baseline assessment of homosexual men with and without human immunodeficiency virus infection: III neurologic and neuropsychological findings. *Archives of General Psychiatry* **48**, 131–8.

Stern, Y., Marder, K. and Mayeux, R. (1992). Reply to Miller et al (1992). *Archives General Psychiatry* **49**: 587–9.

Sternberg, S. (1969). High-speed-scanning in human memory. *Science*, 652–4.

Stevenson, Y., Kalichman, S., Sikkema, K., Kelly, J., Adair, V., Bulto, M. et al (1994). Outcome of brief behavioural intervention for chronic mentally ill outpatients at risk of HIV. *IInd International Conference on the Biopsychosocial aspects of HIV infection*, Brighton, 1994.

Stewart, A.L., Hays, R.D. and Ware, J.E. (1988). The MOS short form general health survey: reliability and validity in a patient population. *Medical Care*, **26**, 724–35.

Stewart, K., Haley, W. and Saag, M. (1993). Effects of caregiving tasks, social network and patient functioning on informal caregivers of HIV infected men. *IXth International Conference on AIDS*, Berlin, 1993.

Stimson, G. (1991). Risk reduction by drug users with regard to HIV infection. *International Review of Psychiatry*, **3**, 401–15.

St Lawrence, J.S., Kelly, J.A., Owens, T.D., Hogan, I.G. and Wilson, R.A. (1988).

Mental health providers' stigmatization toward persons with AIDS. *IVth International Conference on AIDS*, Stockholm, 1988.
St Lawrence, J., Brasfield, T. and Kelly, J.A. (1990). Factors which predict relapse to unsafe sex by gay men. *VIth International Conference on AIDS*, San Francisco, 1990.
Stockwell, T., Murphy, D. and Hodgson, R. (1983). The severity of alcohol dependence questionnaire: its use, reliability and validity. *British Journal of Addiction*, **78**, 145–55.
Stone, A.A., Bruce, R. and Neale, J.M. (1987). Changes in daily event frequency precede episodes of physical symptoms. *Journal of Human Stress*, **13**, 70–4.
Strang, J. and Stimson, G. (eds) (1990). *AIDS and drug misuse*. Routledge, London.
Striegel-Moore, R., Nicholson, T. and Tamborlane, W. (1992). Prevalence of eating disorder symptoms in preadolescent and adolescent girls with IDDM. *Diabetes Care*, **15**, 1361–8.
Stromgren, E. (1974). Psychogenic psychosis. In *Themes and variations in European psychiatry* (eds. S.R. Hirsch and M. Shepherd). University Press of Virginia, Charlottesville.
Stuz, T., Steiger, T., Wasswefallen, F., Kent, C. and Somani B., (1991). The role of assessment in the production of a presentation campaign. *VIIth International Conference*
on AIDS, Florence, 1991.
Su, T., Pagliaro, M., Schmidt, P., Pickar, D., Wolkowitz, O. and Rubinow, D. (1993). Neuropsychiatric effects of anabolic steroids in male normal volunteers. *Journal of the American Medical Association*, **269**, 2760–4.
Sullivan, J., Kessler, H. and Sha, B. (1993). False-positive HIV test: implications for the patient. *Journal of the American Medical Association*, **269**, 2847.
Summerbell, C., Youle, M., McDonald, V., Catalán, J. and Gazzard, B.G. (1992). Megestrol acetate versus cyproheptadine in the treatment of weight loss associated with HIV infection. *International Journal of STD and AIDS*, **3**, 278–80.
Susser, E., Valencia, E. and Conover, S. (1993). Prevalence of HIV infection among psychiatric patients in a New York City men's shelter. *American Journal of Public Health* **83**, 568–70.
Tait, D.R., Pudifin, D.J., Gathiram, V. and Windsor, I.M. (1992). HIV seroconversions in health care workers, Natal, South Africa. *VIIIth International Conference on AIDS*, Amsterdam, 1992
Takigiku, S., Brubaker, T. and Hennon, C. (1993). A contextual model of stress among parent caregivers of gay sons with AIDS. *AIDS Education and Prevention*, **5**, 25–42.
Tannock, C. and Collier, C. (1989). *We're just in time–AIDS, brain damage and psychiatric hospital closures*. The Bow Group, London.
Tapsfield, W. and Amis, P. (1992). Euthanasia. *British Medical Journal*, **305**, 951.
Tarasoff v. Regents of the University of California, **551**, P 2d, 334 (Cal, 1974).
Tarlov, A., Ware J.E., Greenfield S., Nelson E.C., Perrin E. and Zubkoff, M. (1989). The Medical Outcomes Study: an application of methods for monitoring the results of medical care. *Journal of the American Medical Association*, **262**, 925–30
Taylor, M., Sierles, F. and Abrams, R. (1985). *General hospital psychiatry*. The Free Press, New York and London.
Teguis, A. (1992). Dying with AIDS. In *Living and Dying with AIDS* (ed. P Ahmed). Plenum Press, New York and London.
Temoshok, L., Mandel, J., Moulton, J., Solomon G. and Zich, J. (1986). A longitudinal study of AIDS and ARC in San Francisco. *Annual Meeting of the American Psychiatric Association*, Washington, DC.
Temple, T.M., Leigh, C.B. and Schafer, J. (1993). Unsafe behaviour and alcohol use at the event level: results of a national survey. *Journal of Acquired Immune Deficiency Syndromes*, **6**, 393–401.

Tennison, M.B., Messenheimer J, Whaley, R, Gold, S.,Burchinal M, Hall, C. et al (1992). Neurologic status of HIV-positive hemophiliac children. *International Conference on the Neuroscience of HIV Infection*, Amsterdam, 1992.

Terragna, A., Mazzarello, G., Anselmo, M., Canessa, A. and Rossi, E. (1990). Suicidal attempts with zidovudine. *AIDS*, **4**, 88.

Tessier, S., Remy, G., Louis, J. and Trebucq, A. (1993). The frontline of HIV1 diffusion in the central African region: a geographical and epidemiological perspective. *International Journal of Epidemiology*, **22**, 127–33.

Thomas, C. and Szabadi, E. (1987). Paranoid psychosis as the first presentation of a fulminating lethal case of AIDS. *British Journal of Psychiatry*, **151**, 693–5.

Thomas, C., Toone, B., Komy, A.E., Harwin, B. and Farthing, C. (1985). HTLV-III and psychiatric disturbance. *Lancet*, **ii**, 359–60.

Thompson, C. (ed.) (1989). *The instruments of psychiatric research*. John Wiley and Sons, Chichester.

Thompson, C. and McIver, A. (1988). HIV counselling: change in trends in public concern. *Health Bulletin*, **46**, 237–45.

Thornton, S. and Catalán, J. (1993). Preventing the sexual spread of HIV infection—what have we learned? *International Journal of STD and AIDS*, **4**, 311–16.

Thornton, S., Tallis, F., Flynn, R., Catalán, J. and Aroney, R. (1994). Applying the cognitive behavioural model to interventions for HIV sexual risk reduction. *IInd International Conference on the Biopsychosocial aspects of HIV infection*, Brighton, 1994.

Thucydides (1993). *History of the Peloponnesian war* (trans. R. Crawley). Everyman, London.

Thuluvath, P., Connolly, G.M., Forbes, A. and Gazzard, B.G. (1991). Abdominal pain in HIV infection. *Quarterly Journal of Medicine*, **78**, 275–85.

Tindall, B., Forde, S. and Cooper, D. (1992). Self-reported sexual dysfunction in advanced HIV disease. *VIIIth International Conference on AIDS*, Amsterdam, 1992

Tindall, B., Forde, S., Carr, A., Barker, S. and Cooper, D.A. (1993). Attitudes to euthanasia and assisted suicide in a group of homosexual men with advanced HIV disease. *Journal of Acquired Immune Deficiency Syndromes*, **6**, 1069–70.

Tindall, B., Forde, S., Goldstein, D., Ross, M.W. and Cooper, D.A. (1994). Sexual dysfunction in advanced HIV disease. *AIDS Care*, **6**, 105–7.

Tinuper, P., de Carolis, P. and Galeotti, M. (1990). Electroencephalogram and HIV infection: a prospective study in 100 patients. *Clinical Electroencephalography*, **21**, 145–50.

Titmuss, R.M. (1971). *The gift relationship: from human blood to social policy*. Allen and Unwin, London.

Todd, J. (1989). AIDS as a current psychopathological theme: a report on five heterosexual patients. *British Journal of Psychiatry*, **154**, 253–5.

Tokars, J.I., Marcus, R., Culver D.H., Schable, C.A., McKibben, P.S. et al. for the CDC Cooperative Needlestick Surveillance Group (1993). Surveillance of HIV infection and zidovudine use among health care workers after occupational exposure to HIV-infected blood. *Annals of Internal Medicine*, **118**, 913–18.

Tolley, K. and Kennelly, J. (1993). Cost of compulsory HIV testing. *British Medical Journal*, **306**, 1202.

Tomkins, C. (1993). Lawful withdrawal of life support. *Journal of the Medical Defence Union*, **1**, (suppl.).

Townsend, J., Frank, A., Fermont, D., Dyer, S., Karran, O., Walgrove, A. and Piper M. (1990). Terminal cancer care and patients' preference for place of death: a prospective study. *British Medical Journal*, **301**, 415–17.

Tozzi, V., Narcisco, P., Galgani, S., Sette, P., Balestra, P., Gerace, C. et al (1993). Effects of zidovudine in 30 patients with mild to end-stage AIDS dementia complex. *AIDS*, **7**, 683–92.

Tran Dinh, Y.R., Hulbert, M., Cervoni, J., Caulin, C. and Saimot, A.C. (1990). Disturbances in the cerebral perfusion of human immune deficiency virus-1 seropositive asymptomatic subjects: a quantitative tomography study of 18 cases. *Journal of Nuclear Medicine*, **31**, 1601–7.

Troop, M., Easterbrook, P.J., Flynn, R., Thornton, S., Mee, L., Catalán, J. et al (1994). Perceptions of reasons for non-progression in HIV–1 infection. *IInd International Conference on the Biopsychosocial aspects of HIV infection*, Brighton, 1994.

Tross, S., Hirsch, D., Rabkin, B., Barry, C. and Holland, J. (1987). Determinants of current psychiatric disorder in AIDS-spectrum patients. *IIIrd International Conference on AIDS*, Washington, DC, 1987.

Tross, S., Price, R.W., Navia, B.A., Thaler, H., Gold, J., Hirsch, D. and Sidtis J.J. (1988). Neuropsychological characterisation of the AIDS dementia complex: a preliminary report. *AIDS*, **2**, 81–8.

Trujillo, J.R., Worth, J. and McLane, M.F. (1991). GP120 antibodies in AIDS dementia complex (ADC). *International Conference on the Neuroscience of HIV Infection*, Padua, 1991.

Tsiantis, J. and Meyer, M. (1992). Counselling HIV positive young people with thalassemia and haemophilia and their families. *Bereavement Care*, **11**, 30–4.

Turnbull, P. and Stimpson, G.V. (1994). Drug use in prison. *British Medical Journal*, **308**, 1716.

Turnbull, O., Saling, M.M., Kaplan-Solms, T., Cohn, R. and Schoub, B. (1990). Neuropsychological deficit in haemophiliacs with human immunodeficiency virus. *Journal of Neurology, Neurosurgery and Psychiatry*, **54**, 175–7.

Turnbull, P., Dolan, K. and Stimson, G. (1993). HIV testing, and the care and treatment of HIV positive people in English prisons. *AIDS Care*, **5**, 199–206.

Uhlenhuth, E.H. and Paykel, E.S. (1973). Symptom configuration and life events. *Archives of General Psychiatry* **28**, 744–8.

Ussher, J. (1990). Cognitive behaviourial couples therapy with gay men referred for counselling in an AIDS setting: a pilot study. *AIDS Care*, **2**, 43–51.

Vachon, M. (1993). Emotional problems in palliative medicine. In Oxford textbook of palliative medicine (eds. D. Doyle, G. Hanks and N. MacDonald). Oxford University Press, Oxford.

Vago, L., Castangna, A., Lazzarin, A., Trabattoni, G., Cinque, P., Costanzi, G. et al (1993). Reduced frequency of HIV-induced brain lesions in AIDS patients treated with zidovudine. *Journal of Acquired Immune Deficiency Syndromes*, **6**, 42–5.

Valdiserri, E. (1986). Fear of AIDS. *American Journal of Orthopsychiatry*, **56**, 634–8.

Valdiserri, R., Lyter, D., Leviton, L., Callahan, C., Kingsely, L. and Rinaldo, C. (1988). Variables influencing condom use in a cohort of gay and bisexual men. *American Journal of Public Health* **78**, 801–5.

Valdiserri, R., Lyter, D., Leviton, L., Callahan, C., Kingsley, L. and Rinaldo, C. (1989). AIDS prevention in homosexual and bisexual men: results of a randomized trial evaluating two risk reduction interventions. *AIDS*, **3**, 21–6.

Valdiserri, R., Moore, M., Gerber, A., Campbell, C., Dillon, B. and West, G. (1993). A study of clients returning for counselling after HIV testing: implications for improving rates of return. *Public Health Reports*, **108**, 12–18.

Van den Boom, F.M.L.G., Mead, C., Gremmen, T. and Roozenburg, H. (1991). *AIDS, euthanasia and grief. VIIth International Conference on AIDS*, Florence, 1991.

Van den Hoek, J., van Haastrecht, H. and Coutinho, R. (1989). Risk reduction among injecting drug users in Amsterdam under the influence of AIDS. *American Journal of Public Health* **79**, 1355–7.

Van der Maas, P.J., van Delede, J.J.M., Pijnenborg, L. and Looman, C.W.N. (1991). Euthanasia and other medical decisions concerning the end of life. *Lancet*, **338**, 669–74.

Van der Wal, G. (1994). Euthanasia in the Netherlands. *British Medical Journal*, **308**, 1346–9.

Van der Wal, G., van Eiik, J.T., Leenen, H.J., Spreeuwenberg, C. (1992). Euthanasia and assisted suicide II. Do Dutch family doctors act prudently? *Family Practice*, **9**, 135–40.

Van Eerdewegh, M., Bieri, M., Parilla, I. and Clayton, P. (1982). The bereaved child. *British Journal of Psychiatry*, **14**, 23–9.

Van Gorp, W.G., Miller, E.N., Satz, P. and Visscher, B. (1989). Neuropsychological performance in HIV-1 immunocompromised patients: a preliminary study. *Journal of Clinical and Experimental Neuropsychology*, **11**, 763–73.

Van Haastrecht, H., Fennema, J., Coutinho, R., Van der Helm, T., Kint, J. and van den Hoek, J., (1993). HIV prevalence and risk behaviour among prostitutes and clients in Amsterdam: migrants at increased risk for HIV infection. *Genitourinary Medicine*, **69**, 251–6.

Van Hemert, A., Hawton, K., Bolk, J. and Fagg, J. (1993a). Key symptoms in the detection of affective disorder in medical patients. *Journal of Psychosomatic Research*, **37**, 397–404.

Van Hemert, A., van der Mast, R., Hengeveld, M. and Vorsterbosch, M. (1993b). Excess mortality in general hospital patients with delirium: a 5 year follow-up of 519 patients seen in psychiatric consultation. *Journal of Psychosomatic Research*, **38**, 339–46.

Veitch, A. (1988). Princess Anne calls AIDS own goal. *The Guardian*, 27th January 1988.

Velentgas, P., Bynum, C. and Zierler, S. (1990). The buddy volunteer committment in AIDS care. *American Journal of Public Health* 80, 1378–80.

Viney, l., Henry, R., Walker, B. and Crooks, L. (1989). The emotional reactions of HIV positive men. *British Journal of Medical Psychology*, **62**, 153–61.

Viney, L., Allwood, K. and Stillson, L. (1991). Reconstructive group therapy with HIV-affected people. Counselling Psychology Quarterly, **4**, 247–58.

Viney, L., Henry, R., Walker, B. and Crooks, L. (1992). The psychosocial impact of multiple deaths from AIDS. *Omega*, **24**, 151–63.

Victor, B.W. (1989). *Review of six HIV/AIDS home care programme in Uganda and Zambia*. WHO, General Programme on AIDS/IDS/HCS/91.3.

Vogel-Scibilia, S., Mulsant, B. and Keshavan, M. (1988). HIV infection presenting as psychosis: a critique. *Acta Psychiatrica Scandinavica*, **78**, 652–6

Volberding, P.A. (1989). Supporting the health care team in caring for patients with AIDS. *Journal of American Medical Association*, **261**, 747–748.

Volberding, P.A, Lagakos, S.W., Koch, M.A, Pettinelli, C., Myers, M.W., Booth, D.K. et al (1990). Zidovudine in asymptomatic human immunodeficiency virus infection. A controlled trial in persons with fewer than 500 CD4-positive cells per cubic millimeter. The AIDS Clinical Trials Group of the National Institute of Allergy and Infectious Diseases. *New England Journal of Medicine*, **322**, 941–9.

Von Reyn, C.F., Gilbert, T.T., Shaw, F.E., Kathy, C.P., Abramson, J.E. and Smith, M.G. (1993). Absence of HIV transmission from an infected orthopedic surgeon. *Journal of the American Medical Association*, **269**, 1807–11.

Von Roenn, J., Murphy, R., Weber, K., Williams, L. and Weitzman, S. (1988). Megestrol acetate for the treatment of cachexia associated with HIV infection. *Annals of Internal Medicine*, **109**, 840–1.

Wachter, R.M., Luce, J.M., Turner, J., Volberding, P.A. and Hopewell, P.C. (1988). Intensive care of patients with the acquired immunodeficiency syndrome. *American Review of Respiratory Diseases*, **134**, 891–6.

Wald, N. (1993). Ethical issues in randomised prevention trials. *British Medical Journal*, **306**, 563–5.

Walsh, K. (1987). *Neuropsychology: a clinical approach* (2nd edn). Churchill Livingstone, London.

Walter, H. and Vaughan, R. (1993). AIDS risk reduction among a multiethnic sample of urban high school students. *Journal of the American Medical Association*, **270**, 725–30.

Walter, H., Vaughan, R. and Cohall, A. (1991). Psychological influences on acquired immunodeficiency syndrome-risk behaviours among high school students. *Paediatrics*, **88**, 846–52.

Ward, B.J. and Tate, P.A. (1994). Attitudes among NHS doctors to requests for euthanasia. *British Medical Journal*, **308**, 1332–4.

Ward, J.W., Deepe, D.A., Samson, S., Perkins, H., Holland, P., Fernando, L. et al (1987). Risk of human immunodeficiency virus infection from blood donors who later developed the acquired immunodeficiency syndrome. *Annals of Internal Medicine*, **106**, 61–2.

Ward, J.W., Darke, S., Hall, W. and Mattick, R. (1992). Methadone maintenance and HIV: current issues in treatment and research. *British Journal of Addiction*, **87**, 447–53.

Ward, H., Day, S., Mezzone, J., Dunlop, L., Donegan, C., Farrar, S. et al (1993). Prostitution and risk of HIV: female prostitutes in London. *British Medical Journal*, **307**, 356–8.

Warwick, H. (1989). AIDS hypochondriasis. *British Journal of Psychiatry*, **155**, 125–6.

Watters, J., Cheng, Y. and Segal, M. (1991). Syringe exchange in San Francisco: preliminary results. *VIIth International Conference on AIDS*, Florence, 1991.

Watters, J., Estilo, M., Clark, G. and Lorvick, J. (1994). Syringe and needle exchange as HIV/AIDS prevention for injection users. *Journal of the American Medical Association*, **271**, 115–20.

Wawer, M., Sewankambo, N., Berkley, S., Serwadda, D., Musgrave, S., Gary, R. et al (1994). Incidence of HIV-1 infection in a rural region of Uganda. *British Medical Journal*, **308**, 171–3.

Weber, J.N. and Weiss, R.A. (1988). The virology of human immunodeficiency viruses. *British Medical Bulletin*, **44**, 20–37.

Wechsler, D.A. (1981). *The Wechsler Adult Intelligence Scale—revised*. The Psychological Corporation, New York.

Wechsler, D.A. (1987). *The Wechsler Memory Scale—revised*. Psychological corporation, Harcourt Brace Jovanovich, San Antonio.

Wedler, H. (1991). Suicidal behaviour in the HIV-infected population: the actual situation in the FRG. In *HIV and AIDS-related suicidal behaviour* (ed. J.E. Beskow, M. Bellini, J.G.S. Faria and A.J.F.M. Kerkhof). Monduzzi Editore, Bologna.

Weil-Halpern, F. (1989). Problems psycho-sociaux poses par les familles ayant unnourrisson victime de l'infection au HIV ou du SIDA, *Annales de Pediatrie*, **36**, 409–12.

Weinstock, H., Lindan, C., Bolan, G., Kegeles, H. and Hearst N., (1993). Factors associated with condom use in a high risk heterosexual population. *Sexually Transmitted Diseases*, **20**, 14–20.

Weissman, I.L. (1993). The whole body view—New insights into HIV pathogenesis are coming from studies of how the virus spreads within lymphoid organs in vivo and damages them. *Current Biology*, **3**, 766–7.

Wells, R. (1987). Aspects of palliative care. *Palliative Medicine*, **1**, 49–52.

Welsby, P. and Richardson, A. (1993). Palliative care aspects of adult AIDS. In *Oxford textbook of palliative medicine* (ed. D. Doyle, G. Hanks and N. MacDonald). Oxford University Press, Oxford.

Wenstrom, K.D. and Zuidema, L.J. (1989). Determination of the seroprevalence of HIV infection in gravida by non-anonymous versus anonymous screening. *Obstetics and Gynaecology*, **74**, 558–61.

Wermuth, L., Ham J. and Robbins, R. (1992). Women don't wear condoms; AIDS risk among sexual partners of IV drug users. In *The social context of AIDS*, (ed. J. Huber and B.E. Schneder). Sage, London.

Werner, E., Fuchs, D. and Hausen, A. (1988). Tryptophan degradation in patients infected by HIV. *Biological Chemistry*, **369**, 337–40.

White, D., Phillips, K., Mulleady, G. and Cuppit, C. (1993). Sexual issues and condom use among injecting drug users. *AIDS Care*, **5**, 427–37.

Whiteman, M.L., Post, J.D., Berger, J.R., Tate, L.G., Bell, M.D. and Limonte, L.P. (1993). Progressive multifocal leukoencephalopathy in 47 HIV seropositive patients: neuroimaging with clinical and pathologic correlation. *Radiology*, **187**, 223–40.

Whitlock, F.A. (1986). Suicide and physical illness. In *Suicide* (ed. A. Roy), Williams and Williams, Baltimore.

Whitt, J.K., Hooper, S.R., Tennison, M.B., Robertson, W.T., Gold, S.H., Burchinal, M. et al (1993). Neuropsychologic functioning of human immunodeficiency virus-infected children with haemophilia. *Journal of Pediatrics*, **122**, 52–9.

Widman, M., Light, D. and Platt, J. (1994). Barriers to out of hospital care for AIDS patients. *AIDS Care*, **6**, 59–67.

Wielandt, H. (1993). Have the AIDS campaigns changed the pattern of contraceptive usage among adolescents? *Acta Obstetrica and Gynecologica Scandanavica*, **72**, 111–15.

Wiley, C.A,. Masliah, E. and Morey, M. (1991). NeocorticaL damage during HIV infection. *Annals of Neurology*, **29**, 651–7.

Wiley, C.A., Achim, C.L., Schrier, R.D., Heyes, M.P., McCutchan, J. and Grant I. (1992). Relationship of cerebrospinal fluid immune activation associated factors to HIV encephalitis. *AIDS*, **6**, 1299–307.

Wilkie, F., Eisdorfer, C., Morgan, R., Loewenstein, D. and Szapocznik, J. (1990b). Cognition in early human immunodeficiency virus infection. *Archives of Neurology*, **47**, 433–40.

Wilkins, J., Robertson, K., van der Horst, C., Robertson, W., Fryer, J. and Hall, C.D. (1990). The importance of confounding factors in the evaluation of neuropsychological changes in patients infected with human immunodeficiency virus. *Journal of Acquired Immune Deficiency Syndromes*, **3**, 938–42.

Wilkins, J., Robertson, K., Snyder, C., Robertson, W., van der Horst, C., Hall, C. et al (1991). Implications of self-reported cognitive and motor dysfunction in HIV positive patients. *American Journal of Psychiatry*, **148**, 641–3.

Williams, M.J. (1988). Gay men as buddies to persons living with AIDS and ARC. *Smith's College Studies in Social Work*, **59**, 38–52.

Williams, N. (1991). Surgeons and the risks of contamination during operations. *Journal of the Royal Society of Medicine*, **84**, 327–8.

Williams, W. and Polak, P. (1979). Follow-up research in primary prevention. *Journal of Clinical Psychology*, **35**, 35–45.

Williams, J., Rabkin, J., Remien, R., Gorman, J. and Ehrhardt, A. (1991). Multi-disciplinary baseline assessment of homosexual men with HIV infection—II: standardized clinical assessment of current and lifetime psychopathology. *Archives of General Psychiatry* **48**, 124–30.

Willis, L.A.M. (1992). Euthanasia. *British Medical Journal*, **305**, 952.

Winiarski, M. (1993). Integrating mental health services with primary care. *AIDS Patient Care*, **7**, 322–6.

Windgassen E. and Soni, S. (1987). AIDS panic. *British Journal of Psychiatry*, **151**, 126–7.

Wing, J., Cooper, J. and Sartorious, N. (1974). *The measurement and classification of Psychiatric Symptoms*. Cambridge University Press, London.

Winn, R.E., Bower, M.J. and Richards, M.J. (1979). Acute toxic delirium: neurotoxicity of intrathecal amphoteracin B. *Archives of Internal Medicine*, **139**, 706.

Wofsy, C.B. (1987). Use of trimethoprim-sulphamethoxasole in the treatment of pneumocystis carinii pneumonitis. *Review of Infectious Diseases*, **9**, 184–94.

Wofsy, C.B. (1988). AIDS care: providing care for the HIV infected. *Journal of Acquired Immune Deficiency Syndromes*, **1**, 274–83.

Wolcott, D., Namir, S., Fawzy, F., Gottlieb, M. and Mitsuyasu, R. (1986a). Illness concerns, attitudes towards homosexuality and social supports in gay men with AIDS. *General Hospital Psychiatry*, **8**, 395–403.

Wolcott, D., Fawzy, F., Landsverk, J. and McCombs, M. (1986b). AIDS patients' needs for psychosocial services and their use of community service organizations. *Journal of Psychosocial Oncology*, **4**, 135–46.

Wolters, P., Brouwers, P., Moss, H., El-Amin, D., Balis, F., Butler, K. et al (1991). The effects of dideoxyinosine (ddI) on the cognitive functioning of children with HIV infection after 6 and 12 months of treatment. *VIIth International Conference on AIDS*, Florence, 1991.

Woolley, H., Stein, A., Forrest, G. and Baum, J. (1989). Imparting the diagnosis of life-threatening illness in children. *British Medical Journal*, **298**, 1623–6.

Woolley, P.D., Palfreeman, A.J., Patel, R., Talbot, M.D and Samarasinghe, P.L. (1991). Blood-taking practices and needle-stick injuries in house officers. *International Journal of STD and AIDS*, **2**, 46–8.

Worden, J.W. (1991). Grieving a loss from AIDS. *Hospice Journal*, **7**, 143–50.

Worden, J.W. (1992). Grief counselling and grief therapy: a handbook for the mental health practitioner. Routledge, London.

Working Group of the Royal College of Pathologists (1992). *HIV infection: hazards of transmission to patients and health care workers during invasive procedures*. Royal College of Pathologists, London.

World Health Organisation (1987). *Statement from the consultation on prevention and control of AIDS in prisons*. World Health Organisation, Geneva.

World Health Organisation (1988). AIDS: discrimination and public health. *IVth International Conference on AIDS*, Stockholm, 1988.

World Health Organisation (1989). *Statement form the consultation on HIV epidemiology and prostitution*. World Health Organisation. Geneva.

World Health Organisation (1990a). *Drug abusers in prisons: managing their problems*. WHO regional publication, no. 27, Copenhagen.

World Health Organisation (1990b). *Report of the Second Consultation on the Neuropsychiatric Aspects of HIV-1 infection*, Geneva.

World Health Organisation (1993). *Statement from the consultation on testing and counselling for HIV infection*. Global Programme on AIDS, Geneva.

Wright, J.M., Sachdev, P.S., Perkins, R.J. and Rodriguez, P. (1989). Zidovudine-related mania. *The Medical Journal of Australia*, **150**, 339–41.

Wu, A.W., Rubin, H.R., Mathews, W.C., Ware, J.E., Brysk, L.T., Hardy, W.D., et al (1989). A Health Status Questionnaire using 30 items from the medical Outcomes Study. *Medical Care*, **29**, 786–98.

Wu, A.W., Mathews, W.C., Brysk, L.T., Atkinson, J.H., Grant, I., Abramson, I. et al (1990). Quality of life in a placebo-controlled trial of zidovudine in patients with AIDS and AIDS-related complex. *Journal of Acquired Immune Deficiency Syndromes*, **3**, 683–90.

Wu, A.W., Rubin, H.R., Bozette, S.A., Mathews, W.C., Snyder, R., Wright, B. et al (1991). A longitudinal study of quality of life in asymptomatic HIV infection. *VIIth International Conference on AIDS*, Florence, 1991.

Yarchoan, R., Berg, G., Brouwers, P., Fischl, M., Spitzer, A.R., Wichman, A. et al (1987). Response of human immuno-deficiency-virus-associated neurological disease to 3′-azido–3′-deoxythymidine. *Lancet*, **1**, 132–5.

Yarchoan, R., Thomas, R.V., Grafman, J., Wichman, A., Dalakas, M., McAtee, M. et al (1988). Long-term administration of 3′-azido–2′,3′-dideoxythimidine to patients with AIDS-related neurological disease. *Annals of Neurology*, **23** (suppl.), S82–S87.

Youle, M., Clarbour, J., Farthing, C., Connolly G.M., Hawkins D.A. et al (1989). Treatment of resistant aphthous ulceration with Thalidomide in patients positive for HIV antibody. *British Medical Journal*, **298**, 432.

Young, R.C., Biggs, J., Ziegler, V. and Meyer, D. (1978). A rating scale for mania: reliability, validity and sensitivity. *British Journal of Psychiatry*, **133**, 429–31.

Zealberg, J., Lydiard, R. and Christie, S. (1991). Exacerbation of panic disorder in a woman treated with trimethoprin-sulphamethoxazole. *Journal of Clinical Psychopharmacology*, **11**, 144–5.

Zenilman, J., Erickson, B., Fox, R., Reichart, C. and Hook, E. (1992). Effect of HIV post-test counselling on STD incidence. *Journal of Americcan Medical Association*, **267**, 843–5.

Ziegler, P. (1969). *The black death*. Penguin, London.

Ziegler, J. (1993). Breast feeding and HIV. The Lancet, 342, 1437–8.

Zierler, S., Feingold, L., Laufer, D., Velentgas, P., Kantrowitz-Gordon, I. and Mayer, K. (1991). Adult survivors of sexual abuse and subsequent risk of HIV infection. *American Journal of Public Health* **81**, 572–5.

Zigmond, A.S. and Snaith, P. (1983). The hospital Anxiety and Depression Scale. *Acta Psychiatrica Scandinavica*, **67**, 361–70.

Zuger, A., Louie, E., Holzman, R.S., Simberkoff M.S. and Rahal, J.J. (1986). Cryptococcal disease in patients with the acquired immunodeficiency syndrome; diagnostic features and treatment. *Annals of Internal Medicine*, **104**, 234–40.

Zumwaldt, R., McFeeley, P. and Maito, J. (1987). Fraudulent AIDS. *Journal of the American Medical Association*, **257**, 3231.

Index